Clinical Coding Workout:

Practice Exercises for Skill Development Without Answers

2013 Edition

Ann Barta, MSA, RHIA

Angie Comfort, RHIT, CDIP, CCS

Kathy DeVault, RHIA, CCS, CCS-P

Melanie Endicott, MBA/HCM, RHIA, CDIP, CCS, CCS-P

Karen Kostick, RHIT, CCS, CCS-P

Theresa Rihanek, MHA, RHIA, CCS

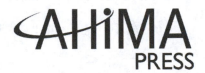

AHIMA

PRESS

ISBN: 978-1-58426-418-7
AHIMA Product No. AC201614

AHIMA Staff:
Jessica Block, MA, Assistant Editor
Jason O. Malley, Director, Creative Content Development
Ashley Sullivan, Production Development Editor

For more information, including updates, about AHIMA Press publications, visit http://www.ahima.org/publications/updates.aspx.

American Health Information Management Association
233 North Michigan Avenue, 21st Floor
Chicago, Illinois 60601-5800

http://www.ahima.org

Contents

Preface

The *Clinical Coding Workout* is designed to challenge coding professionals and students alike to develop expert skills in the assignment of clinical codes required for administrative use.

The coding process requires a range of skills that combines knowledge and practice. Someone new to this discipline must conquer the basic principles of using the required code sets. A student at the intermediate level learns to apply code set conventions, guidelines, and principles in various combinations, settings, and scenarios. A person with advanced coding skills analyzes complex health data and determines what needs to be reported to accurately reflect each patient's condition and treatment. Like a violinist or a gymnast, the coding professional develops virtuosity step-by-step through systematic exercise. At each level of skill development, practice enhances performance.

The AHIMA Practice Resources team has gathered coding scenarios and case studies together to create a resource for skill development and review of guidelines and conventions applied in code selection. Practice exercises take the user from beginning concepts and selection of codes, through intermediate applications using short code assignment scenarios, to advanced case studies that are based on excerpts from health records and that require complex clinical analysis skills and multiple code assignments. The user is encouraged to reference the American Hospital Association's *Coding Clinic*; National Center for Health Statistics' *ICD-9-CM Official Guidelines for Coding and Reporting (ICD-9-CM)*, *ICD-10-CM Official Guidelines for Coding and Reporting*, and *ICD-10-PCS Official Guidelines for Coding and Reporting*; and American Medical Association's *CPT Assistant* (cited within select case scenarios to further enhance learning). Coding challenges in the final chapter include exercises for ICD-10-CM and ICD-10-PCS, CPT modifiers, HCPCS Level II modifiers, home health, LTAC coding, and rehabilitation and SNF cases.

How to Use This Book

Unlike coding instructional books that are based on one coding classification system, *Clinical Coding Workout* uses the full range of administrative code sets applicable in today's healthcare environment for reporting diagnoses, procedures, and services in various settings and specialty practice areas.

The actual codes used in the exercises for this book are those that were confirmed or already in effect at the time of publication, as follows:

- *International Classification of Diseases, 9th Revision, Clinical Modification (ICD-9-CM)*, 2013 edition, codes effective October 1, 2012

- *International Classification of Diseases, 10th Revision, Clinical Modification (ICD-10-CM)*, 2013 draft edition

- *International Classification of Diseases, 10th Revision, Procedure Coding System (ICD-10-PCS)*, 2013 draft edition

- *Current Procedural Terminology (CPT)*, 2013 edition, codes effective January 1, 2013

- *Healthcare Common Procedural Coding System Level II (HCPCS)*, 2013 edition, codes effective January 1, 2013

As in actual practice, ICD-9-CM codes are used for diagnoses and inpatient procedures for hospital reporting in this book; whereas for ambulatory facility and physician service reporting, ICD-9-CM codes are used for diagnoses and HCPCS/CPT codes are used for procedures and services.

The Centers for Medicare and Medicaid Services (CMS) and the National Center for Health Statistics (NCHS) provide the *ICD-9-CM and ICD-10-CM/PCS Official Guidelines for Coding and Reporting*, which should be used as a companion document to the official version. The guidelines have been approved by the four organizations that make up the Cooperating Parties for the ICD-9-CM: the American Hospital Association (AHA), the American Health Information Management Association (AHIMA), CMS, and NCHS.

The guidelines are a set of rules that have been developed to accompany and complement the official conventions and instructions provided within ICD-9-CM and ICD-10-CM/PCS. The guidelines are based upon the coding and sequencing instructions found in ICD-9-CM and ICD-10-CM/PCS, and they provide additional instruction. Adherence to the guidelines is required under the Health Insurance Portability and Accountability Act (HIPAA). The guidelines for ICD-9-CM and ICD-10-CM are organized into sections. Section I includes the structure and conventions of the classification, general guidelines that apply to the entire classification, and chapter-specific guidelines that correspond to the chapters as they are arranged in the classification. This section is applicable to all healthcare settings unless otherwise indicated. Section II includes guidelines for selecting principal diagnoses for nonoutpatient settings. Section III includes guidelines for reporting additional diagnoses in nonoutpatient settings. Section IV is for outpatient coding (including physician) and reporting. The guidelines for ICD-10-PCS are organized into three sections. Section A includes the structure and conventions of the classification. Section B includes the Medical and Surgical section guidelines. Section C includes Obstetrics section guidelines.

The ICD-9-CM and ICD-10-CM guidelines are regularly updated and are available at http://www.cdc.gov/nchs/icd.htm. The ICD-10-PCS guidelines are available at http://www.cms.gov/ICD10/.

Federal Register notices and other regulatory updates are available from the Centers for Medicare and Medicaid Services at http://www.cms.gov. HCPCS Level II codes are updated each quarter and are available by download from https://www.cms.gov/HCPCSRelease CodeSets/. CPT code sets are generally released in mid-September for implementation by January 1 of the following year.

Refer to the instructions in each chapter for additional information. Please report any potential inconsistencies or inaccuracies in this book to https://secure.ahima.org/contact/contact.aspx.

Acknowledgments

AHIMA Press appreciates all readers who challenge the material and request clarification on items presented in this book. A special note of appreciation is warranted to the coding professionals who assist in reviewing the manuscript.

AHIMA thanks the following authors for their contributions to prior editions of this book:

Kathy Giannangelo, MA, RHIA, CCS, CPHIMS, FAHIMA
Anita C. Hazelwood, MLS, RHIA, FAHIMA
Carol A. Venable, MPH, RHIA, FAHIMA

Part I
Beginning Coding Exercises

Chapter 1

Basic Principles of ICD-9-CM and ICD-10-CM/PCS Coding

The following exercises are designed to review ICD-9-CM and ICD-10-CM/PCS coding guidelines and to provide practice in assigning ICD-9-CM and ICD-10-CM/PCS codes. Because ICD-9-CM and ICD-10-CM/PCS index diagnoses and procedures in many different ways, the rationale for the selection of a particular code may be different from the approach that you use. The information included in the rationale is not meant to describe the only way to obtain an appropriate code but to represent one possible way.

Note: The exercises in this chapter are based on the 2013 edition of ICD-9-CM and the 2013 draft editions of ICD-10-CM and ICD-10-PCS but are suitable for other editions in most instances.

Instructions: Circle the correct answer, fill in the blank, or assign the correct code(s) for each of the following exercise items.

Characteristics and Conventions of the ICD-9-CM Classification System

1.1. Nonessential modifiers are enclosed in:

    a. Brackets
    b. Parentheses
    c. Slanted brackets
    d. Boxes

1.2. A diagnostic descriptor that is listed in italics is a(n):

    a. Manifestation code
    b. Inappropriate principal diagnosis
    c. CC exclusion
    d. Code that must be reported first

1.3. The abbreviation UHDDS refers to the _____.

1.4.   Diagnoses described as "suspected," "possible," "probable," "likely," and "still to be ruled out" are reported if present at the time of discharge for _____ records.

1.5.   For patients receiving therapeutic services in the outpatient setting for chemotherapy, radiation therapy, or rehabilitation, the first listed reported diagnosis is:

a. The diagnosis toward which the treatment is directed
b. The appropriate V code
c. Either a or b
d. The diagnosis that the physician lists first on the order

1.6.   When multiple burns are present, the first sequenced diagnosis is the:

a. Burn that is treated surgically
b. Burn that is closest to the head
c. Highest degree burn
d. Any of the above

1.7.   A coding professional may assume a cause-and-effect relationship between hypertension and which of the following complications?

a. Hypertension and heart disease
b. Hypertension and chronic kidney disease
c. Hypertension and heart and chronic kidney disease
d. None of the above

1.8.   Codes that describe the behavior of cells in neoplasms are called

_____.

1.9.   New ICD-9-CM codes go into effect on _____ of each year.

1.10.   Supplementary classifications include:

a. V codes
b. V codes and E codes
c. V codes, E codes, and M codes
d. None of the above

1.11.   The neoplasm table includes:

a. The nature and status (primary, secondary, in situ) for malignancies
b. A listing of the morphology codes
c. The stage of benign neoplasms
d. E codes for reactions to chemotherapy

1.12. V codes can be used as:

    a. Principal diagnosis only
    b. Secondary diagnosis only
    c. Either principal diagnosis or secondary diagnosis, depending on the code
       and the circumstances of the admission
    d. Secondary diagnosis only on inpatient stays and principal diagnosis only
       on outpatient visits

1.13. Terms listed in the Alphabetic Index in boldface type are known as

_____.

1.14. Manifestation codes:

    a. Can never be reported first
    b. Are printed in italics in the Tabular List
    c. Describe a condition that results from another, underlying condition
    d. All of the above

1.15. Codes that contain the descriptive abbreviation NOS are to be used:

    a. When the record itself is not available for review
    b. When the coder lacks sufficient information to assign a more specific code
    c. When only outpatient diagnostic records are being coded
    d. All the time

Infectious and Parasitic Diseases

1.16. Meningitis due to ECHO virus

    ICD-9-CM Code(s): _____

    ICD-10-CM Code(s): _____

1.17. Chickenpox

    ICD-9-CM Code(s): _____

    ICD-10-CM Code(s): _____

1.18. Pulmonary anthrax

    ICD-9-CM Code(s): _____

    ICD-10-CM Code(s): _____

1.19. *Aerobacter aerogenes* is an example of a gram-_____
bacterial organism.

1.20. Genital herpes

    ICD-9-CM Code(s): _____

    ICD-10-CM Code(s): _____

1.21.   Patients with any known prior diagnosis of an HIV–related illness should be reported with this ICD-9-CM code: _____.

ICD-10-CM Code(s): _____

1.22.   Acute salpingitis due to gonococcal infection

ICD-9-CM Code(s): _____

ICD-10-CM Code(s): _____

1.23.   A patient with known AIDS is admitted to the hospital for treatment of *Pneumocystis carinii* pneumonia. Assign the principal ICD-9-CM diagnosis code.

a. 042
b. 486
c. 136.3
d. Any of the above

1.24.   A patient with known chronic hepatitis C is seen in the outpatient department for interferon treatment. Assign the primary diagnosis.

ICD-9-CM Code(s):

a. 070.51
b. 070.44
c. 070.54
d. 070.32

ICD-10-CM Code(s): _____

1.25.   Paratyphoid fever A

ICD-9-CM Code(s): _____

ICD-10-CM Code(s): _____

1.26.   Salmonella gastroenteritis due to food poisoning

ICD-9-CM Code(s): _____

ICD-10-CM Code(s): _____

1.27.   Infectious diarrhea due to Proteus Morganii

ICD-9-CM Code(s): _____

ICD-10-CM Code(s): _____

1.28.   Pulmonary tuberculosis, bacilli identified with microscopy

ICD-9-CM Code(s): _____

ICD-10-CM Code(s): _____

1.29. Scarlatina

ICD-9-CM Code(s): _____

ICD-10-CM Code(s): _____

1.30. Pneumococcal septicemia

ICD-9-CM Code(s): _____

ICD-10-CM Code(s): _____

1.31. Dermatophytosis of scalp

ICD-9-CM Code(s): _____

ICD-10-CM Code(s): _____

1.32. Pneumonia as a complication of measles

ICD-9-CM Code(s): _____

ICD-10-CM Code(s): _____

1.33. Mumps

ICD-9-CM Code(s): _____

ICD-10-CM Code(s): _____

1.34. Plantar wart

ICD-9-CM Code(s): _____

ICD-10-CM Code(s): _____

1.35. Infectious mononucleosis

ICD-9-CM Code(s): _____

ICD-10-CM Code(s): _____

1.36. Condyloma acuminata

ICD-9-CM Code(s): _____

ICD-10-CM Code(s): _____

1.37. Infection with Shiga toxin-producing *Escherichia coli O157*

ICD-9-CM Code(s): _____

ICD-10-CM Code(s): _____

Neoplasms

1.38. Hodgkin's sarcoma of thoracic lymph nodes

ICD-9-CM Code(s): _____

ICD-10-CM Code(s): _____

1.39.   Malignant neoplasm of bronchus

ICD-9-CM Code(s): _____

ICD-10-CM Code(s): _____

1.40.   When a patient is admitted to the hospital for radiation therapy for a primary malignancy that is still present, what code is reported as the principal diagnosis?

ICD-9-CM Code(s): _____

ICD-10-CM Code(s): _____

1.41.   A patient is admitted as an inpatient to receive radiation and chemotherapy for distal esophageal carcinoma. What is the appropriate principal diagnosis?

ICD-9-CM Code(s):

a. V58.0
b. V58.11
c. 150.5
d. Either a or b

ICD-10-CM Code(s): _____

1.42.   Carcinoma of the broad ligament (confined to this location)

ICD-9-CM Code(s): _____

ICD-10-CM Code(s): _____

1.43.   Adenoma of the islet cells of the pancreas

ICD-9-CM Code(s): _____

ICD-10-CM Code(s): _____

1.44.   Neoplasms at the cellular level that are incapable of spreading to distant sites are called _____ neoplasms.

1.45.   Malignant melanoma of the skin of the chest wall

ICD-9-CM Code(s): _____

ICD-10-CM Code(s): _____

1.46.   Adenocarcinoma of the lesser curvature of the stomach

ICD-9-CM Code(s): _____

ICD-10-CM Code(s): _____

1.47.   Secondary carcinoma of the submandibular salivary gland

ICD-9-CM Code(s): _____

ICD-10-CM Code(s): _____

1.48. Benign neoplasm of the appendix

ICD-9-CM Code(s): _____

ICD-10-CM Code(s): _____

1.49. Carcinoma in situ of right breast

ICD-9-CM Code(s): _____

ICD-10-CM Code(s): _____

1.50. Which of the following neoplasm types is correct for sympathicoblastoma?

a. Benign
b. Malignant
c. Uncertain behavior
d. Unspecified

1.51. Myxofibrosarcoma is a malignant neoplasm that affects what type of tissue?

_____

1.52. The site at which a malignant neoplasm originated is known as the _____ site.

1.53. Bronchogenic carcinoma

ICD-9-CM Code(s): _____

ICD-10-CM Code(s): _____

1.54. Carcinoma in situ of the uterine cervix

ICD-9-CM Code(s): _____

ICD-10-CM Code(s): _____

1.55. In ICD-9-CM, neoplasm coding of the lymphatic and hematopoietic systems (200–202), a fifth digit of 5 refers to which organs?

a. Lymph nodes of inguinal region and lower limb
b. Lymph nodes of head, face, and neck
c. Lymph nodes of axilla and upper limb
d. Intrapelvic lymph nodes

1.56. Merkel cell carcinoma of the neck

ICD-9-CM Code(s): _____

ICD-10-CM Code(s): _____

1.57. Acute plasma cell leukemia in relapse

ICD-9-CM Code(s): _____

ICD-10-CM Code(s): _____

1.58. Carcinoma of the ureteric orifice of bladder

ICD-9-CM Code(s): _____

ICD-10-CM Code(s): _____

1.59. Squamous cell carcinoma of skin of the left eyelid

ICD-9-CM Code(s): _____

ICD-10-CM Code(s): _____

Endocrine, Nutritional, and Metabolic Diseases and Immunity Disorders

1.60. Hereditary hemochromatosis

ICD-9-CM Code(s): _____

ICD-10-CM Code(s): _____

1.61. Hypernatremia

ICD-9-CM Code(s): _____

ICD-10-CM Code(s): _____

1.62. Primary hypercholesterolemia

ICD-9-CM Code(s): _____

ICD-10-CM Code(s): _____

1.63. Bartter's syndrome is a form of which of the following?

a. Diabetic neuropathy
b. Hyperaldosteronism
c. Hypertriglyceridemia
d. Polycystic ovarian disease

1.64. Type I diabetes mellitus with diabetic renal nephrosis, out of control

ICD-9-CM Code(s): _____

ICD-10-CM Code(s): _____

1.65. Secondary diabetes mellitus caused by Cushing's syndrome

ICD-9-CM Code(s): _____

ICD-10-CM Code(s): _____

1.66. Type I diabetes mellitus with moderate nonproliferative retinopathy and macular edema

ICD-9-CM Code(s): _____

ICD-10-CM Code(s): _____

1.67. Type I diabetes mellitus with ketoacidosis

ICD-9-CM Code(s): _____

ICD-10-CM Code(s): _____

1.68. Type I diabetes mellitus with ophthalmic manifestations

ICD-9-CM Code(s): _____

ICD-10-CM Code(s): _____

1.69. Hypoinsulinemia following total pancreatectomy

ICD-9-CM Code(s): _____

ICD-10-CM Code(s): _____

1.70. ICD-9-CM code 255.2 (adrenogenital disorders) includes which of the following?

    a. Achard–Thiers syndrome
    b. Macrogenitosomia praecox in the male
    c. Congenital adrenal hyperplasia
    d. All of the above

1.71. Hypophyseal gigantism

ICD-9-CM Code(s): _____

ICD-10-CM Code(s): _____

1.72. Hypopotassemia

ICD-9-CM Code(s): _____

ICD-10-CM Code(s): _____

1.73. Cystic fibrosis with pulmonary manifestations

ICD-9-CM Code(s): _____

ICD-10-CM Code(s): _____

1.74. Hurler's syndrome, gargoyle syndrome, and Sanfilippo's syndrome are all forms of _____.

1.75. Adult morbid obesity with a BMI of 45.5

ICD-9-CM Code(s): _____

ICD-10-CM Code(s): _____

1.76. Polycystic ovaries

ICD-9-CM Code(s): _____

ICD-10-CM Code(s): _____

1.77.   Renal glycosuria

ICD-9-CM Code(s): _____

ICD-10-CM Code(s): _____

1.78.   Uninodular goiter with thyrotoxicosis

ICD-9-CM Code(s): _____

ICD-10-CM Code(s): _____

1.79.   Hypothyroidism following irradiation therapy

ICD-9-CM Code(s): _____

ICD-10-CM Code(s): _____

1.80.   Hereditary systemic amyloidosis

ICD-9-CM Code(s): _____

ICD-10-CM Code(s): _____

Disorders of the Blood and Blood-Forming Organs

1.81.   Iron-deficiency anemia secondary to chronic blood loss

ICD-9-CM Code(s): _____

ICD-10-CM Code(s): _____

1.82.   Sickle cell anemia and thalassemia are both types of:

a. Iron-deficiency anemias
b. Hereditary hemolytic anemias
c. Aplastic anemia
d. Coagulation defects

1.83.   Sickle cell trait

ICD-9-CM Code(s): _____

ICD-10-CM Code(s): _____

1.84.   Anemia due to acute blood loss

ICD-9-CM Code(s): _____

ICD-10-CM Code(s): _____

1.85.   Anemia due to antineoplastic chemotherapy

ICD-9-CM Code(s): _____

ICD-10-CM Code(s): _____

1.86. Which of the following is (are) not an example(s) of constitutional red blood cell aplasia?

    a. Fanconi's anemia
    b. Familial hypoplastic anemia
    c. Blackfan-Diamond syndrome
    d. All of the above

1.87. von Willebrand's disease

ICD-9-CM Code(s): _____

ICD-10-CM Code(s): _____

1.88. Agranulocytosis is a disease of the _____ blood cells.

1.89. Aplastic anemia

ICD-9-CM Code(s): _____

ICD-10-CM Code(s): _____

1.90. Dietary folate deficiency anemia

ICD-9-CM Code(s): _____

ICD-10-CM Code(s): _____

1.91. Amino-acid deficiency anemia

ICD-9-CM Code(s): _____

ICD-10-CM Code(s): _____

1.92. Osteosclerotic anemia

ICD-9-CM Code(s): _____

ICD-10-CM Code(s): _____

1.93. Posttransfusion purpura

ICD-9-CM Code(s): _____

ICD-10-CM Code(s): _____

1.94. Thrombocytopenic purpura

ICD-9-CM Code(s): _____

ICD-10-CM Code(s): _____

1.95. Thrombocytopenia following massive blood transfusions

ICD-9-CM Code(s): _____

ICD-10-CM Code(s): _____

1.96. Anemia

ICD-9-CM Code(s): _____

ICD-10-CM Code(s): _____

1.97. Congenital aplastic anemia

ICD-9-CM Code(s): _____

ICD-10-CM Code(s): _____

1.98. Eosinophilic leukocytosis

ICD-9-CM Code(s): _____

ICD-10-CM Code(s): _____

1.99. Anemia secondary to vitamin B_{12} deficiency

ICD-9-CM Code(s): _____

ICD-10-CM Code(s): _____

1.100. Christmas disease

ICD-9-CM Code(s): _____

ICD-10-CM Code(s): _____

1.101. Neutropenic fever

ICD-9-CM Code(s): _____

ICD-10-CM Code(s): _____

1.102. Aplastic anemia due to adverse effect of antineoplastic chemotherapy, initial encounter

ICD-9-CM Code(s): _____

ICD-10-CM Code(s): _____

Mental Disorders

Because the code assignment for mental disorders can have significant impact on the patient, coding professionals must take special care to ensure that codes are based on diagnostic statements clearly provided in physician documentation.

1.103. In ICD-9-CM coding, to report Jakob-Creutzfeldt disease with dementia, you would need:

a. One code
b. Two codes
c. Either one or two codes
d. More than two codes

1.104. Alcoholic dependent chronic brain syndrome

ICD-9-CM Code(s): _____

ICD-10-CM Code(s): _____

1.105. Bipolar disorder currently with moderate depression

ICD-9-CM Code(s): _____

ICD-10-CM Code(s): _____

1.106. Schizoid personality disorder

ICD-9-CM Code(s): _____

ICD-10-CM Code(s): _____

1.107. Panic attack

ICD-9-CM Code(s): _____

ICD-10-CM Code(s): _____

1.108. Which of the following is a synonym for multiple personality disorder?

    a. Dissociative identity disorder
    b. Factitious illness
    c. Adjustment reaction
    d. Multiple psychoses

1.109. Childhood autism

ICD-9-CM Code(s): _____

ICD-10-CM Code(s): _____

1.110. Which of the following is a sexual deviation or disorder per ICD-9-CM?

    a. Bestiality
    b. Pedophilia
    c. Voyeurism
    d. All of the above

1.111. Alcoholism with acute intoxication

ICD-9-CM Code(s): _____

ICD-10-CM Code(s): _____

1.112. Morphine addiction, in remission

ICD-9-CM Code(s): _____

ICD-10-CM Code(s): _____

1.113. Heroin and diazepam addiction

ICD-9-CM Code(s): _____

ICD-10-CM Code(s): _____

1.114. Psychogenic torticollis

ICD-9-CM Code(s): _____

ICD-10-CM Code(s): _____

1.115. Gilles de la Tourette's syndrome

ICD-9-CM Code(s): _____

ICD-10-CM Code(s): _____

1.116. Major depression, recurrent

ICD-9-CM Code(s): _____

ICD-10-CM Code(s): _____

1.117. Separation anxiety disorder

ICD-9-CM Code(s): _____

ICD-10-CM Code(s): _____

1.118. Moderate intellectual disabilities, measured IQ of 42

ICD-9-CM Code(s): _____

ICD-10-CM Code(s): _____

1.119. Attention deficit/hyperactivity disorder

ICD-9-CM Code(s): _____

ICD-10-CM Code(s): _____

1.120. Alcoholic paranoia

ICD-9-CM Code(s): _____

ICD-10-CM Code(s): _____

1.121. DTs due to alcohol withdrawal

ICD-9-CM Code(s): _____

ICD-10-CM Code(s): _____

1.122. Multi–infarct dementia with depression

ICD-9-CM Code(s): _____

ICD-10-CM Code(s): _____

1.123. Passive-aggressive personality disorder

ICD-9-CM Code(s): _____

ICD-10-CM Code(s): _____

1.124. Alzheimer's dementia with aggressive behavior

ICD-9-CM Code(s): _____

ICD-10-CM Code(s): _____

Nervous System and Sense Organs

1.125. Acute endophthalmitis

ICD-9-CM Code(s): _____

ICD-10-CM Code(s): _____

1.126. Duchenne muscular dystrophy

ICD-9-CM Code(s): _____

ICD-10-CM Code(s): _____

1.127. Which of the following are the correct ICD-9-CM codes for proliferative type 1 diabetic retinopathy?

    a. 250.53, 362.01
    b. 362.02, 250.50
    c. 250.51, 362.02
    d. 362.02, 250.01

1.128. Central retinal artery occlusion

ICD-9-CM Code(s): _____

ICD-10-CM Code(s): _____

1.129. Acanthamoeba keratitis

ICD-9-CM Code(s): _____

ICD-10-CM Code(s): _____

1.130. Bilateral retinal detachment, traction type

ICD-9-CM Code(s): _____

ICD-10-CM Code(s): _____

1.131. Senile cataract, posterior subcapsular

ICD-9-CM Code(s): _____

ICD-10-CM Code(s): _____

1.132. Angle closure glaucoma, acute

ICD-9-CM Code(s): _____

ICD-10-CM Code(s): _____

1.133. Tritan defect

ICD-9-CM Code(s): _____

ICD-10-CM Code(s): _____

1.134. Bullous keratopathy, bilateral

ICD-9-CM Code(s): _____

ICD-10-CM Code(s): _____

1.135. Temporal sclerosis

ICD-9-CM Code(s): _____

ICD-10-CM Code(s): _____

1.136. All but one of the following conditions are examples of strabismus (ICD-9-CM category 378). Identify the condition that is not a form of strabismus.

a. Esotropia
b. Exotropia
c. Presbyopia
d. Heterotropia

1.137. Chronic serous otitis media

ICD-9-CM Code(s): _____

ICD-10-CM Code(s): _____

1.138. Acute suppurative otitis media with eardrum rupture due to pressure in right ear

ICD-9-CM Code(s): _____

ICD-10-CM Code(s): _____

1.139. Cholesteatoma involving left middle ear and mastoid

ICD-9-CM Code(s): _____

ICD-10-CM Code(s): _____

1.140. Hyperactive labyrinth, right side

ICD-9-CM Code(s): _____

ICD-10-CM Code(s): _____

1.141. Anisocoria

ICD-9-CM Code(s): _____

ICD-10-CM Code(s): _____

1.142. Malignant otitis externa

ICD-9-CM Code(s): _____

ICD-10-CM Code(s): _____

1.143. Poorly controlled epilepsy

ICD-9-CM Code(s): _____

ICD-10-CM Code(s): _____

1.144. Reflex sympathetic dystrophy, both arms

ICD-9-CM Code(s): _____

ICD-10-CM Code(s): _____

1.145. Parkinson's dementia without behavioral disturbance

ICD-9-CM Code(s): _____

ICD-10-CM Code(s): _____

1.146. Brain death

ICD-9-CM Code(s): _____

ICD-10-CM Code(s): _____

Circulatory System

1.147. Pulmonary aneurysm

ICD-9-CM Code(s): _____

ICD-10-CM Code(s): _____

1.148. Malignant hypertension with hypertensive heart disease and congestive heart failure is coded:

ICD-9-CM Code(s):

a. 402.01
b. 402.01, 428.9
c. 428.0, 402.11
d. 402.01, 428.0

ICD-10-CM Code(s): _____

1.149. Mitral valve stenosis and aortic valve insufficiency

ICD-9-CM Code(s): _____

ICD-10-CM Code(s): _____

1.150. Hospital discharge diagnosis: Acute inferolateral myocardial infarction

ICD-9-CM Code(s): _____

ICD-10-CM Code(s): _____

1.151. In ICD-9-CM, a myocardial infarction is considered to be acute when it is less than _____ weeks old.

ICD-10-CM Answer: _____

1.152. Hypertension

ICD-9-CM Code(s): _____

ICD-10-CM Code(s): _____

1.153. Identify the main term and codes in the diagnostic statement "idiopathic hypertrophic subaortic stenosis (IHSS)."

ICD-9-CM Main Term and Code(s): _____

ICD-10-CM Main Term and Code(s): _____

1.154. Atrial flutter

ICD-9-CM Code(s): _____

ICD-10-CM Code(s): _____

1.155. Ventricular fibrillation

ICD-9-CM Code(s): _____

ICD-10-CM Code(s): _____

1.156. Acute diastolic heart failure

ICD-9-CM Code(s): _____

ICD-10-CM Code(s): _____

1.157. Preinfarction angina

ICD-9-CM Code(s): _____

ICD-10-CM Code(s): _____

1.158. Pulmonary infarction

ICD-9-CM Code(s): _____

ICD-10-CM Code(s): _____

1.159. ASHD of transplanted heart (native artery)

ICD-9-CM Code(s): _____

ICD-10-CM Code(s): _____

1.160. Atherosclerosis of left internal mammary artery bypass graft

ICD-9-CM Code(s): _____

ICD-10-CM Code(s): _____

1.161. Dysarthria secondary to old stroke (cerebrovascular disease)

ICD-9-CM Code(s): _____

ICD-10-CM Code(s): _____

1.162. Cerebral infarct due to stenosis of the vertebral artery

ICD-9-CM Code(s): _____

ICD-10-CM Code(s): _____

1.163. Chronic pulmonary embolism

ICD-9-CM Code(s): _____

ICD-10-CM Code(s): _____

1.164. Orthostatic hypotension

ICD-9-CM Code(s): _____

ICD-10-CM Code(s): _____

1.165. Varicose veins of the left leg with ulceration

ICD-9-CM Code(s): _____

ICD-10-CM Code(s): _____

1.166. Abdominal aortic aneurysm, ruptured

ICD-9-CM Code(s): _____

ICD-10-CM Code(s): _____

1.167. Chronic diastolic congestive heart failure

ICD-9-CM Code(s): _____

ICD-10-CM Code(s): _____

1.168. Chronic embolism of superior vena cava

ICD-9-CM Code(s): _____

ICD-10-CM Code(s): _____

Respiratory System

1.169. Acute bronchitis

ICD-9-CM Code(s): _____

ICD-10-CM Code(s): _____

1.170. Acute laryngitis with airway obstruction

ICD-9-CM Code(s): _____

ICD-10-CM Code(s): _____

1.171. Hypertrophy of tonsils and adenoids

ICD-9-CM Code(s): _____

ICD-10-CM Code(s): _____

1.172. Maxillary sinus polyp(s)

ICD-9-CM Code(s): _____

ICD-10-CM Code(s): _____

1.173. The correct code assignment(s) for pneumonia due to the RSV organism is (are):

ICD-9-CM Code(s):

a. 486 and 079.6
b. 480.1
c. 466.11
d. 079.6

ICD-10-CM Code(s): _____

1.174. Methicillin resistant pneumonia due to Staphylococcus aureus

ICD-9-CM Code(s): _____

ICD-10-CM Code(s): _____

1.175. Acute exacerbation of chronic obstructive pulmonary disease

ICD-9-CM Code(s): _____

ICD-10-CM Code(s): _____

1.176. Emphysema

ICD-9-CM Code(s): _____

ICD-10-CM Code(s): _____

1.177. Bilateral granulomatous hemorrhagic septic pneumonia

ICD-9-CM Code(s): _____

ICD-10-CM Code(s): _____

1.178. Influenza A due to identified 2009 H1N1 influenza virus with pneumonia

ICD-9-CM Code(s): _____

ICD-10-CM Code(s): _____

1.179. Moderate persistent asthma with status asthmaticus

ICD-9-CM Code(s): _____

ICD-10-CM Code(s): _____

1.180. Postoperative pneumothorax

ICD-9-CM Code(s): _____

ICD-10-CM Code(s): _____

1.181. Acute on chronic respiratory failure

ICD-9-CM Code(s): _____

ICD-10-CM Code(s): _____

1.182. Tracheostomy stenosis

ICD-9-CM Code(s): _____

ICD-10-CM Code(s): _____

1.183. Postinfective bronchiectasis

ICD-9-CM Code(s): _____

ICD-10-CM Code(s): _____

1.184. What is the correct code assignment for extrinsic asthma with acute exacerbation and status asthmaticus?

ICD-9-CM Code(s):

a. 493.02
b. 493.00
c. 493.01
d. 493.02, 493.01

ICD-10-CM Code(s): _____

1.185. Spontaneous pneumothorax

ICD-9-CM Code(s): _____

ICD-10-CM Code(s): _____

1.186. Childhood asthma

ICD-9-CM Code(s): _____

ICD-10-CM Code(s): _____

1.187. Radiation pneumonitis due to radioactive isotope, initial encounter

ICD-9-CM Code(s): _____

ICD-10-CM Code(s): _____

1.188. Common cold

ICD-9-CM Code(s): _____

ICD-10-CM Code(s): _____

1.189. Aspiration pneumonia

ICD-9-CM Code(s): _____

ICD-10-CM Code(s): _____

1.190. Methicillin susceptible pneumonia due to Staphylococcus aureus

ICD-9-CM Code(s): _____

ICD-10-CM Code(s): _____

1.191. Respiratory bronchiolitis interstitial lung disease

ICD-9-CM Code(s): _____

ICD-10-CM Code(s): _____

Digestive System

1.192. Submandibular gland abscess

ICD-9-CM Code(s): _____

ICD-10-CM Code(s): _____

1.193. Acute duodenal ulcer with bleeding

ICD-9-CM Code(s): _____

ICD-10-CM Code(s): _____

1.194. Gastric ulcer

ICD-9-CM Code(s): _____

ICD-10-CM Code(s): _____

1.195. Leukoplakia of tongue

ICD-9-CM Code(s): _____

ICD-10-CM Code(s): _____

1.196. Identify the appropriate code for reflux esophagitis.

ICD-9-CM Code(s):

a. 530.81
b. 530.11
c. 530.10
d. 530.89

ICD-10-CM Code(s): _____

1.197. Select the correct code for acute peptic ulcer of stomach with perforation.

ICD-9-CM Code(s):

a. 533.10
b. 531.50
c. 533.60
d. 531.10

ICD-10-CM Code(s): _____

1.198. Angiodysplasia of the stomach

ICD-9-CM Code(s): _____

ICD-10-CM Code(s): _____

1.199. Alcoholic gastritis with hemorrhage

ICD-9-CM Code(s): _____

ICD-10-CM Code(s): _____

1.200. Acute obstructive appendicitis

ICD-9-CM Code(s): _____

ICD-10-CM Code(s): _____

1.201. Incisional hernia

ICD-9-CM Code(s): _____

ICD-10-CM Code(s): _____

1.202. Bilateral inguinal hernia, recurrent

ICD-9-CM Code(s): _____

ICD-10-CM Code(s): _____

1.203. Incarcerated right femoral hernia

ICD-9-CM Code(s): _____

ICD-10-CM Code(s): _____

1.204. Crohn's disease of the large bowel

ICD-9-CM Code(s): _____

ICD-10-CM Code(s): _____

1.205. Ulcerative colitis

ICD-9-CM Code(s): _____

ICD-10-CM Code(s): _____

1.206. Ileus due to gallstones impacting the intestine

ICD-9-CM Code(s): _____

ICD-10-CM Code(s): _____

1.207. Select the correct code for diverticulosis of the colon.

ICD-9-CM Code(s):

a. 562.11
b. 562.00
c. 562.10
d. 562.12

ICD-10-CM Code(s): _____

1.208. Postoperative peritoneal adhesions

ICD-9-CM Code(s): _____

ICD-10-CM Code(s): _____

1.209. Cholelithiasis with acute and chronic cholecystitis

ICD-9-CM Code(s): _____

ICD-10-CM Code(s): _____

1.210. Chronic pancreatitis

ICD-9-CM Code(s): _____

ICD-10-CM Code(s): _____

1.211. Pouchitis

ICD-9-CM Code(s): _____

ICD-10-CM Code(s): _____

1.212. Barrett's esophagus

ICD-9-CM Code(s): _____

ICD-10-CM Code(s): _____

Genitourinary System

1.213. Acute renal failure with lesion of tubular necrosis

ICD-9-CM Code(s): _____

ICD-10-CM Code(s): _____

1.214. Ureterolithiasis

ICD-9-CM Code(s): _____

ICD-10-CM Code(s): _____

1.215. Acute pyelonephritis

ICD-9-CM Code(s): _____

ICD-10-CM Code(s): _____

1.216. Urethrolithiasis

ICD-9-CM Code(s): _____

ICD-10-CM Code(s): _____

1.217. Hydronephrosis

ICD-9-CM Code(s): _____

ICD-10-CM Code(s): _____

1.218. UTI

ICD-9-CM Code(s): _____

ICD-10-CM Code(s): _____

1.219. Overactive bladder

ICD-9-CM Code(s): _____

ICD-10-CM Code(s): _____

1.220. Gross hematuria

ICD-9-CM Code(s): _____

ICD-10-CM Code(s): _____

1.221. Select the appropriate code for urethral stricture.

ICD-9-CM Code(s):

a. 598
b. 598.9
c. 598.00
d. 598.8

ICD-10-CM Code(s): _____

1.222. In the diagnostic statement "urinary tract infection due to *Escherichia coli*," which condition is coded as the principal diagnosis?

a. The *E coli*
b. The urinary tract infection
c. Either may be coded as the principal diagnosis.
d. The circumstances of the admission determine which condition is coded as the principal diagnosis.

1.223. Select the appropriate code for benign prostatic hypertrophy.

ICD-9-CM Code(s):

a. 222.2
b. 600.20
c. 600.00
d. 600.90

ICD-10-CM Code(s): _____

1.224. PIN II

ICD-9-CM Code(s): _____

ICD-10-CM Code(s): _____

1.225. In the diagnostic statement "tuberculous prostatitis," which condition is coded as the principal diagnosis in ICD-9-CM?

a. The tuberculosis
b. The prostatitis
c. Either may be coded as the principal diagnosis.
d. The circumstances of the admission determine which condition is coded as the principal diagnosis.

1.226. Gynecomastia

ICD-9-CM Code(s): _____

ICD-10-CM Code(s): _____

1.227. Acute PID

ICD-9-CM Code(s): _____

ICD-10-CM Code(s): _____

1.228. Endometriosis of the broad ligament

ICD-9-CM Code(s): _____

ICD-10-CM Code(s): _____

1.229. Corpus luteum cyst of ovary

ICD-9-CM Code(s): _____

ICD-10-CM Code(s): _____

1.230. Dysmenorrhea

ICD-9-CM Code(s): _____

ICD-10-CM Code(s): _____

1.231. Postmenopausal atrophic vaginitis

ICD-9-CM Code(s): _____

ICD-10-CM Code(s): _____

1.232. CIN II

ICD-9-CM Code(s): _____

ICD-10-CM Code(s): _____

1.233. Priapism due to trauma

ICD-9-CM Code(s): _____

ICD-10-CM Code(s): _____

1.234. Stenosis of cystostomy

ICD-9-CM Code(s): _____

ICD-10-CM Code(s): _____

Pregnancy, Childbirth, and the Puerperium

1.235. Contracted pelvis, infant delivered vaginally

ICD-9-CM Code(s): _____

ICD-10-CM Code(s): _____

1.236. Gestational diabetes, admitted for control, not delivered

ICD-9-CM Code(s): _____

ICD-10-CM Code(s): _____

1.237. Maternal hypotension syndrome, onset 10 minutes after delivery in third trimester

ICD-9-CM Code(s): _____

ICD-10-CM Code(s): _____

1.238. In ICD-9-CM, the postpartum period begins immediately following delivery and lasts for _____ weeks following delivery.

1.239. By ICD-9-CM definition, an "elderly primigravida" is a woman who is _____ _____ years or older at the time of her first delivery.

1.240. Large-for-dates baby, delivered this admission (maternal record) in third trimester

ICD-9-CM Code(s): _____

ICD-10-CM Code(s): _____

1.241. Twin delivery with two placentae and two amniotic sacs in third trimester (maternal record)

ICD-9-CM Code(s): _____

ICD-10-CM Code(s): _____

1.242. Vaginal delivery with third-degree perineal laceration

ICD-9-CM Code(s): _____

ICD-10-CM Code(s): _____

1.243. Postpartum puerperal sepsis, patient readmitted 2 weeks after delivery

ICD-9-CM Code(s): _____

ICD-10-CM Code(s): _____

1.244. Hyperemesis gravidarum at 16 weeks, with dehydration, not delivered

ICD-9-CM Code(s): _____

ICD-10-CM Code(s): _____

1.245. False labor, 39 weeks, not delivered

ICD-9-CM Code(s): _____

ICD-10-CM Code(s): _____

1.246. Pregnancy in bicornuate uterus, 20 weeks, undelivered this admission

ICD-9-CM Code(s): _____

ICD-10-CM Code(s): _____

1.247. Dehiscence of cesarean section wound requiring readmission 1 week after delivery

ICD-9-CM Code(s): _____

ICD-10-CM Code(s): _____

1.248. Postpartum amniotic fluid embolism occurring while patient is still in the hospital

ICD-9-CM Code(s): _____

ICD-10-CM Code(s): _____

1.249. In ICD-9-CM the fifth digit to describe a delivery that was accompanied by a postpartum complication while the patient was still in the hospital is _____ _____.

1.250. In ICD-9-CM if a patient is admitted for treatment of a postpartum condition following delivery that occurred during a previous episode of care, the appropriate fifth digit is _____.

1.251. Oligohydramnios, reported with ICD-9-CM code 658.0X, is:

    a. Infection of the amniotic fluid
    b. Excessive amount of amniotic fluid
    c. Deficient amount of amniotic fluid
    d. Embolism of amniotic fluid

1.252. Missed abortion

    ICD-9-CM Code(s): _____

    ICD-10-CM Code(s): _____

1.253. In ICD-9-CM when an abortion is complicated by septic shock, the appropriate fourth digit is _____.

1.254. Ectopic pregnancies include which of the following types?

    a. Tubal
    b. Abdominal
    c. Septic
    d. a and b

1.255. Classical hydatidiform mole

    ICD-9-CM Code(s): _____

    ICD-10-CM Code(s): _____

1.256. Spontaneous abortion at 21 weeks of gestation, complete

    ICD-9-CM Code(s): _____

    ICD-10-CM Code(s): _____

Skin and Subcutaneous Tissue

1.257. Carbuncle of the hand

    ICD-9-CM Code(s): _____

    ICD-10-CM Code(s): _____

1.258. Paronychia of right finger

    ICD-9-CM Code(s): _____

    ICD-10-CM Code(s): _____

1.259. Sunburn

    ICD-9-CM Code(s): _____

    ICD-10-CM Code(s): _____

1.260. Cellulitis of chin

ICD-9-CM Code(s): _____

ICD-10-CM Code(s): _____

1.261. Pilonidal cyst with abscess

ICD-9-CM Code(s): _____

ICD-10-CM Code(s): _____

1.262. Poison ivy

ICD-9-CM Code(s): _____

ICD-10-CM Code(s): _____

1.263. Dermatitis due to cat dander

ICD-9-CM Code(s): _____

ICD-10-CM Code(s): _____

1.264. Lupus erythematosus

ICD-9-CM Code(s): _____

ICD-10-CM Code(s): _____

1.265. Keloid scar

ICD-9-CM Code(s): _____

ICD-10-CM Code(s): _____

1.266. Actinic keratosis

ICD-9-CM Code(s): _____

ICD-10-CM Code(s): _____

1.267. Alopecia areata

ICD-9-CM Code(s): _____

ICD-10-CM Code(s): _____

1.268. Hidradenitis suppurativa

ICD-9-CM Code(s): _____

ICD-10-CM Code(s): _____

1.269. Select the correct code(s) for a stage II pressure ulcer of heel.

ICD-9-CM Code(s):

a. 707.15
b. 707.14
c. 707.07, 707.22
d. 707.09, 707.20

ICD-10-CM Code(s): _____

1.270. In the diagnostic statement "diabetic foot ulcer," what condition should be assigned as the principal diagnosis in ICD-9-CM?

    a. The ulcer
    b. The diabetes mellitus
    c. Either condition
    d. The circumstances of the admission will determine which condition is classified as the principal diagnosis.

1.271. Lichen planus, generalized

ICD-9-CM Code(s): _____

ICD-10-CM Code(s): _____

1.272. Contact dermatitis due to new detergent

ICD-9-CM Code(s): _____

ICD-10-CM Code(s): _____

1.273. Abscess of right axilla

ICD-9-CM Code(s): _____

ICD-10-CM Code(s): _____

1.274. Ammonia dermatitis from soiled diapers

ICD-9-CM Code(s): _____

ICD-10-CM Code(s): _____

1.275. Erythema multiforme

ICD-9-CM Code(s): _____

ICD-10-CM Code(s): _____

1.276. Second-degree sunburn

ICD-9-CM Code(s): _____

ICD-10-CM Code(s): _____

1.277. Dermatitis due to base metals in jewelry

ICD-9-CM Code(s): _____

ICD-10-CM Code(s): _____

1.278. Decubitus ulcer of the left elbow, stage III

ICD-9-CM Code(s): _____

ICD-10-CM Code(s): _____

1.279. Pilar cyst

ICD-9-CM Code(s): _____

ICD-10-CM Code(s): _____

1.280. Trichilemmal cyst

ICD-9-CM Code(s): _____

ICD-10-CM Code(s): _____

Musculoskeletal System and Connective Tissue

1.281. Bacterial pyogenic arthritis of the hip

ICD-9-CM Code(s): _____

ICD-10-CM Code(s): _____

1.282. Rheumatoid arthritis involving the hands

ICD-9-CM Code(s): _____

ICD-10-CM Code(s): _____

1.283. Aseptic necrosis of femoral head

ICD-9-CM Code(s): _____

ICD-10-CM Code(s): _____

1.284. Osteoarthritis of the knees

ICD-9-CM Code(s): _____

ICD-10-CM Code(s): _____

1.285. DJD, generalized

ICD-9-CM Code(s): _____

ICD-10-CM Code(s): _____

1.286. Chronic bucket handle tear of the lateral meniscus of the left knee

ICD-9-CM Code(s): _____

ICD-10-CM Code(s): _____

1.287. Chondromalacia patellae

ICD-9-CM Code(s): _____

ICD-10-CM Code(s): _____

1.288. Hemarthrosis of the elbow, chronic

ICD-9-CM Code(s): _____

ICD-10-CM Code(s): _____

1.289. Ankylosing spondylitis

ICD-9-CM Code(s): _____

ICD-10-CM Code(s): _____

1.290. Osteoarthritis of the cervical spine with cord compression documented at surgery

ICD-9-CM Code(s): _____

ICD-10-CM Code(s): _____

1.291. HNP L4–5, with left lower extremity sciatica

ICD-9-CM Code(s): _____

ICD-10-CM Code(s): _____

1.292. Degenerative disk disease of lumbar spine

ICD-9-CM Code(s): _____

ICD-10-CM Code(s): _____

1.293. Low back pain

ICD-9-CM Code(s): _____

ICD-10-CM Code(s): _____

1.294. Synovial cyst of wrist

ICD-9-CM Code(s): _____

ICD-10-CM Code(s): _____

1.295. SLE

ICD-9-CM Code(s): _____

ICD-10-CM Code(s): _____

1.296. Osteomyelitis, acute, of first and second metatarsi

ICD-9-CM Code(s): _____

ICD-10-CM Code(s): _____

1.297. Postmenopausal osteoporosis

ICD-9-CM Code(s): _____

ICD-10-CM Code(s): _____

1.298. Pathologic fracture of neck of femur, initial encounter

ICD-9-CM Code(s): _____

ICD-10-CM Code(s): _____

1.299. Nontraumatic complete tear of right rotator cuff

ICD-9-CM Code(s): _____

ICD-10-CM Code(s): _____

1.300. Kyphosis

ICD-9-CM Code(s): _____

ICD-10-CM Code(s): _____

Newborn/Congenital Disorders

1.301. Spina bifida of lumbar region with congenital hydrocephalus

ICD-9-CM Code(s): _____

ICD-10-CM Code(s): _____

1.302. Branchial cleft cyst

ICD-9-CM Code(s): _____

ICD-10-CM Code(s): _____

1.303. VSD

ICD-9-CM Code(s): _____

ICD-10-CM Code(s): _____

1.304. Coarctation of the aorta

ICD-9-CM Code(s): _____

ICD-10-CM Code(s): _____

1.305. Bilateral complete cleft palate

ICD-9-CM Code(s): _____

ICD-10-CM Code(s): _____

1.306. Hypospadias

ICD-9-CM Code(s): _____

ICD-10-CM Code(s): _____

1.307. Polycystic kidney disease

ICD-9-CM Code(s): _____

ICD-10-CM Code(s): _____

1.308. Congenital dislocation of left hip, with subluxation of right hip

ICD-9-CM Code(s): _____

ICD-10-CM Code(s): _____

1.309. Syndactyly of fingers involving soft tissues only

ICD-9-CM Code(s): _____

ICD-10-CM Code(s): _____

1.310. Congenital spondylolisthesis, L5-S1

ICD-9-CM Code(s): _____

ICD-10-CM Code(s): _____

1.311. Congenital urethral fistula

ICD-9-CM Code(s): _____

ICD-10-CM Code(s): _____

1.312. Klinefelter's syndrome

ICD-9-CM Code(s): _____

ICD-10-CM Code(s): _____

1.313. Osteogenesis imperfecta

ICD-9-CM Code(s): _____

ICD-10-CM Code(s): _____

1.314. Congenital CMV infection

ICD-9-CM Code(s): _____

ICD-10-CM Code(s): _____

1.315. Meconium aspiration syndrome

ICD-9-CM Code(s): _____

ICD-10-CM Code(s): _____

1.316. Hemolytic disease of newborn due to Rh maternal/fetal incompatibility

ICD-9-CM Code(s): _____

ICD-10-CM Code(s): _____

1.317. Omphalocele

ICD-9-CM Code(s): _____

ICD-10-CM Code(s): _____

1.318. Drug withdrawal syndrome in newborn due to heroin dependence in mother

ICD-9-CM Code(s): _____

ICD-10-CM Code(s): _____

1.319. In the diagnostic statement "newborn male with meconium aspiration syndrome, subarachnoid hemorrhage, and neonatal jaundice due to prematurity," what is the ICD-9-CM principal diagnosis?

a. 772.2
b. V30.00
c. 770.1
d. 774.2

1.320. Necrotizing enterocolitis of the newborn, stage 1

ICD-9-CM Code(s): _____

ICD-10-CM Code(s): _____

1.321. Supernumerary cervical rib

ICD-9-CM Code(s): _____

ICD-10-CM Code(s): _____

1.322. Pulmonary artery coarctation and atresia

ICD-9-CM Code(s): _____

ICD-10-CM Code(s): _____

1.323. Pulmonary arteriovenous malformation

ICD-9-CM Code(s): _____

ICD-10-CM Code(s): _____

1.324. Hemolytic disease in newborn due to ABO antibodies; baby has jaundice

ICD-9-CM Code(s): _____

ICD-10-CM Code(s): _____

1.325. Crack baby

ICD-9-CM Code(s): _____

ICD-10-CM Code(s): _____

Symptoms, Signs, and Ill-Defined Conditions

1.326. Anorexia

ICD-9-CM Code(s): _783.0_

ICD-10-CM Code(s): _R63.0_

1.327. Failure to thrive, 35-year-old patient

ICD-9-CM Code(s): _783.7_

ICD-10-CM Code(s): _R62.7_

1.328. Fussy infant

ICD-9-CM Code(s): _780.91_

ICD-10-CM Code(s): _R68.12_

1.329. Posttransfusion fever

ICD-9-CM Code(s): _780.66_

ICD-10-CM Code(s): _R50.84_

1.330. Syncope

ICD-9-CM Code(s): _780.2_

ICD-10-CM Code(s): _R55_

1.331. Chronic fatigue syndrome

ICD-9-CM Code(s): _780.71_

ICD-10-CM Code(s): _R53.82_

1.332. Chest wall pain

ICD-9-CM Code(s): _786.50_

ICD-10-CM Code(s): _R07.9_

1.333. Post-traumatic seizure

ICD-9-CM Code(s): _780.33_

ICD-10-CM Code(s): _R56.1_

1.334. Concentration deficit

ICD-9-CM Code(s): _799.51_

ICD-10-CM Code(s): _R41.840_

1.335. Abnormal GTT

ICD-9-CM Code(s): ___790.29___

ICD-10-CM Code(s): ___R73.09___

1.336. Nausea and vomiting

ICD-9-CM Code(s): ___787.01___

ICD-10-CM Code(s): ___R11.2___

1.337. Infant colic

ICD-9-CM Code(s): ___789.7___

ICD-10-CM Code(s): ___R10.83___

1.338. Urinary frequency

ICD-9-CM Code(s): ___788.41___

ICD-10-CM Code(s): ___R35.0___

1.339. RUQ abdominal pain

ICD-9-CM Code(s): ___789.01___

ICD-10-CM Code(s): ___R10.11___

1.340. LGISIL found on cervical pap smear

ICD-9-CM Code(s): ___795.03___

ICD-10-CM Code(s): ___R87.612___

1.341. Nonvisualization of gallbladder on x-ray examination

ICD-9-CM Code(s): ___793.3___

ICD-10-CM Code(s): ___R93.2___

1.342. Abnormal mammogram

ICD-9-CM Code(s): ___793.80___

ICD-10-CM Code(s): ___R92.8___

1.343. SIDS

ICD-9-CM Code(s): ___798.0___

ICD-10-CM Code(s): ___R99___

1.344. Cachexia

ICD-9-CM Code(s): ___799.4___

ICD-10-CM Code(s): ___R64___

1.345. Hyperventilation

ICD-9-CM Code(s): _786.01_

ICD-10-CM Code(s): _R06.4_

1.346. Dysphagia, pharyngeal phase

ICD-9-CM Code(s): _787.23_

ICD-10-CM Code(s): _R13.13_

1.347. Altered mental status

ICD-9-CM Code(s): _780.97_

ICD-10-CM Code(s): _R41.82_

1.348. Acute idiopathic pulmonary hemorrhage in a 2-month-old infant

ICD-9-CM Code(s): _786.31_

ICD-10-CM Code(s): _R04.81_

1.349. Fecal incontinence

ICD-9-CM Code(s): _787.60_

ICD-10-CM Code(s): _R15.90_

1.350. Abnormality of gait

ICD-9-CM Code(s): _781.2_

ICD-10-CM Code(s): _R26.9_

1.351. Elevated blood pressure reading without diagnosis of hypertension

ICD-9-CM Code(s): _796.2_

ICD-10-CM Code(s): _R03.0_

Trauma/Poisoning

1.352. Open skull fracture with subarachnoid and subdural hemorrhage, expired without regaining consciousness, initial encounter

ICD-9-CM Code(s): _____

ICD-10-CM Code(s): _____

1.353. Fracture of C3 with complete transection of spinal cord at that level, initial encounter

ICD-9-CM Code(s): _____

ICD-10-CM Code(s): _____

1.354. Fracture ribs 2 to 4 right and 2 to 5 left, initial encounter

ICD-9-CM Code(s): _____

ICD-10-CM Code(s): _____

1.355. Multiple open fractures of pelvis with loss of continuity of pelvic circle, initial encounter

ICD-9-CM Code(s): _____

ICD-10-CM Code(s): _____

1.356. Comminuted, impacted fracture of surgical neck of right humerus, initial encounter

ICD-9-CM Code(s): _____

ICD-10-CM Code(s): _____

1.357. Torus fracture of upper radius and ulna, left arm, initial encounter

ICD-9-CM Code(s): _____

ICD-10-CM Code(s): _____

1.358. Nursemaid's elbow, initial encounter

ICD-9-CM Code(s): _____

ICD-10-CM Code(s): _____

1.359. Missile fracture of left patella due to bullet, initial encounter

ICD-9-CM Code(s): _____

ICD-10-CM Code(s): _____

1.360. Dislocation of jaw, initial encounter

ICD-9-CM Code(s): _____

ICD-10-CM Code(s): _____

1.361. Sprained wrist, initial encounter

ICD-9-CM Code(s): _____

ICD-10-CM Code(s): _____

1.362. Pneumothorax with puncture wound of anterior thoracic cavity due to knife, initial encounter

ICD-9-CM Code(s): _____

ICD-10-CM Code(s): _____

1.363. Mosquito bite, buttocks, with secondary skin infection, initial encounter

ICD-9-CM Code(s): _____

ICD-10-CM Code(s): _____

1.364. Third-degree burns of palm of hand, initial encounter

ICD-9-CM Code(s): _____

ICD-10-CM Code(s): _____

1.365. Intentional overdose of Prozac, initial encounter

ICD-9-CM Code(s): _____

ICD-10-CM Code(s): _____

1.366. Anaphylactic shock due to ingestion of pecans, initial encounter

ICD-9-CM Code(s): _____

ICD-10-CM Code(s): _____

1.367. Frostbite of face, initial encounter

ICD-9-CM Code(s): _____

ICD-10-CM Code(s): _____

1.368. Leakage of prosthetic heart valve, initial encounter

ICD-9-CM Code(s): _____

ICD-10-CM Code(s): _____

1.369. Rejection of transplanted liver

ICD-9-CM Code(s): _____

ICD-10-CM Code(s): _____

1.370. Accidental laceration of aorta during laminectomy procedure

ICD-9-CM Code(s): _____

ICD-10-CM Code(s): _____

1.371. Confirmed battered spouse (wife seeking care), initial encounter

ICD-9-CM Code(s): _____

ICD-10-CM Code(s): _____

1.372. Retained cholelithiasis following cholecystectomy

ICD-9-CM Code(s): _____

ICD-10-CM Code(s): _____

1.373. Anaphylactic reaction due to vaccination, initial encounter

ICD-9-CM Code(s): _____

ICD-10-CM Code(s): _____

1.374. Aspiration pneumonia following surgery

ICD-9-CM Code(s): _____

ICD-10-CM Code(s): _____

1.375. Complete transection right common femoral artery, initial encounter

ICD-9-CM Code(s): _____

ICD-10-CM Code(s): _____

ICD-9-CM and ICD-10-CM External Causes of Morbidity

1.376. A patient was injured due to a tackle in a football game. The injury occurred on a football field, and the patient is a student who is on a recreational football team, initial encounter.

Assign the applicable ICD-9-CM and ICD-10-CM External Cause, Place of Occurrence, Activity, and Status Codes.

ICD-9-CM Code(s): *E000.8; E849.4; E007.0; E886.0*

ICD-10-CM Code(s): _____

1.377. A patient fell from a ladder inside a building construction site. Patient is an employed construction worker, initial encounter.

Assign the applicable ICD-9-CM and ICD-10-CM External Cause, Place of Occurrence, Activity, and Status Codes.

ICD-9-CM Code(s): *E000.0; E016.2; E849.3; E881.0*

ICD-10-CM Code(s): _____

1.378. Assign the appropriate external cause codes for burns due to ignition of clothing from fireplace in restaurant, initial encounter. Do not assign an external cause code for place of occurrence.

ICD-9-CM Code(s): *E893.1*

ICD-10-CM Code(s): _____

1.379. Assign the appropriate main external cause code for injury from rattlesnake bite, initial encounter.

ICD-9-CM Code(s): *E905.0*

ICD-10-CM Code(s): _____

1.380. Assign the appropriate main external cause code for injury in an avalanche, initial encounter.

ICD-9-CM Code(s): *E909.2*

ICD-10-CM Code(s): _____

1.381. A patient injured her toe due to bumping into a table while performing household maintenance in the kitchen of her single family home. The patient is an unemployed homeowner, initial encounter.

Assign the applicable ICD-9-CM and ICD-10-CM main External Cause, Place of Occurrence, Activity, and Status Codes.

ICD-9-CM Code(s): *E000.8; E013.9; E849.0; E917.3*

ICD-10-CM Code(s): _____

1.382. Assign the appropriate main external cause code for drowning in the bathtub, initial encounter.

ICD-9-CM Code(s): *E910.4*

ICD-10-CM Code(s): _____

1.383. Assign the appropriate main external cause code for injury from fireworks, initial encounter.

ICD-9-CM Code(s): *E923.0*

ICD-10-CM Code(s): _____

1.384. Assign the appropriate activity code involving rappelling.

ICD-9-CM Code(s): *E004.1*

ICD-10-CM Code(s): _____

1.385. Laceration of hand from assault with knife. Assign both the diagnosis code and the main external cause code, initial encounter.

ICD-9-CM Code(s): *882.0; E966*

ICD-10-CM Code(s): _____

1.386. Cervical strain due to car accident, secondary to loss of control and collision with tree. Patient was the restrained driver. Assign both the diagnosis code and the main external cause code, initial encounter.

ICD-9-CM Code(s): *847.0; E816.0*

ICD-10-CM Code(s): _____

1.387. Closed fracture of right ulna due to fall from motorcycle when sitting in driveway. Patient was a passenger on the back of the motorcycle, initial encounter. Assign both the diagnosis code and the main external cause code.

ICD-9-CM Code(s): *813.82; E818.3*

ICD-10-CM Code(s): _____

1.388. Assign the appropriate activity code for an injury that occurred while practicing drumming.

ICD-9-CM Code(s): *E018.1*

ICD-10-CM Code(s): _____

1.389. Assign the appropriate main external cause code for injury from dog bite, initial encounter.

ICD-9-CM Code(s): _E906.0_____

ICD-10-CM Code(s): _____

1.390. What is the appropriate place of occurrence code for an accident occurring on a street or highway?

ICD-9-CM Code(s): _E849.5_____

ICD-10-CM Code(s): _____

1.391. Assign the appropriate main external cause code for clamp left inside a patient during a surgical procedure.

ICD-9-CM Code(s): _E871.0_____

ICD-10-CM Code(s): _____

1.392. Assign the appropriate main external cause code for injury during a tornado, initial encounter.

ICD-9-CM Code(s): _E908.1_____

ICD-10-CM Code(s): _____

1.393. Assign the appropriate main external cause code for injury from a metalworking lathe, initial encounter.

ICD-9-CM Code(s): _E919.3_____

ICD-10-CM Code(s): _____

1.394. While at work, a patient was shot by another person, with the intent to injure using a shotgun. The accident occurred on the employer factory premises, initial encounter.

Assign the applicable ICD-9-CM and ICD-10-CM External Cause, Place of Occurrence, Activity, and Status Codes.

ICD-9-CM Code(s): _E000.0; E849.3; E965.1_____

ICD-10-CM Code(s): _____

1.395. Laceration of pinna of the ear from accidental human bite, with secondary skin infection. Assign both the diagnosis code and the main external cause code, initial encounter.

ICD-9-CM Code(s): _872.11 ; E928.3_____

ICD-10-CM Code(s): _____

ICD-9-CM V Codes/ICD-10-CM Z Codes

1.396. Encounter for artificial insemination

ICD-9-CM Code(s): _____

ICD-10-CM Code(s): _____

1.397. Hepatitis B carrier

ICD-9-CM Code(s): _____

ICD-10-CM Code(s): _____

1.398. History of carcinoma of the breast

ICD-9-CM Code(s): _____

ICD-10-CM Code(s): _____

1.399. History of colonic polyps

ICD-9-CM Code(s): _____

ICD-10-CM Code(s): _____

1.400. Family history of lung cancer

ICD-9-CM Code(s): _____

ICD-10-CM Code(s): _____

1.401. Well-baby visit, baby is 30 days old

ICD-9-CM Code(s): _____

ICD-10-CM Code(s): _____

1.402. Incidental pregnancy

ICD-9-CM Code(s): _____

ICD-10-CM Code(s): _____

1.403. Liveborn male twin, delivered by cesarean section

ICD-9-CM Code(s): _____

ICD-10-CM Code(s): _____

1.404. Encounter for amniocentesis for screening for chromosomal anomalies

ICD-9-CM Code(s): _____

ICD-10-CM Code(s): _____

1.405. Body mass index (BMI) 23.0 adult

ICD-9-CM Code(s): _____

ICD-10-CM Code(s): _____

1.406. Renal dialysis status

ICD-9-CM Code(s): _____

ICD-10-CM Code(s): _____

1.407. Cardiac pacemaker status, without complications

ICD-9-CM Code(s): _____

ICD-10-CM Code(s): _____

1.408. Encounter for reprogramming of AICD

ICD-9-CM Code(s): _____

ICD-10-CM Code(s): _____

1.409. Aftercare for pathological fracture of L4 vertebra, routine healing

ICD-9-CM Code(s): _____

ICD-10-CM Code(s): _____

1.410. Admission for change of tracheostomy tube and stoma revision

ICD-9-CM Code(s): _____

ICD-10-CM Code(s): _____

1.411. Admission for planned colostomy closure

ICD-9-CM Code(s): _____

ICD-10-CM Code(s): _____

1.412. Admission for chemotherapy

ICD-9-CM Code(s): _____

ICD-10-CM Code(s): _____

1.413. Patient status is "do not resuscitate (DNR)"

ICD-9-CM Code(s): _____

ICD-10-CM Code(s): _____

1.414. Observation of child post-MVA with no apparent injury and no complaints

ICD-9-CM Code(s): _____

ICD-10-CM Code(s): _____

1.415. Encounter for screening mammogram

ICD-9-CM Code(s): _____

ICD-10-CM Code(s): _____

1.416. History of gestational diabetes

ICD-9-CM Code(s): _____

ICD-10-CM Code(s): _____

1.417. Exposure to uranium

ICD-9-CM Code(s): _____

ICD-10-CM Code(s): _____

1.418. Homicidal ideation

ICD-9-CM Code(s): _____

ICD-10-CM Code(s): _____

ICD-9-CM Procedure Coding

1.419. Vasectomy

ICD-9-CM Code(s): _____

1.420. Stapling of left atrial appendage (LAA)

ICD-9-CM Code(s): _____

1.421. Right thyroid lobectomy

ICD-9-CM Code(s): _____

1.422. Lamellar keratoplasty with donor corneal tissue

ICD-9-CM Code(s): _____

1.423. Myringotomy with placement of pressure equalization tube

ICD-9-CM Code(s): _____

1.424. Cleft palate repair

ICD-9-CM Code(s): _____

1.425. Lung volume reduction surgery

ICD-9-CM Code(s): _____

1.426. Open-heart surgery for repair of atrial septal defect with mesh

ICD-9-CM Code(s): _____

1.427. Right coronary artery PTCA

ICD-9-CM Code(s): _____

1.428. Coronary artery bypass grafting using left and right internal mammary arteries

ICD-9-CM Code(s): _____

1.429. Bilateral radical neck dissection

ICD-9-CM Code(s): _____

1.430. Total intra-abdominal colectomy performed by laparoscope

ICD-9-CM Code(s): _____

1.431. Whipple procedure

ICD-9-CM Code(s): _____

1.432. Laparoscopic bilateral direct inguinal herniorrhaphy with mesh

ICD-9-CM Code(s): _____

1.433. Transplant nephrectomy

ICD-9-CM Code(s): _____

1.434. Paraurethral suspension utilizing Pereyra suture

ICD-9-CM Code(s): _____

1.435. Pelvic exenteration for ovarian cancer

ICD-9-CM Code(s): _____

1.436. Repair of fourth-degree laceration of rectum during delivery

ICD-9-CM Code(s): _____

1.437. Right total hip replacement

ICD-9-CM Code(s): _____

1.438. Reattachment of arm amputated through humerus

ICD-9-CM Code(s): _____

1.439. Mid-forceps extraction with episiotomy

ICD-9-CM Code(s): _____

1.440. Retropubic prostatectomy

ICD-9-CM Code(s): _____

1.441. Subtotal jejunectomy with end-to-end anastomosis

ICD-9-CM Code(s): _____

1.442. Percutaneous transmyocardial revascularization

ICD-9-CM Code(s): _____

1.443. Insertion of drug-eluting coronary artery stent

ICD-9-CM Code(s): _____

ICD-10-PCS Coding

1.444. Bilateral vasectomy, open.

ICD-10-PCS Code(s): _____

1.445. Ventriculoperitoneostomy: The operative report indicates that a synthetic shunt is placed to allow passage of the cerebral spinal fluid to the peritoneal cavity.

ICD-10-PCS Code(s): _____

1.446. Right thyroid lobectomy: The operative report indicates that the entire right thyroid lobe was excised using an open approach.

ICD-10-PCS Code(s): _____

1.447. Percutaneous lamellar keratoplasty, left cornea, with donor corneal tissue.

ICD-10-PCS Code(s): _____

1.448. Right myringotomy with placement of pressure equalization tube.

ICD-10-PCS Code(s): _____

1.449. Left below knee amputation, proximal tibia and fibula.

ICD-10-PCS Code(s): _____

1.450. Mitral valve replacement using porcine tissue, open.

ICD-10-PCS Code(s): _____

1.451. Right coronary artery PTCA.

ICD-10-PCS Code(s): _____

1.452. Fulguration of sigmoid colon polyp, endoscopic.

ICD-10-PCS Code(s): _____

1.453. Thrombectomy of arteriovenous dialysis graft. The operative report indicates that the AV graft is located in the right upper arm with the right cephalic vein being obstructed with the thrombus. An incision was performed as the approach to the procedure.

ICD-10-PCS Code(s): _____

1.454. Bilateral direct inguinal herniorrhaphy, open.

ICD-10-PCS Code(s): _____

1.455. Right kidney transplant, organ donor match.

ICD-10-PCS Code(s): _____

1.456. Laparoscopic left carpal tunnel release.

ICD-10-PCS Code(s): _____

1.457. Open reduction with internal fixation, left fibula.

ICD-10-PCS Code(s): _____

1.458. Right total hip replacement. The operative report indicated that the procedure was performed via an incision and the devices implanted were ceramic-on-ceramic and cemented in.

ICD-10-PCS Code(s): _____

1.459. Posterior spinal fusion of the anterior column at L2–L4 with Bak cage interbody fusion device, open.

ICD-10-PCS Code(s): _____

1.460. Diagnostic arthroscopy of the right knee.

ICD-10-PCS Code(s): _____

1.461. Revision of left knee replacement with readjustment of prosthesis, open.

ICD-10-PCS Code(s): _____

1.462. EGD with duodenal biopsy.

ICD-10-PCS Code(s): _____

1.463. Laparoscopic-assisted total vaginal hysterectomy.

ICD-10-PCS Code(s): _____

1.464. Hysteroscopy with diagnostic D&C.

ICD-10-PCS Code(s): _____

1.465. Extracorporeal shockwave lithotripsy (EWSL) of right ureter.

ICD-10-PCS Code(s): _____

Chapter 2

Basic Principles of CPT Coding

The following exercises are designed to review CPT coding guidelines and to provide practice in assigning CPT codes. Because CPT indexes procedures in many different ways, the rationale for the selection of a particular code may be different from the approach that you use. The information included in the rationale is not meant to describe the only way to obtain an appropriate code but to represent one possible way. Unless the coder is specifically instructed to assign modifiers, no modifiers will appear in the rationale.

Note: These exercises were developed to be used with the 2013 edition of CPT but are suitable for other editions in most cases.

Instructions: Circle the correct answer, fill in the blank, or assign the correct code(s) for each of the following exercise items.

CPT Organization, Structure, and Guidelines

2.1. Category II codes cover all but one of the following topics. Which is not addressed by Category II codes?

    a. Patient management
    b. New technology
    c. Therapeutic, preventive, or other interventions
    d. Patient safety

2.2. In CPT, the symbols ▶◀ are used to indicate:

    a. Changes in verbiage within code descriptions
    b. A new code
    c. Changes in verbiage other than that in code descriptions; for example, changes in coding guidelines or parenthetical notes
    d. A code for which there is a corresponding HCPCS Level II code

2.3.   During the performance of a femoral angioplasty, a patient develops additional areas of occlusion. A diagnostic angiogram of the affected artery is performed. Is it appropriate to code this diagnostic study in addition to the therapeutic procedure?

a. No. All diagnostic procedures are included in therapeutic interventional procedures.
b. Yes. Per revised coding guidelines, if there is a clinical change during an interventional procedure that requires further diagnostic study, the diagnostic angiogram may be reported in addition to the therapeutic procedure.

2.4.   Per CPT coding guidelines, a "complete" diagnostic ultrasound of the retroperitoneum includes at least the following organs:

a. Kidneys, abdominal aorta, common iliac artery origins, inferior vena cava
b. Kidneys, abdominal aorta, common iliac artery origins, inferior vena cava, urinary bladder
c. Liver, gallbladder, common bile duct, pancreas, spleen, kidneys, upper aorta, inferior vena cava
d. Kidneys, abdominal aorta, common iliac artery origins

2.5.   A list of codes describing procedures that include conscious sedation, if administered by the same surgeon as performs the procedure, can be found in:

a. Appendix E
b. Appendix F
c. Appendix G
d. Appendix J

2.6.   True or false? Category II codes may be used as the first-listed CPT code when the patient is seen only for counseling.

a. True
b. False

2.7.   Which of the appendices would a neurologist's practice consult to determine the nerve conduction code to assign for a study of the suprascapular motor nerve to the infraspinatus?

a. Appendix I
b. Appendix J
c. Appendix K
d. Appendix L

2.8.   In order to be included in the CPT manual, a procedure must meet which of the following criteria?

a. It must be commonly performed by many physicians across the country.
b. It must be consistent with contemporary medical practice.
c. It must be covered by Medicare.
d. Both a and b

2.9.   Which of the following statements about CPT Category III codes is false?

a. They are updated only once every 2 years.
b. They were developed to reflect emerging technologies and procedures.
c. They are archived after 5 years if the code has not been accepted for inclusion in the main body of CPT.
d. Reimbursement for these services is dependent on individual payer policy.

2.10.   Per CPT guidelines, a separate procedure:

a. Is coded when it is performed as a part of another, larger procedure
b. Is considered to be an integral part of another, larger service
c. Is never coded under any circumstances
d. Both a and b above

2.11.   Which of the following statements is (are) true of CPT codes?

a. They are numeric.
b. They describe nonphysician services.
c. They are updated annually by CMS.
d. All of the above

2.12.   What does the symbol ▲ before a code in the CPT manual signify?

a. The code is new for this year.
b. The code is exempt from bundling requirements.
c. The code can only be used as an add-on code, never reported alone or first.
d. The code has been revised in some way this year.

2.13.   What does the symbol ● before a code in the CPT manual signify?

a. The code is new for this year.
b. The code is exempt from bundling requirements.
c. The code can only be used as an add-on code, never reported alone or first.
d. The code has been revised in some way this year.

2.14.   CPT was developed and is maintained by:

a. CMS
b. AMA
c. The Cooperating Parties
d. WHO

2.15.   CPT is updated:

a. Annually for the main body of codes and every 6 months for Category III codes
b. Annually
c. Every 6 months
d. As often as required by new technology

2.16.   The Alphabetic Index to CPT includes listings for:

    a. Procedures/services
    b. Examinations/tests
    c. Anatomic sites
    d. All of the above

2.17.   The use of the term "for" followed by a diagnosis in CPT means that:

    a. The procedure must be reported for that diagnosis.
    b. The procedure can only be reported for that diagnosis.
    c. The diagnosis is an example of the types of diagnoses for which this procedure could be done.
    d. None of the above

2.18.   If a surgeon performs a procedure for which there is no CPT code and no HCPCS Level II code, what code should be reported on the CMS 1500 form?

    a. CPT code 99999
    b. An unlisted procedure code from the appropriate chapter of CPT
    c. An ICD-9-CM procedure code
    d. A procedure that does not have a valid CPT code should not be reported.

2.19.   There are six sections to CPT: E/M, laboratory/pathology, surgery, radiology, medicine, and _____.

2.20.   The symbol + before a code in CPT means that:

    a. This code can never be reported alone.
    b. This code can never be reported first.
    c. This is an add-on code.
    d. All of the above

2.21.   A listing of all current modifiers is found in which appendix of CPT?

    a. Appendix A
    b. Appendix B
    c. Appendix C
    d. Appendix D

2.22.   The codes in the musculoskeletal section of CPT may be used by:

    a. Orthopedic surgeons only
    b. Orthopedic surgeons and emergency department physicians
    c. Any physician
    d. Orthopedic surgeons and neurosurgeons

Evaluation and Management (E/M) Services

2.23. A nursing facility patient develops an acute illness and is seen by her attending physician. He performs a detailed interval history and a detailed physical examination and performs medical decision making of moderate complexity. What code should the physician use to report these services?

    a. 99304
    b. 99305
    c. 99309
    d. 99310
    e. 99318

2.24. For reporting of physician services, E/M codes are usually based on:

    a. Documentation of history, physical examination, and medical decision making
    b. The final diagnosis for the visit
    c. The amount of time spent with the patient
    d. Documentation of medical decision making

2.25. Select the appropriate E/M code for a new patient office visit in which a comprehensive history and comprehensive physical examination were performed and medical decision making was of moderate complexity.

_____

2.26. Select the appropriate E/M code for a new patient office visit in which a comprehensive history and comprehensive physical examination were performed and medical decision making was of straightforward complexity. _____

2.27. Select the appropriate E/M code for an established patient visit in which a comprehensive history and expanded problem-focused physical examination were performed and medical decision making was of low complexity.

_____

2.28. When counseling consumes more than half the total visit time, _____ may be used as the criterion for assigning the E/M code.

2.29. Observation E/M codes (99218–99220) are used when:

    a. A patient is admitted and discharged on the same date.
    b. A patient is admitted for routine nursing care following surgery.
    c. A patient does not meet admission criteria.
    d. A patient is placed in designated observation status.

2.30. A physician sees a patient in his office in the morning, then again in the early afternoon, at which time he sends the patient to the hospital in observation status. Later that day he visits the patient in the hospital and admits him as a full inpatient. What E/M codes should be assigned for this day of care?

    a. Two E/M codes for the office visits, one for the observation care, and one for the inpatient admission

    b. One code combining the two office visits, one for the observation care, and one for the inpatient admission

    c. One code for the observation care and one for the inpatient admission

    d. One code for the inpatient admission only

2.31. History, physical examination, and medical decision making are the _____ components considered in assigning an E/M code.

2.32. Which of the following are considered components of the social history?

    a. Occupational history

    b. Marital history

    c. Allergic history

    d. a and b above

2.33. Documentation in history of use of drugs, alcohol, and/or tobacco is considered part of the_____.

    a. Past medical history

    b. Social history

    c. Systems review

    d. History of present illness

2.34. Per CPT guidelines, a presenting problem of moderate severity is one that:

    a. May not require the presence of a physician, but for which care is provided under the supervision of a physician

    b. Runs a definite and prescribed course, is transient in nature and is not likely to permanently alter health status, or has a good prognosis with management and compliance

    c. Has a low risk of morbidity without treatment, little or no risk of mortality without treatment, with full recovery expected without functional impairment

    d. Has a moderate risk of morbidity without treatment, a moderate risk of mortality without treatment, uncertain prognosis, or increased probability of functional impairment

2.35. Pediatric inpatient critical care, patient 6 months of age, first day

Code(s): _____

2.36. Dr. Smith sees a patient in consultation in the hospital at the request of Dr. Jones. He renders an opinion. He then takes over the management of a portion of the patient's care. What codes should Dr. Smith use to bill for his subsequent hospital visits?

    a. Inpatient consultation codes
    b. Initial inpatient hospital care codes
    c. Subsequent hospital care codes
    d. No codes; the initial consultation includes all subsequent visits

2.37. Assign the appropriate E/M code for an outpatient office consultation in which the physician performed a detailed history, a comprehensive physical examination, and medical decision making of moderate complexity.

_____

2.38. Per CPT guidelines, a concise statement describing the symptom, problem, condition, diagnosis, or other factor that is the reason for the encounter, usually stated in the patient's words, is the definition of the:

    a. History of present illness
    b. Chief complaint
    c. Admission diagnosis
    d. Past history

2.39. Which of the following are parts of medical decision making?

    a. Number of possible diagnoses or management options that must be considered
    b. Amount or complexity of medical record, diagnostic tests, or other information that must be obtained, reviewed, and analyzed
    c. Risk of significant complications, morbidity, and/or mortality associated with the patient's presenting problem, the diagnostic procedures, and/or the management options
    d. All of the above

2.40. Which E/M codes are used to report services to patients in a facility that provides room, board, and other personal assistance services, generally on a long-term basis?

    a. Outpatient services
    b. Nursing facility care
    c. Domiciliary, rest home, or custodial care services
    d. Care plan oversight services

2.41. Preventive medicine services are based on which of the following criteria?

    a. Documentation of history, physical examination, and medical decision making
    b. Age of the patient
    c. Amount of time spent with the patient
    d. The final diagnosis for the visit

2.42.   AHIMA Hospital has a "fast-track" department attached to the emergency department. This area is staffed by emergency department physicians on a rotating basis, treats minor problems, and is open from 5:00 a.m. until 8:00 p.m. What codes should be used to report services rendered in this department?

a. Emergency department services codes
b. Office or other outpatient services codes
c. These are not codable services because the department is not open 24 hours per day.
d. Either office or emergency department codes may be used.

2.43.   In order to report a critical care code, a physician must spend at least _____ minutes with a critically ill patient.

Anesthesia Services

2.44.   Per CPT guidelines, anesthesia time begins when the anesthesiologist begins to prepare the patient for induction, and ends:

a. When the patient leaves the operating room
b. When the anesthesiologist is no longer in personal attendance
c. When the patient has fulfilled postanesthesia care unit criteria for recovery
d. When the patient leaves the postanesthesia care unit

2.45.   A physical status anesthesia modifier of P2 means that a patient:

a. Has a mild systemic disease
b. Has a severe systemic disease
c. Has a severe systemic disease that is a constant threat to life
d. Is moribund

2.46.   Qualifying circumstances anesthesia codes are used:

a. In addition to the anesthesia codes
b. To describe provision of anesthesia under particularly difficult circumstances
c. To describe circumstances that impact the character of the anesthesia
d. All of the above

2.47.   The qualifying circumstance code to assign when anesthesia services are provided under emergency circumstances is _____.

2.48.   Anesthesia for total repair of cleft palate, patient 4 years of age

Code(s): _____

2.49.   Anesthesia for tracheal reconstruction, patient 6 months of age

Code(s): _____

2.50.   Anesthesia for permanent transvenous pacemaker insertion

Code(s): _____

2.51. Anesthesia for lumbar laminectomy with fusion and insertion of rods and hooks

Code(s): _____

2.52. Anesthesia for ventral hernia repair, patient a 76-year-old female

Code(s): _____

2.53. Anesthesia for donor nephrectomy

Code(s): _____

2.54. Anesthesia for left knee arthroscopy with medial meniscectomy

Code(s): _____

2.55. Anesthesia for total hip replacement

Code(s): _____

2.56. Anesthesia for vasectomy

Code(s): _____

2.57. Anesthesia for cesarean section following failed attempt at vaginal delivery under spinal anesthesia

Code(s): _____

2.58. Anesthesia for emergency completion of near-total amputation through the midthigh with laceration of femoral artery with imminent exsanguination

Code(s): _____

2.59. Anesthesia for ORIF of fracture of the distal tibia and fibula

Code(s): _____

2.60. Anesthesia for left ventricular reduction surgery with heart–lung bypass and systemic hypothermia

Code(s): _____

2.61. Anesthesia for Whipple procedure

Code(s): _____

2.62. Anesthesia for direct coronary artery bypass grafting with pump oxygenator

Code(s): _____

2.63. Anesthesia for laparoscopically assisted vaginal hysterectomy

Code(s): _____

Integumentary System

2.64.   A patient undergoes placement of brachytherapy after loading of catheters into her right breast under conscious sedation. The physician who performs the procedure administers the Versed himself, and a nurse is present throughout the procedure to monitor the patient. Is it appropriate for the surgeon to report the conscious sedation for this procedure?

   a. Yes
   b. No

2.65.   Tissue transplanted from one individual to another of the same species but different genotype is called a(n):

   a. Autograft
   b. Xenograft
   c. Allograft or allogeneic graft
   d. Heterograft

2.66.   True or false? Per coding guidelines, skin grafting codes cannot be used unless there is surgical fixation of the graft to the recipient tissue.

   a. True
   b. False

2.67.   When a malignant lesion is excised and the resultant skin defect is closed with a Z-plasty, what code(s) should be reported?

   a. A code for the Z-plasty only (14000–14061)
   b. A code for the malignant lesion excision (11600–11646) and a code for the Z-plasty (14000–14061)
   c. A code for the malignant lesion excision only (11600–11646)
   d. A code for the complex repair only (13100–13160)

2.68.   When lesions are excised from multiple sites, which of the following is the correct coding protocol?

   a. Add all the dimensions and assign one code based on the total area.
   b. Code each lesion separately.
   c. Code only the largest lesion.
   d. Add all the dimensions for each body part, such as arms, legs, and so on, and assign as many codes as there are body parts treated.

2.69.   A patient presents with a palpable lump in the left breast. The surgeon dissects down to the mass and removes it entirely. The procedure is described as "Biopsy of mass of left breast." Assign the appropriate CPT code (omitting modifiers).

   a. 19120
   b. 19101
   c. 19125
   d. 19301

2.70. When calculating dimensions for assigning a lesion excision code, which of the following is the appropriate method?

    a. Measurement of the lesion documented by the surgeon preexcision

    b. Measurement of the lesion plus circumferential margins documented by the surgeon preexcision

    c. Measurement of the lesion documented by the pathologist postexcision

    d. Measurement of the lesion plus circumferential margins documented by the pathologist postexcision

2.71. "The sharp removal by transverse incision or horizontal slicing to remove epidermal and dermal lesions without a full-thickness dermal excision" is the CPT definition of_____.

2.72. Debridement of skin, subcutaneous tissue, muscle, and bone. A total surface area of 18 sq cm was debrided down to and including removal of subcutaneous tissue.

    Code(s): _____

2.73. Excision of 2.5-cm solar keratosis of the cheek with no significant margins

    Code(s): _____

2.74. Excision of basal cell carcinoma, abdominal wall, 1.2 cm in diameter, with 1-cm skin margin all around

    Code(s): _____

2.75. Excision of skin and subcutaneous tissue from the right groin for hidradenitis, with layered closure

    Code(s): _____

2.76. Insertion and injection of tissue expander, scalp

    Code(s): _____

2.77. Repair of 5.2-cm laceration of the left hand, dorsum, with layered closure

    Code(s): _____

2.78. Repair of 3.4-cm laceration of the left forearm, single-layer closure with 4-0 Dexon; repair of 2.0-cm laceration of the left upper arm, single-layer closure

    Code(s): _____

2.79. Repair of 3.0-cm laceration of the scalp, 2.5-cm laceration of the left foot, and 6.0-cm laceration of the left lower leg

    Code(s): _____

2.80. Repair of 5.0-cm laceration of the left cheek, 3.2-cm laceration of the forehead, and 16.0-cm complex laceration of the left chest wall, utilizing multilayered closure

Code(s): _____

2.81. Incision and drainage of complicated pilonidal cyst

Code(s): _____

2.82. A wound repair that involves layered closure of one or more of the deeper layers of subcutaneous tissue and superficial (nonmuscle) fascia or extensive cleaning of heavily contaminated wounds is a (an) _____ repair.

2.83. Open excisional biopsy of breast lesion identified by preoperative placement of radiological marker

Code(s): _____

2.84. Mohs micrographic surgery involves the surgeon acting as:

   a. Both plastic surgeon and general surgeon
   b. Both surgeon and pathologist
   c. Both plastic surgeon and dermatologist
   d. Both dermatologist and pathologist

2.85. Excision of two nonpalpable suspicious area of possible microcalcification identified on mammogram (needle identifying the site placed at an outside radiologist's suite)

Code(s): _____

2.86. Excision of 2-cm squamous cell carcinoma from left chest with repair of resultant 8-cm^2 defect using V-Y plasty

Code(s): _____

2.87. Insertion of breast expander in post-mastectomy patient for breast reconstruction

Code(s): _____

2.88. Debridement down to and including removal of muscle and subcutaneous system; total surface area is 22 sq cm.

Code(s): _____

2.89. Complex wound repair (13100–13160) may require extensive undermining, placement of stents, or retention sutures.

   a. True
   b. False

2.90. Debridement is always considered a separate procedure and should always be reported.

    a. True
    b. False

2.91. Simple repair of a 3.0-cm laceration cheek with extensive removal of gravel and debris.

    Code(s): _____

Musculoskeletal System

2.92. Per coding guidelines, the type of fracture does not have a coding correlation to the type of treatment provided.

    a. True
    b. False

2.93. True or false? If a bone biopsy is performed in conjunction with a kyphoplasty procedure, it is separately coded.

    a. True
    b. False

2.94. Per the description of code 22523, fracture reduction and bone biopsy, if performed, are included in the procedure and are not separately coded. 3D reconstruction is not to be reported with which of the following base modalities?

    a. CT angiography
    b. MR angiography
    c. PET scans
    d. All of the above

2.95. Which of the following terms does not describe an open fracture?

    a. Missile
    b. Comminuted
    c. Infected
    d. Compound

2.96. Open fracture treatment includes which of the following scenarios?

    a. The fractured bone is exposed to the environment.
    b. The bone ends are visualized and internal fixation inserted.
    c. The fractured bone is opened remote from the fracture site and an intramedullary nail is inserted across the fracture site.
    d. All of the above

2.97. If an orthopedic surgeon attempted to reduce a fracture but was unsuccessful in obtaining acceptable alignment, what type of code should be assigned for the procedure?

a. A "with manipulation" code
b. A "without manipulation" code
c. An unlisted procedure code
d. An E/M code only

2.98. Keller bunionectomy

Code(s): _____

2.99. Diagnostic arthroscopy, left knee, with medial meniscectomy

Code(s): _____

2.100. Open reduction of knee dislocation with repair of the anterior cruciate ligament by anchor suture

Code(s): _____

2.101. Percutaneous vertebroplasty, T10. (Do not assign radiological supervision and interpretation code.)

Code(s): _____

2.102. Incision and drainage of infected shoulder bursa

Code(s): _____

2.103. Putti-Platt procedure, left shoulder

Code(s): _____

2.104. Open reduction, internal fixation humerus shaft fracture with cast application

Code(s): _____

2.105. Wrist fusion with bone graft from iliac crest

Code(s): _____

2.106. Closed reduction of distal radial wrist fracture

Code(s): _____

2.107. Total hip arthroplasty

Code(s): _____

2.108. Casting is separately reported:

    a. When a cast is replaced for stabilization or for patient comfort, by a separate physician

    b. For initial application by a physician who does not perform the fracture care

    c. When recasting is done during fracture follow-up

    d. All of the above

2.109. Anterior removal of artificial cervical disc

Code(s): _____

2.110. Open bone biopsy obtained from iliac crest

Code(s): _____

2.111. Application of short leg walking cast for severe sprain of ankle

Code(s): _____

2.112. Arthroscopy of shoulder with complete rotator cuff repair

Code(s): _____

2.113. Midthigh amputation of leg

Code(s): _____

2.114. Closed reduction, temporomandibular joint dislocation

Code(s): _____

2.115. Which of the following terms is used to describe the reduction of a fracture?

    a. Manipulation

    b. Traction

    c. Percutaneous fixation

    d. External fixation

2.116. Hip arthroscopy to perform a femoroplasty

Code(s): _____

2.117. Open treatment of 2 lumbar vertebral fractures, posterior approach

Code(s): _____

2.118. Segmental instrumentation is defined as fixation at each end of the construct and at least one additional interposed bony attachment.

    a. True

    b. False

2.119. Cranial halo application with seven pins placed for thin skull osteology

Code(s): _____

2.120. Excision of a 2.3-cm soft tissue tumor of the hand

Code(s): _____

2.121. Incision and drainage of infected bursa of the left shoulder.

Code(s): _____

2.122. Removal of 19 skin tags.

Code(s): _____

Respiratory System

2.123. A pulmonologist performed a diagnostic bronchoscopy with biopsy. The endoscope was introduced into the bronchus, and attachments were used to perforate the bronchial wall. Tissue was obtained and submitted to the pathologist, who identified it as "lung parenchyma." What type of biopsy was performed?

    a. Transbronchial lung biopsy
    b. Bronchial biopsy
    c. Bronchoalveolar lavage
    d. Protected specimen brush biopsy

2.124. Submucous resection of nasal turbinates

Code(s): _____

2.125. Control of epistaxis, anterior, by packing and silver nitrate cautery

Code(s): _____

2.126. Nasal sinus endoscopy with total ethmoidectomy

Code(s): _____

2.127. Total laryngectomy with left radical neck dissection

Code(s): _____

2.128. Direct laryngoscopy with vocal cord stripping using the operating microscope

Code(s): _____

2.129. Bronchoscopy with transbronchial lung biopsy

Code(s): _____

2.130. Thoracentesis without imaging guidance

Code(s): _____

2.131. Thoracoscopy of the pericardial sac with biopsy

Code(s): _____

2.132. Open Caldwell-Luc procedure of maxillary sinuses

Code(s): _____

2.133. Emergency endotracheal intubation

Code(s): _____

2.134. Flexible bronchoscopy with placement of catheters for afterloading of radiotherapeutic agents

Code(s): _____

2.135. Right lung middle lobectomy

Code(s): _____

2.136. Double-lung transplant with cardiopulmonary bypass

Code(s): _____

2.137. Functional endoscopic sinus surgery (FESS) with frontal sinus polyp removal

Code(s): _____

2.138. Endoscopic control of nasal hemorrhage

Code(s): _____

2.139. When a bronchoscopy is performed under fluoroscopic guidance, how are the codes assigned per CPT coding guidelines?

    a. The fluoroscopy guidance code is assigned as a secondary procedure code with the bronchoscopy code.
    b. The fluoroscopy guidance code is assigned as the first procedure code.
    c. The fluoroscopy is included in the bronchoscopy and no code is assigned for it.
    d. Individual hospital coding guidelines determine whether the fluoroscopy is separately coded.

2.140. Talc pleurodesis for pneumothorax

Code(s): _____

2.141. Laryngoplasty for reconstruction following third-degree chemical burns of the larynx

Code(s): _____

2.142. Anterovertical hemilaryngectomy

Code(s): _____

2.143. A surgical thoracoscopy always includes a diagnostic thoracoscopy.

    a. True
    b. False

2.144. Nasal endoscopy with dilation of frontal sinus ostium

Code(s): _____

2.145. Thoracotomy with removal of foreign body in the lung

Code(s): _____

2.146. Clagett procedure of chest wall

Code(s): _____

Cardiovascular System

2.147. Codes describing endovascular repair of the descending thoracic aorta include all of the following procedures except one. Which procedure is not included in the repair code?

    a. Arterial embolization
    b. Angiography of the thoracic aorta
    c. Fluoroscopic guidance in delivery of the endovascular components
    d. Preprocedure diagnostic imaging

2.148. True or false? A combination code exists for ligation and stripping of the long saphenous vein and ligation and stripping of the short saphenous vein.

    a. True
    b. False

2.149. In coding arterial catheterizations, when the tip of the catheter is manipulated from the insertion into the aorta and then out into another artery, this is called:

    a. Selective catheterization
    b. Nonselective catheterization
    c. Manipulative catheterization
    d. Radical catheterization

2.150. Complete pericardiectomy without cardiopulmonary bypass

Code(s): _____

2.151. Insertion of permanent pacemaker with ventricular transvenous leads

Code(s): _____

2.152. When coding a selective catheterization, how are codes assigned?

    a. One code for each vessel entered
    b. One code for the point of entry vessel
    c. One code for the final vessel entered
    d. One code for the vessel of entry and one for the final vessel, with intervening vessels not coded

2.153. Replacement of the mitral valve with cardiopulmonary bypass

    Code(s): _____

2.154. CABG using saphenous vein to the LAD

    Code(s): _____

2.155. LIMA graft to the circumflex coronary artery and sequentially to the right coronary artery

    Code(s): _____

2.156. Removal of intra-aortic balloon pump, percutaneous

    Code(s): _____

2.157. Introduction of catheter into the aorta

    Code(s): _____

2.158. Venipuncture by cutdown, patient 32 years of age

    Code(s): _____

2.159. A 4-year-old patient required implantation of a tunneled central venous catheter with insertion of a Life-Port vascular access device (VAD).

    Code(s): _____

2.160. Creation of Brescia-Cimino fistula for chronic hemodialysis

    Code(s): _____

2.161. Ligation and stripping of long and short saphenous veins

    Code(s): _____

2.162. Laparoscopic splenectomy

    Code(s): _____

2.163. Injection for identification of sentinel node

Code(s): _____

2.164. Temporal artery biopsy

Code(s): _____

2.165. A tunneled centrally-inserted central venous catheter is placed in a 57-year-old patient.

Code(s): _____

2.166. Blood transfusion

Code(s): _____

2.167. Aortobifemoral bypass graft

Code(s): _____

2.168. Revascularization by percutaneous transluminal popliteal angioplasty

Code(s): _____

2.169. The physician documents that he replaced the cardiac pacemaker "battery." The physician is actually referring to the:

a. Lead
b. Generator
c. Electrode
d. Cardioverter

2.170. Replacement of a peripherally inserted central venous catheter (PICC) through same access

Code(s): _____

2.171. Percutaneous endovascular revascularization of the right femoral vessel with transluminal stent placement and atherectomy

Code(s): _____

2.172. Application of right and left pulmonary artery bands

Code(s): _____

Digestive System

2.173. Primary repair of bilateral cleft lip, one-stage procedure

Code(s): _____

2.174. Laparoscopic repair of paraesophageal hernia with mesh

Code(s): _____

2.175. Uvulopalatopharyngoplasty for sleep apnea

Code(s): _____

2.176. T&A, 10-year-old patient

Code(s): _____

2.177. Upper gastrointestinal endoscopy with biopsy of lesion of esophagus

Code(s): _____

2.178. Per CPT coding guidelines, if a lesion is biopsied and then the remainder of the lesion is removed, what code(s) is (are) assigned?

   a. A code for the biopsy and one for the lesion excision
   b. A code for the lesion excision only
   c. A code for the biopsy only
   d. Hospital-specific coding procedures determine what is coded.

2.179. Rigid esophagoscopy with removal of impacted food

Code(s): _____

2.180. EGD with esophageal dilation over guidewire

Code(s): _____

2.181. When the physician does not specify the method used to remove a lesion during an endoscopy, what is the appropriate procedure?

   a. Assign the removal by snare technique code.
   b. Assign the removal by hot biopsy forceps code.
   c. Assign the ablation code.
   d. Query the physician as to the method used.

2.182. ERCP with sphincterotomy

Code(s): _____

2.183. Laparoscopic Nissen fundoplication

Code(s): _____

2.184. Laparoscopic gastric banding

Code(s): _____

2.185. Endoscopic percutaneous gastrostomy tube placement

Code(s): _____

2.186. Incision and drainage perianal abscess

Code(s): _____

2.187. Laparoscopic partial colectomy with end colostomy (Hartmann procedure)

Code(s): _____

2.188. Placement of seton

Code(s): _____

2.189. Small bowel endoscopy with control of hemorrhagic site in ileum using bipolar cautery

Code(s): _____

2.190. Colonoscopy with removal of five colonic polyps using hot biopsy forceps

Code(s): _____

2.191. Flexible sigmoidoscopy with decompression of volvulus

Code(s): _____

2.192. Laparoscopic cholecystectomy with cholangiography duct

Code(s): _____

2.193. Destruction of 2 groups of internal hemorrhoids with the use of infrared coagulation

Code(s): _____

2.194. Proctosigmoidoscopy with multiple biopsies and removal of foreign body

Code(s): _____

2.195. Complete esophagogastric fundoplasty via thoracotomy

Code(s): _____

Urinary System

2.196. Percutaneous needle biopsy of kidney

Code(s): _____

2.197. Donor nephrectomy, live donor open procedure

Code(s): _____

2.198. Surgical laparoscopy with ablation of renal cysts

Code(s): _____

2.199. Extracorporeal sound wave lithotripsy of large kidney stone

Code(s): _____

2.200. Change of ureterostomy tube

Code(s): _____

2.201. Complex cystometrogram with voiding pressure studies

Code(s): _____

2.202. Placement of indwelling bladder catheter

Code(s): _____

2.203. Cystourethroscopy with fulguration of three bladder tumors ranging in size from 0.4 to 1.6 cm

Code(s): _____

2.204. Cystourethroscopy with insertion of permanent urethral stent

Code(s): _____

2.205. Cystourethroscopy with insertion of double-J ureteral stent

Code(s): _____

2.206. Percutaneous cryoablation of two moderate-sized renal tumors

Code(s): _____

2.207. Transurethral resection of prostate with control of postoperative bleeding

Code(s): _____

2.208. Insertion of inflatable urethra–bladder neck sphincter

Code(s): _____

2.209. Repeat dilation of urethral stricture with filiforms and followers, male patient

Code(s): _____

2.210. Laparoscopic ureterolithotomy

Code(s): _____

2.211. Insertion of temporary prostatic urethral stent

Code(s): _____

2.212. Anterior vesicourethropexy by Marshall-Marchetti-Krantz procedure

Code(s): _____

2.213. Cystourethroscopy with biopsy of bladder wall

Code(s): _____

2.214. Cystourethroscopy with diagnostic ureteroscopy and removal of ureteral stones

Code(s): _____

2.215. Repeat transurethral resection of prostate tissue 4 years after original procedure

Code(s): _____

2.216. Transurethral radiofrequency micro-remodeling of the female bladder neck and proximal urethra

Code(s): _____

2.217. Closure of nephrovisceral fistula via thoracic approach

Code(s): _____

2.218. Backbench preparation of cadaver renal donor prior to transplantation including dissection of fat and other attachments, excision of adrenal gland, and preparation of ureters and vascular structures

Code(s): _____

Male/Female Genital System and Laparoscopy

2.219. Laser destruction of condylomata of penis

Code(s): _____

2.220. Insertion of inflatable penile prosthesis

Code(s): _____

2.221. Removal and replacement of semi-rigid penile prosthesis from infected site, with irrigation and debridement of infected and necrotic tissue

Code(s): _____

2.222. Laparoscopic orchiopexy for undescended (intra-abdominal) testicle

Code(s): _____

2.223. Vasectomy

Code(s): _____

2.224. Needle biopsy of prostate

Code(s): _____

2.225. Radical retropubic prostatectomy

Code(s): _____

2.226. Incision and drainage of Bartholin's abscess

Code(s): _____

2.227. Colposcopy of cervix with cervical curettage

Code(s): _____

2.228. Total abdominal hysterectomy with concurrent Marshall-Marchetti-Krantz urethropexy

Code(s): _____

2.229. Vaginal hysterectomy (weight of uterus, 283 g) with bilateral salpingo-oophorectomy

Code(s): _____

2.230. Biopsy of right ovary

Code(s): _____

2.231. Laparoscopic myomectomy with removal of eight intramural myomas

Code(s): _____

2.232. Ligation of fallopian tubes for elective sterilization

Code(s): _____

2.233. Laparoscopic sterilization procedure with fulguration, bilateral

Code(s): _____

2.234. Bilateral salpingo-oophorectomy for ovarian malignancy with pelvic lymph node and peritoneal biopsies

Code(s): _____

2.235. Catheterization with dye injection for hysterosalpingogram

Code(s): _____

2.236. Eight-day-old male infant surgically circumcised per parents' request

Code(s): _____

2.237. Testicular torsion repair

Code(s): _____

2.238. Laparoscopic fulguration of endometrial implants on the peritoneum and broad ligament

Code(s): _____

2.239. What is the correct CPT code assignment for hysteroscopy with lysis of intrauterine adhesions?

a. 58559
b. 58558, 58559
c. 58559, 58558, 58740
d. 58559, 58740

2.240. Insertion of a radiation afterloading apparatus into the vagina for brachytherapy

Code(s): _____

2.241. Repair of an incomplete circumcision

Code(s): _____

2.242. One stage urethroplasty using local skin flaps; patient has hypospadias

Code(s): _____

2.243. Excision of hydrocele, bilateral

Code(s): _____

2.244. Incision and drainage of a vulvar abscess

Code(s): _____

2.245. Hysteroscopy, with sampling of endometrium with D&C

Code(s): _____

Endocrine System

2.246. Incision and drainage of infected thyroglossal duct cyst

Code(s): _____

2.247. Percutaneous needle biopsy of thyroid gland

Code(s): _____

2.248. Excision of adenoma of thyroid

Code(s): _____

2.249. Partial right-sided thyroidectomy

Code(s): _____

2.250. Partial right-sided thyroid lobectomy with isthmusectomy and subtotal resection of left thyroid

Code(s): _____

2.251. Left total thyroid lobectomy

Code(s): _____

2.252. Total right-sided thyroid lobectomy with isthmusectomy and subtotal resection of left thyroid

Code(s): _____

2.253. Total thyroidectomy

Code(s): _____

2.254. Total thyroidectomy for thyroid carcinoma with partial neck dissection

Code(s): _____

2.255. Thyroidectomy for thyroid carcinoma with radical neck dissection

Code(s): _____

2.256. Parathyroidectomy

Code(s): _____

2.257. Thyroidectomy (with sternal portion of thyroid) via cervical approach

Code(s): _____

2.258. Excision of recurrent thyroglossal duct cyst

Code(s): _____

2.259. Parathyroidectomy with mediastinal exploration

Code(s): _____

2.260. Transthoracic thymectomy

Code(s): _____

2.261. Exploration and biopsy of adrenal glands, transabdominal

Code(s): _____

2.262. Laparoscopic adrenalectomy

Code(s): _____

2.263. Excision of carotid body tumor and carotid artery

Code(s): _____

2.264. Transthoracic thymectomy with radical mediastinal dissection

Code(s): _____

2.265. Aspiration of thyroid gland cyst

Code(s): _____

2.266. Thyroidectomy, total with removal of all thyroid tissue following a previous removal of a portion of the thyroid

Code(s): _____

2.267. Total thymectomy via transcervical approach

Code(s): _____

Nervous System

2.268. Cranial burr holes for drainage of subdural hematoma

Code(s): _____

2.269. Decompression craniectomy for treatment of intracranial hypertension

Code(s): _____

2.270. Excision of posterior fossa meningioma tumor via craniectomy

Code(s): _____

2.271. Percutaneous transcatheter embolization, spinal cord

Code(s): _____

2.272. Stereotactic radiosurgery for eradication of a 2.0-cm pituitary tumor

Code(s): _____

2.273. Ventriculoperitoneal shunt procedure

Code(s): _____

2.274. Therapeutic lumbar spinal tap for drainage of fluid

Code(s): _____

2.275. Implantation of cranial neurostimulator pulse generator

Code(s): _____

2.276. Excision neuroma, digital nerve, right fourth finger. Assign the CPT code and appropriate modifier.

Code(s): _____

2.277. Subtemporal decompression procedure for pseudotumor cerebri

Code(s): _____

2.278. Repair of 20-mm aneurysm, vertebrobasilar circulation

Code(s): _____

2.279. Stereotactic biopsy of intracranial lesion with magnetic resonance (MR) guidance. (Do not assign the radiological supervision and interpretation code.)

Code(s): _____

2.280. Intracranial neuroendoscopy with excision of pituitary tumor, transnasal approach

Code(s): _____

2.281. Reprogramming of programmable cerebrospinal fluid shunt

Code(s): _____

2.282. Anterior diskectomy, T2–3 interspace

Code(s): _____

2.283. Injection of lidocaine, brachial plexus

Code(s): _____

2.284. Suture of digital nerves to the left third and fourth fingers. Assign the appropriate modifier(s) in addition to the CPT code.

Code(s): _____

2.285. Phenol injection for destruction of the infraorbital branch of the trigeminal nerve

Code(s): _____

Eye/Ocular Adnexa

2.286. Removal of corneal foreign body without slit lamp

Code(s): _____

2.287. Penetrating keratoplasty, aphakic eye

Code(s): _____

2.288. Removal ocular implant

Code(s): _____

2.289. Extracapsular cataract extraction by phacoemulsification with placement of posterior chamber IOL

Code(s): _____

2.290. Scleral buckle for retinal detachment

Code(s): _____

2.291. YAG laser photocoagulation of diabetic retinopathy

Code(s): _____

2.292. Strabismus surgery with recession of lateral and medial rectus muscles

Code(s): _____

2.293. Strabismus surgery with recession of superior oblique muscle

Code(s): _____

2.294. Strabismus surgery with 6-mm recession of superior rectus muscle and 3-mm recession of inferior rectus muscle, with placement of adjustable suture at inferior rectus

Code(s): _____

2.295. Repair of blepharoptosis by frontalis muscle fascial sling

Code(s): _____

2.296. Repair of entropion by suture

Code(s): _____

2.297. Dacryocystorhinostomy

Code(s): _____

2.298. Probing of nasolacrimal duct with stent placement

Code(s): _____

2.299. Excision of chalazions (three) from left upper and left lower eyelids

Code(s): _____

2.300. Laser photocoagulation of retina for prophylaxis of retinal detachment

Code(s): _____

2.301. Trabeculectomy ab externo

Code(s): _____

2.302. Enucleation of eyeball with implant, muscle controlled

Code(s): _____

2.303. Removal of foreign body from posterior chamber using magnet

Code(s): _____

2.304. Excision of pterygium with normal conjunctival tissue graft

Code(s): _____

2.305. Subtotal vitrectomy with endolaser panretinal photocoagulation

Code(s): _____

2.306. Placement of self-retaining amniotic membrane on the eye for wound healing

Code(s): _____

2.307. Excision of 1.3-cm conjunctival lesion

Code(s): _____

2.308. Photocoagulation, iridoplasty, 3 sessions

Code(s): _____

Auditory System

2.309. Removal of exostosis, external ear canal

Code(s): _____

2.310. Myringotomy with aspiration under general anesthesia

Code(s): _____

2.311. Myringotomy with PE tube insertion

Code(s): _____

2.312. Tympanoplasty with mastoidectomy with ossicular chain reconstruction

Code(s): _____

2.313. Decompression of internal auditory canal

Code(s): _____

2.314. Drainage of abscess of external ear canal

Code(s): _____

2.315. Removal of bead from a toddler's external ear canal using conscious sedation

Code(s): _____

2.316. Biopsy external ear

Code(s): _____

2.317. Removal of impacted cerumen, bilateral

Code(s): _____

2.318. Tympanoplasty without mastoidectomy, with placement of PORP

Code(s): _____

2.319. Tympanostomy with ventilation tube insertion under general anesthesia

Code(s): _____

2.320. Transmastoid excision of glomus tumor of ear

Code(s): _____

2.321. Repair of tympanic membrane perforation using synthetic patch

Code(s): _____

2.322. Stapedotomy with footplate drillout

Code(s): _____

2.323. Implantation of cochlear device

Code(s): _____

2.324. Oval window fistula repair

Code(s): _____

2.325. Transcanal labyrinthectomy with mastoidectomy

Code(s): _____

2.326. Removal and replacement of electromagnetic hearing aid in temporal bone

Code(s): _____

2.327. Debridement of mastoid cavity under general anesthesia

Code(s): _____

2.328. Removal of ventilation tubes under general anesthesia

Code(s): _____

Radiology Services

2.329. True or false? Code 76857 Ultrasound, pelvic (nonobstetrical), real time with image documentation, limited or follow up, can be used to describe examinations of either the male or female pelvis.

a. True
b. False

2.330. X-ray of mandible, three views

Code(s): _____

2.331. X-ray, including fluoroscopy, of pharynx for foreign body

Code(s): _____

2.332. CT scan of the brain, with and without contrast

Code(s): _____

2.333. Chest x-ray, AP and lateral

Code(s): _____

2.334. Whole-body PET scan

Code(s): _____

2.335. X-ray, neck, six views, including oblique and flexion

Code(s): _____

2.336. Thoracic myelogram, radiological supervision and interpretation

Code(s): _____

2.337. Shoulder arthrogram, radiological supervision and interpretation

Code(s): _____

2.338. X-ray of fractured hip in the operating room to confirm reduction

Code(s): _____

2.339. Barium enema with KUB

Code(s): _____

2.340. Percutaneous transhepatic cholangiography, radiological supervision and interpretation

Code(s): _____

2.341. Intravenous pyelogram with KUB and tomograms

Code(s): _____

2.342. Angiography, radiological supervision and interpretation

Code(s): _____

2.343. Ultrasound, pregnant uterus, second trimester

Code(s): _____

2.344. Nonselective pulmonary angiography, radiological supervision and interpretation

Code(s): _____

2.345. SPECT bone scan

Code(s): _____

2.346. Mammographic guidance for preoperative needle placement in breast, radiological supervision and interpretation

Code(s): _____

2.347. Retroperitoneal ultrasound

Code(s): _____

2.348. Acute gastrointestinal blood loss imaging scan

Code(s): _____

2.349. CT scan of the abdomen and pelvis without contrast material would be coded:

    a. 72192, 74176
    b. 74178
    c. 74176
    d. 74178, 74177

2.350. A physician administers the injection for a retrograde urethrocystogram. He also provided supervision and interpretation services. What is the correct code(s)?

Code(s): _____

2.351. Ultrasonic guidance for amniocentesis, imaging supervision and interpretation

Code(s): _____

Pathology/Laboratory Services

2.352. The symbol ⊁ added to the Laboratory and Pathology section means:

    a. This is an add-on laboratory code.
    b. The code is sex specific.
    c. This code should only be reported for Medicare patients.
    d. FDA approval of the vaccine is pending.

2.353. Mr. Smith is seen in his primary care physician's office for his annual physical examination. He has a digital rectal examination and is given three small cards to take home and return with fecal samples to screen for colorectal cancer. Assign the appropriate CPT code to report this occult blood sampling.

    a. 82270
    b. 82271
    c. 82272
    d. 82274

2.354. True or false? Code 80048, basic metabolic panel, can be assigned with a modifier of 52, reduced services, if only seven of the eight tests are performed.

    a. True
    b. False

2.355. Code 87900, infectious agent drug susceptibility phenotype prediction using regularly updated genotypic bioinformatics, is used in the management of patients with what disease?

    a. Cancer patients on toxic chemotherapy agents
    b. HIV patients on antiretroviral therapy
    c. Tuberculosis patients on rifampin therapy
    d. Organ transplant patients on immunosuppressive therapy

2.356. Creatine phosphokinase isoenzymes

    Code(s): _____

2.357. Histamine

    Code(s): _____

2.358. Free prostate-specific antigen

    Code(s): _____

2.359. Spinal fluid pH

    Code(s): _____

2.360. Hepatic function panel

    Code(s): _____

2.361. Plasma sodium

Code(s): _____

2.362. Automated CBC with automated differential

Code(s): _____

2.363. Urine pregnancy test

Code(s): _____

2.364. Prothrombin time

Code(s): _____

2.365. Antinuclear antibody titer

Code(s): _____

2.366. VDRL

Code(s): _____

2.367. HBsAb

Code(s): _____

2.368. Chlamydia antibody, IgM

Code(s): _____

2.369. Erythrocyte sedimentation rate, automated

Code(s): _____

2.370. Surgical pathology, examination (gross and microscopic) of arterial biopsy

Code(s): _____

2.371. Surgical pathology, examination (gross and microscopic) of breast from mastectomy and regional lymph nodes

Code(s): _____

2.372. Lyme disease antibody

Code(s): _____

2.373. Automated urinalysis by dip stick with microscopy

Code(s): _____

2.374. Annual Pap test, smear manually obtained under physician supervision and examined by independent laboratory, test results reported using the Bethesda system

Code(s): _____

2.375. Bacterial blood culture

Code(s): _____

2.376. Antigen testing of donor blood using reagent serum

Code(s): _____

2.377. Infectious agent genotype analysis by nucleic acid, HIV-1, integrase regions

Code(s): _____

Medicine

2.378. An infusion that lasts less than 15 minutes would be reported with a(n) _____ code.

    a. Intravenous infusion
    b. Intravenous piggyback
    c. Intravenous push
    d. Intravenous hydration

2.379. Codes 96360 and 96361 are used to report infusion of:

    a. Chemotherapeutic agents
    b. Sequential drugs of the same drug family
    c. Hormonal antineoplastics
    d. Prepackaged fluids and/or electrolytes

2.380. A 7-year-old patient is seen for a minor routine therapeutic service that required the administration of moderate sedation for 40 minutes performed by a physician other than the physician performing the therapeutic service. Assign the appropriate CPT code(s).

    a. 99143
    b. 99144
    c. 99149
    d. 99149, 99150

2.381. A prostate cancer patient is seen in the office for infusion of luteinizing hormone-releasing hormone agonist therapy, given subcutaneously. Assign the appropriate CPT code.

    a. 96401
    b. 96402
    c. 96413
    d. 96405

2.382. True or false? When reported by the physician, the "initial service" code under Hydration, Infusions and Chemotherapy is chosen based on the first substance infused.

    a. True

    b. False

2.383. Select the appropriate code(s) to report an injection of rabies immune globulin performed under direct physician supervision.

    a. 96372

    b. 90471

    c. 90375, 96372

    d. 90375, 90473

2.384. Psychotherapy that involves the use of physical aids and nonverbal communication to overcome barriers to therapeutic intervention is called _____ psychotherapy.

2.385. Individual psychotherapy, inpatient hospital, 50 minutes

Code(s): _____

2.386. Duodenal manometry

Code(s): _____

2.387. Fluorescein angiography

Code(s): _____

2.388. Reprogramming of cochlear implant device, patient 11 years of age

Code(s): _____

2.389. Transcatheter placement of coronary artery stent, right coronary artery

Code(s): _____

2.390. EKG, physician interpretation and report, using hospital equipment

Code(s): _____

2.391. Combined right heart catheterization and retrograde left heart catheterization for congenital cardiac anomalies

Code(s): _____

2.392. Electronic analysis of pacing cardioverter-defibrillator, dual chamber, with reprogramming

Code(s): _____

2.393. Duplex scan of left lower extremity arteries

Code(s): _____

2.394. Pulmonary stress testing with measurements of CO_2 production, O_2 uptake, and electrocardiographic recordings

Code(s): _____

2.395. EEG, awake and asleep

Code(s): _____

2.396. Therapeutic exercises, 35 minutes

Code(s): _____

2.397. Chiropractic manipulation of the spine, thoracic, and lumbar regions

Code(s): _____

2.398. EMG testing of both upper extremities and related paraspinal musculature

Code(s): _____

2.399. Bronchospasm provocation evaluation

Code(s): _____

2.400. Lymphatic drainage (15 minutes of manual traction)

Code(s): _____

2.401. Chemotherapy administration via IV push

Code(s): _____

2.402. Comprehensive electrophysiologic testing with induction of arrhythmia

Code(s): _____

2.403. Vaccine for influenza virus, pandemic formulation, split virus for IM use; patient is 20 years old

Code(s): _____

2.404. Computerized ophthalmic diagnostic imaging, posterior segment, of the right retina

Code(s): _____

2.405. A cardiac clinic performs several cardiac catheterization procedures. Which of the following would be correct to report a right heart catheterization with measurement of oxygen saturation?

    a. 93451, 93455
    b. 93456
    c. 93453
    d. 93451

2.406. Coronary angiography, left ventriculography through left heart catheterization

Code(s): _____

2.407. Chemotherapy administered into the peritoneal cavity via indwelling port

Code(s): _____

Modifiers

2.408. In physician professional fee coding, when multiple procedures other than E/M services are provided on the same date by the same provider, modifier _____ should be appended to the second and all subsequent procedures.

2.409. The modifier used to report therapeutic interventional procedures on the right coronary artery is_____.

2.410. Which of the following circumstances can be described by the use of a HCPCS modifier?

    a. A service has been increased or reduced.
    b. Only part of a service was performed.
    c. A service was provided more than once.
    d. All of the above

2.411. A radiologist interprets x-rays for a community hospital. The equipment belongs to the hospital. What modifier should the radiologist append to his CPT codes? _____

2.412. A patient underwent repair of an ectropion of the left upper eyelid by tarsal wedge technique. Assign the appropriate CPT code and modifier(s).

_____

2.413. A pediatric thoracic and cardiovascular surgeon performs a curative procedure on an infant but does not see the child again. Instead, a pediatric cardiologist does all follow-up. What modifier should the surgeon append to his CPT procedure code? _____

2.414. A surgeon performs a palmar fasciotomy for Dupuytren's contracture of the right hand by open technique. Assign the appropriate CPT code(s) and modifier(s). _____

2.415. A patient is scheduled for a colonoscopy, but due to a sudden drop in blood pressure, the procedure is canceled just as the scope is introduced into the rectum. Because of moderately severe mental retardation, the patient is given a general anesthetic prior to the procedure. How should this procedure be coded by the hospital?

    a. Assign the code for a colonoscopy with modifier 74.
    b. Assign the code for a colonoscopy with modifier 52.
    c. Assign no code because no procedure was performed.
    d. Assign an anesthesia code only.

2.416. When clinical laboratory tests are repeated on the same day, what modifier should be assigned? _____

2.417. When a surgeon performs a procedure and a separately identifiable E/M service on the same date, how should codes and modifiers be assigned?

    a. Assign a code for the procedure only.
    b. Assign a code for the procedure and one for the E/M service without any modifiers.
    c. Assign a code for the procedure and one for the E/M service, with modifier 25 appended to the E/M code.
    d. Assign a code for the procedure and one for the E/M service, with modifier 25 appended to both the E/M code and the procedure code.

2.418. When absolutely identical procedures are performed on both members of a set of paired organs, such as kidneys, what modifier is assigned?

_____

2.419. Planned rigid proctosigmoidoscopy with removal of foreign body under conscious sedation, procedure not completed due to hypotension. How would the physician report this?

Code(s): _____

2.420. When a separately identifiable evaluation and management service is performed by the same physician on the same day of a procedure of their service, what modifier should be reported with the E/M code?

_____

2.421. When a physician performs a consultation as a required second opinion for an HMO, what modifier should be appended to the consultation code?

_____

2.422. When a patient is seen in two hospital outpatient departments in 1 day, what modifier should be appended to the second E/M code to ensure appropriate reimbursement? _____

2.423. When ambulance services are furnished directly by a provider of services, what modifier should be appended to the codes for ambulance services? _____

2.424. When a procedure or service is performed on the same day as other non-E/M services that are not normally reported together, but are appropriate under certain circumstances, modifier _____ should be appended to indicate that the procedure/service was distinct or independent.

2.425. In addition to the claim submitted by the surgeon, the assistant surgeon also bills for his or her services. What modifier does the assistant surgeon attach to the procedure code? _____

2.426. When two surgeons work together as primary surgeons performing distinct parts of a procedure, each surgeon should report which modifier to the procedure code(s)? _____

2.427. Some reconstructive plastic surgical procedures are performed in multiple stages. What modifier should the surgeon report when the patient is returned to surgery for a planned-staged procedure? _____

Category III Codes

2.428. Which of the following statements about Category III CPT codes is true?

    a. They are temporary.
    b. They are updated more frequently than the rest of CPT.
    c. They are intended to allow for the coding of new technologies, services, and procedures.
    d. All of the above

2.429. Both a regular CPT unlisted procedure code and a Category III code may exist to report the same procedure. Which code(s) should be reported?

    a. Report the CPT unlisted procedure code.
    b. Report the Category III code.
    c. Report both the CPT unlisted procedure code and the Category III code.
    d. Report the Category III code with modifier 59.

2.430. After 5 years, all Category III codes:

    a. Will be archived unless there is evidence that a temporary code is still needed
    b. Will be automatically renewed for another 5 years
    c. Will be automatically retired
    d. Will be replaced with a regular CPT code

2.431. Fistulization of sclera for glaucoma, through ciliary body

    Code(s): _____

2.432. Holotranscobalamin, quantitative

    Code(s): _____

2.433. Excision of rectal tumor via TEMS approach

Code(s): _____

2.434. Lumbar discectomy and arthrodesis utilizing pre-sacral interbody fusion technique

Code(s): _____

2.435. How frequently are Category III codes updated?

    a. Annually
    b. Semiannually
    c. Every two years
    d. Every four months

2.436. Removal of intracardiac ischemia monitoring device

Code(s): _____

2.437. Remote real-time interactive video-conferenced critical care, evaluation, and management of a critically ill patient for 60 minutes

Code(s): _____

2.438. Suprachoroidal delivery of pharmacologic agent

Code(s): _____

2.439. Anterior diskectomy and total arthroplasty, utilizing artificial disk, of C3 and C4

Code(s): _____

2.440. Category III codes can be used by what groups of providers?

    a. Hospital outpatient providers only
    b. Physicians only
    c. Hospitals, physicians, insurers, health services researchers
    d. Medicare-approved providers only

2.441. 64-lead electrocardiogram with tracing and graphics, without interpretation and report

Code(s): _____

2.442. Extracorporeal shock wave for integumentary wound healing, high energy for initial wound

Code(s): _____

2.443. Near-infrared spectroscopy studies of a lower extremity wound for oxyhemoglobin measurement

Code(s): _____

2.444. Speech audiometry threshold, automated

Code(s): _____

2.445. Cerebral perfusion study using CT with contrast

Code(s): _____

2.446. Open treatment of 3 rib fractures using internal fixation

Code(s): _____

2.447. Automated comprehensive audiometry threshold evaluation and speech recognition

Code(s): _____

Chapter 3

HCPCS Level II Coding

> **Note:** These exercises are intended for use with the 2013 version of the Healthcare Common Procedure Coding System (HCPCS) Level II codes. HCPCS codes are revised annually by the Centers for Medicare and Medicaid Services (CMS) and become effective January 1 each calendar year. Books are available from a variety of publishers. An electronic file is available for downloading from the Internet at https://www.cms.gov/HCPCSReleaseCodeSets/ANHCPCS/list.asp.
>
> **Instructions:** Circle the correct answer, fill in the blank, or assign the correct code(s) for each of the following exercise items.

205

Drugs

3.1. HCPCS Level II contains codes for drugs that are administered:

   a. Subcutaneously
   b. Intramuscularly
   c. Intravenously
   (d.) All of the above

3.2. Injection Unasyn, 1.5 g

   Code(s): __J0295__

3.3. Injection baclofen, 50 mcg intrathecal trial

   Code(s): __J0476__

3.4. Injection Botox, two units

   Code(s): __J0585 x 2__   why x3 ?

3.5. Injection Dilaudid, 2 mg

   Code(s): __J1170__

3.6.   Injection RhoGam, 300 mcg

Code(s): _J2790_

3.7.   Injection Cytosar–U, 100 mg

Code(s): _J9100_

3.8.   Injection mitomycin, 5 mg

Code(s): _J9280_

3.9.   Injection digoxin, 0.3 mg

Code(s): _J1160_

3.10.   Intra-articular injection of Synvisc, 16 mg, left knee

Code(s): _J7325   why not x 16_

3.11.   Injection adrenalin, 0.1 mg

Code(s): _J0171_

3.12.   Injection Bicillin CR, 200,000 mg

Code(s): _J0558   why not x2_

3.13.   Injection ARZERRA, 10 mg

Code(s): _J9302_

Supplies

3.14.   CPAP device

Code(s): _____

3.15.   Blood tubing, venous, for hemodialysis

Code(s): _____

3.16.   Urinary ostomy pouch with barrier attached

Code(s): _____

3.17.   Alginate dressing, 36-in^2 pad

Code(s): _____

3.18.   Radiopharmaceutical technetium medronate (Tc-99m), 30 millicuries

Code(s): _____

3.19. Two-way Foley catheter

Code(s): _____

3.20. Tracheal suction, closed system, for 72 or more hours of use

Code(s): _____

3.21. Blood glucose reagent strips for home glucose monitor, bottle of 50 strips

Code(s): _____

3.22. Distilled water used with nebulizer, 1,000 mL

Code(s): _____

3.23. Surgical trays used in physician-office surgery

Code(s): _____

Ambulance

3.24. Advanced life support IV drug therapy disposable supplies

Code(s): _____

3.25. The two-character modifier to indicate that a patient was taken from the acute hospital to a skilled nursing facility by ambulance is:

Code(s): _____

3.26. Basic life support ambulance services

Code(s): _____

3.27. Ground ambulance transport services are reported:

    a. Per trip
    b. Per mile
    c. Per minute of travel time
    d. Per hour of travel time

3.28. Helicopter transport, per mile

Code(s): _____

3.29. Because of the patient's condition, an additional EMT is required for the transport. What is the code for the presence of the extra attendant?

Code(s): _____

3.30. Ambulance waiting time is measured in:

    a. Minutes
    b. Hours
    c. Half hours
    d. 10-minute increments

3.31. Routine disposable supplies used during a basic life support transport

Code(s): _____

3.32. Neonatal transport

Code(s): _____

3.33. Oxygen administered during advanced life support transport

Code(s): _____

3.34. Advanced life support defibrillation

Code(s): _____

Durable Medical Equipment

3.35. Rental of portable liquid oxygen system

Code(s): _____

3.36. Totally electric hospital bed, without mattress, and alternating pressure mattress for hospital bed

Code(s): _____

3.37. Cycler dialysis machine for peritoneal dialysis

Code(s): _____

3.38. Portable whirlpool

Code(s): _____

3.39. Wheelchair, amputee, with detachable arms and detachable, swing-away footrests

Code(s): _____

3.40. Adult transport chair for a patient with a weight of 350 pounds

Code(s): _____

3.41. Pulse oximeter

Code(s): _____

3.42. Eggcrate dry pressure pad

Code(s): _____

3.43. Four-lead TENS unit

Code(s): _____

3.44. Recording apnea monitor

Code(s): _____

3.45. Skin protection wheelchair seat cushion, adjustable, 28 inches in width

Code(s): _____

3.46. Breast pump, electric

Code(s): _____

Procedures/Services

3.47. True or false? Code G0118 should be assigned when an ophthalmologist screens a high-risk patient for glaucoma.

    a. True
    b. False

3.48. Colorectal cancer screening by barium enema

Code(s): _____

3.49. Diagnostic mammography, unilateral

Code(s): _____

3.50. PET scanning, whole body, for diagnosis of esophageal carcinoma, for restaging

Code(s): _____

3.51. Direct hospital observation referral for a patient with diagnosis of congestive heart failure (CHF), chest pain, or asthma

Code(s): _____

3.52. Transcatheter placement of drug-eluting stent, coronary artery, percutaneous

Code(s): _____

3.53.   Sacroiliac joint injection for arthrography

Code(s): _____

3.54.   Diabetes self-management training, group session, per 30 minutes

Code(s): _____

3.55.   Trimming of dystrophic nails

Code(s): _____

3.56.   Hepatitis B vaccine

Code(s): _____

3.57.   Implantable silicone breast prosthesis

Code(s): _____

3.58.   Auditory osseointegrated device abutment, replacement

Code(s): _____

3.59.   Screening for prostate cancer, digital rectal examination

Code(s): _____

Part II
Intermediate Coding Exercises

Chapter 4

Case Studies from Inpatient Health Records

Note: Even though the specific cases are divided by setting, most of the information pertaining to the diagnosis is applicable to most settings. If you practice or apply codes in a particular type of setting, you may find additional information in other sections of this publication that may be pertinent to you.

Every effort has been made to follow current recognized coding guidelines and principles, as well as nationally recognized reporting guidelines. The material presented may differ from some health plan requirements for reporting. The ICD-9-CM codes used are effective October 1, 2012, through September 30, 2013. The current standard transactions and code sets named in HIPAA have been utilized, which require ICD-9-CM Volume III procedure codes for inpatients. The 2013 draft editions of ICD-10-CM and ICD-10-PCS are utilized in this chapter.

Instructions: Cases are presented as either multiple choice or fill in the blank.

- For multiple-choice cases:
  - Select the letter of the appropriate code set.
- For the fill-in-the-blank cases:
  - Assign the MS-DRG, where indicated.
  - Assign present on admission (POA) indicator for each ICD-9-CM diagnosis code.
    - Y: Yes (POA)
    - N: No (Not POA)
    - U: Unknown (Documentation is insufficient to determine if condition is POA.)
    - W: Clinically undetermined (Provider is unable to clinically determine whether or not the condition was POA.)
    - Leave blank for the exercises in this book all codes that are exempt from POA reporting. See the Exempt List as published in the *ICD-9-CM Official Guidelines for Coding and Reporting.* These codes are exempt because they represent circumstances regarding healthcare encounters or factors influencing health status that do not represent a current disease or injury, or are always present on admission.

ICD-9-CM Coding Instructions:

- Sequence the ICD-9-CM principal diagnosis in the first diagnosis position.
- Assign all reportable secondary diagnosis codes including V codes and E codes (both cause of injury and place of occurrence).
- Sequence the ICD-9-CM principal procedure code in the first procedure position.
- Assign all reportable secondary ICD-9-CM procedure codes.

ICD-10-CM and ICD-10-PCS Coding Instructions:

- Sequence the ICD-10-CM principal diagnosis code in the first diagnosis position.
- Assign all reportable secondary ICD-10-CM codes.
- Sequence the principal ICD-10-PCS code in the first procedure position.
- Assign all reportable secondary ICD-10-PCS codes.

The scenarios are based on selected excerpts from health records. In practice, the coding professional should have access to and refer to the entire health record. Health records are analyzed and codes assigned based on physician documentation. Documentation for coding purposes must be assigned based on medical record documentation. A physician may be queried when documentation is ambiguous, incomplete, or conflicting. The queried documentation must be a permanent part of the medical record.

The objective of the cases and scenarios reproduced in this publication is to provide practice in assigning correct codes, not necessarily to emulate complete coding, which can be achieved only with the complete medical record. For example, the reader may be asked to assign codes based on only an operative report when in real practice, a coder has access to the entire medical record.

The *ICD-9-CM Official Guidelines for Coding and Reporting*, published by the National Center for Health Statistics (NCHS), includes Present on Admission (POA) Reporting Guidelines in Appendix I. These guidelines supplement the official conventions and instructions provided within ICD-9-CM. Adherence to these guidelines when assigning ICD-9-CM diagnosis codes is required under the Health Insurance Portability and Accountability Act (HIPAA) of 1996. Additional official coding guidance can be found in the American Hospital Association (AHA)'s *Coding Clinic for ICD-9-CM* publication.

Disorders of the Blood and Blood-Forming Organs

4.1.   This 45-year-old man underwent colon resection for carcinoma of the transverse colon. The physician progress note on postoperative day 2 states anemia. Hemoglobin and hematocrit levels dropped significantly after surgery, and a blood transfusion was ordered. How is the anemia coded?

ICD-9-CM Code(s):

a. 285.1
b. 998.11
c. 998.11, 285.1
d. Query the physician because opportunity exists to improve documentation of etiology of anemia

ICD-10-CM Code(s): _____

4.2. This 82-year-old female was admitted for acute exacerbation of chronic obstructive pulmonary disease. The progress notes indicate that the patient received a transfusion for anemia. The discharge diagnoses state acute exacerbation of chronic obstructive pulmonary disease and pancytopenia. Transfusion of nonautologous packed red blood cells was given via peripheral vein. What codes are assigned for this case?

ICD-9-CM Code(s):

a. 491.21, 284.19, 99.04
b. 491.21, 284.19, 285.9, 99.04
c. 496, 284.19, 99.04
d. 491.21, 284.19, 285.9, 99.02

ICD-10-CM Code(s): _____

ICD-10-PCS Code(s): _____

4.3. This 35-year-old female patient has carcinoma of the upper-outer left breast. On this admit she had a lumpectomy performed and a sentinel lymph node biopsy of the axillary lymph node. The pathology report for the lymph node states no pathological change. What codes are assigned in this case?

ICD-9-CM Diagnosis Code(s) with POA Indicator: _____

ICD-9-CM Procedure Code(s): _____

ICD-10-CM Code(s): _____

ICD-10-PCS Code(s): _____

ICD-10-PCS Note: Assign only the procedure codes for the lumpectomy and excision of left axillary lymph node for biopsy.

4.4. An 8-year-old male hemophiliac is admitted with acute blood loss anemia following uncontrolled bleeding. He was given 4 units of packed red blood cells via the peripheral vein. While in the hospital he also received his regular preventive infusion of clotting factors. Which of the following answers would be correct?

ICD-9-CM Code(s):

a. 286.0, 99.06, 99.03
b. 285.1, 286.0, 99.04, 99.06
c. 286.0, 285.1, 99.06, 99.03
d. 285.1, 99.06, 99.03

ICD-10-CM Code(s): _____

ICD-10-PCS Code(s): _____

4.5. What code(s) is/are assigned for a patient admitted for an azathioprine I drug-induced aplastic anemia (initial encounter)? The patient has peripheral neuropathy of multiple joints of the lower extremities secondary to severe rheumatoid arthritis.

ICD-9-CM Diagnosis Code(s) with POA Indicator and MS-DRG:

_____

ICD-9-CM Procedure Code(s): _____

ICD-10-CM Code(s): _____

ICD-10-PCS Code(s): _____

Disorders of the Cardiovascular System

4.6.   When a diagnostic statement lists hypertension and chronic kidney disease, which of the following coding guidelines applies?

ICD-9-CM

a. The conditions are reported with two separate codes unless the physician specifically states that there is a cause-and-effect relationship.
b. Code 403.9X is assigned, with an additional code to identify the stage of chronic kidney disease.
c. A cause-and-effect relationship is never assumed.
d. Code 403.9X is assigned, with an additional code to specify the type of hypertension.

ICD-10-CM

a. The conditions are reported with two separate codes unless the physician specifically states that there is a cause-and-effect relationship.
b. A code from category I12.9 is assigned, with an additional code from category N18 to identify the stage of chronic kidney disease.
c. A cause-and-effect relationship is never assumed.
d. Code I12.9 is assigned, with an additional code to specify the type of hypertension.

4.7.   This 52-year-old male stayed one week in Hospital A for an ST elevation lateral wall myocardial infarction (STEMI) and was then transferred to Hospital B for further treatment. A cardiac catheterization was performed at Hospital B, which revealed severe occlusive disease, and a coronary bypass grafting was carried out. The physician's final diagnostic statement at Hospital B listed, "Acute lateral wall STEMI due to severe coronary atherosclerosis." What is the appropriate principal diagnosis for Hospital B?

ICD-9-CM Diagnosis Code(s): _____

ICD-10-CM Code(s): _____

4.8.   A patient is readmitted to the acute care hospital from a long-term care facility for treatment of heart failure. She had an acute non-ST anterior wall myocardial infarction (MI) 5 weeks ago. She was placed in the intensive care unit and monitored on telemetry. She was also found to have urinary tract infection (UTI) due to *Escherichia coli*. After intense drug therapy, she continued to improve and was transferred back to the long-term care facility. The acute systolic and diastolic heart failure was improved, but she will be monitored. What codes are assigned in this case?

ICD-9-CM Code(s):

a. 428.21, 428.31, 410.12, 599.0, 041.49, 89.54
b. 428.41, 410.72, 599.0, 041.49, 89.54
c. 428.0, 412, 599.0, 041.49, 89.54
d. 428.41, 410.11, 599.0, 041.49, 89.54

ICD-10-CM Code(s): _____

ICD-10-PCS Code(s): _____

4.9. A patient with severe arteriosclerotic heart disease (ASHD) of native arteries, unstable angina and severe chronic obstructive pulmonary disease (COPD) was admitted for coronary artery bypass graft (CABG) with cardiopulmonary bypass for two hours. An open 3-vessel CABG with the left internal mammary artery anastomosed to the left anterior descending coronary artery and separate greater saphenous vein grafts, harvested endoscopically from the left leg, to the obtuse marginal branch and posterior descending coronary artery. Postoperatively, the patient developed pulmonary arterial embolus that required treatment and extended the inpatient stay.

ICD-9-CM Diagnosis Code(s) with POA Indicator and MS-DRG:

_____

ICD-9-CM Procedure Code(s): _____

ICD-10-CM Code(s): _____

ICD-10-PCS Code(s): _____

4.10. The following was documented in the history and physical:

This patient was admitted with a diagnosis of acute myocardial infarction. He was hospitalized for pneumonia last year and 2 years ago had surgery for a bleeding gastric ulcer. Additional history is that he was diagnosed 5 years ago with Parkinson's disease, which is getting progressively worse. He is being treated with levodopa. History also notes emphysema being treated with bronchodilators and corticosteroids.

Discharge Summary: The discharge summary repeats the information in the history and physical examination (H&P), plus adds the following information. During the hospital stay, the patient developed congestive heart failure confirmed by x-ray and started Lasix p.o.

Discharge Diagnoses: Acute ST elevation myocardial infarction, Parkinson's disease, congestive heart failure, emphysema, history of pneumonia, and history of bleeding gastric ulcer. What conditions are coded in this example?

a. Acute ST elevation myocardial infarction, congestive heart failure, Parkinson's disease, emphysema
b. Acute ST elevation myocardial infarction, congestive heart failure
c. Acute ST elevation myocardial infarction, congestive heart failure, Parkinson's disease, emphysema, pneumonia, bleeding ulcer
d. Acute ST elevation myocardial infarction, pneumonia, congestive heart failure, emphysema

4.11. The following documentation is from the health record of a cardiac service patient.

Discharge Summary

Admit Date:	1/9/XX
Discharge Date:	1/12/XX
Final Diagnoses:	1. Coronary artery disease (CAD)
	2. Sick sinus syndrome
Procedures:	1. Permanent dual chamber pacemaker insertion
	2. Percutaneous transluminal coronary angioplasty (PTCA) with stent insertion

History of Present Illness: The patient is a 60-year-old female who was admitted to another hospital on 1/8/XX, after experiencing tachycardia. There she underwent a cardiac catheterization, showing the presence of severe single-vessel coronary artery disease. The patient does not have any history of a CABG in the past. The patient has a history of sick sinus syndrome. She was transferred to our hospital to undergo a percutaneous transluminal angioplasty.

Physical Examination: No physical abnormalities were found on the cardiovascular examination. Pulse 50, blood pressure 100/66. HEENT: PERRLA, faint carotid bruits. Lungs: Clear to percussion and auscultation. Heart: Normal sinus rhythm with a 2.6 systolic ejection murmur. Extremities and abdomen were negative.

Laboratory Data: Unremarkable

Hospital Course: To manage the patient's sick sinus syndrome, a permanent dual chamber pacemaker with atrial and ventricular leads was implanted on 1/9. An incision was made into the left chest wall with the dual chamber pacemaker being placed in the subcutaneous pocket. Next, a small incision was made in the skin and the leads were percutaneously passed into the right ventricle and right atrium.

On 1/10, the patient underwent a PTCA with insertion of a drug-eluting stent in the right coronary artery without complications, and good results were obtained.

Postoperatively, the patient was stable and was subsequently discharged. Patient was discharged on the following medications: Cardizem, 30 mg p.o. q. 6 hours; ASA, 5 grains q. a.m.; Metamucil and Colace p.r.n.; Nitro paste 1/2 inch q. 6 hours.

ICD-9-CM Diagnosis Code(s) with POA Indicator and MS-DRG:

_____

ICD-10-CM Code(s): _____

4.12.   This 62-year-old male patient was admitted to the hospital with progressive episodes of chest pain determined to be crescendo angina. He had myocardial infarction 5 years ago and progressively has been having more frequent episodes of chest pain. During the hospital stay, he was given IV nitroglycerin and was subsequently placed on Cardizem for further treatment of his angina. He is scheduled for cardiac catheterization next week because he refused to have it performed during this admission. No other complications arose during the hospitalization. What is the code assignment?

ICD-9-CM Diagnosis Code(s): _____

ICD-9-CM Procedure Code(s): _____

ICD-10-CM Code(s): _____

ICD-10-PCS Code(s): _____

4.13. This 55-year-old female patient is admitted with occlusion of the cerebral arteries resulting in an infarction. The patient suffered a stroke 2 years ago with residual hemiplegia affecting her left dominant side. What would be the correct code assignment for this case?

ICD-9-CM Diagnosis Code(s) with POA Indicator and MS-DRG:

_____

ICD-10-CM Code(s): _____

4.14. A 75-year-old male patient was admitted for an acute exacerbation of chronic systolic congestive heart failure and severe mitral regurgitation and aortic stenosis. What would be the correct code assignment for this case?

ICD-9-CM Code(s):

a. 428.23, 396.2
b. 428.23, 428.0, 396.2
c. 428.0, 394.1, 424.1
d. 391.8, 396.2

ICD-10-CM Code(s): _____

4.15. What code(s) is/are assigned for percutaneous transluminal coronary angioplasty of two arteries, RCA with bare metal stent and LAD without stent?

ICD-9-CM Procedure Code(s): _____

ICD-10-PCS Code(s): _____

Disorders of the Digestive System

4.16. This 44-year-old male patient was admitted for evaluation of melena. This patient is known to have diverticulitis of the colon. He has noticed melena occasionally for the past week. The initial impression was that this is bleeding from diverticulitis. Patient was scheduled for colonoscopy. Colonoscopy identified the cause of the bleeding to be angiodysplasia of the ascending colon. What are the codes assigned for this case?

ICD-9-CM Diagnosis Code(s) with POA Indicator and MS-DRG:

_____

ICD-9-CM Procedure Code(s): _____

ICD-10-CM Code(s): _____

ICD-10-PCS Code(s): _____

4.17. The patient was admitted because of severe abdominal pain. There has been a history of abdominal pain and some bleeding, but never this severe. Because of the symptoms, the patient underwent emergency laparotomy to repair the perforation in the antrum of the stomach by suturing. The physician states: acute peptic ulcer with perforation and bleeding. What codes are assigned for this case?

ICD-9-CM Diagnosis Code(s) with POA Indicator and MS-DRG:

_____

ICD-9-CM Procedure Code(s): _____

ICD-10-CM Code(s): _____

ICD-10-PCS Code(s): _____

4.18. This patient with chronic systolic and diastolic congestive heart failure was admitted because of melena. Patient had EGD with biopsy of the stomach and duodenum. No findings were found to determine the source of the melena. What codes are assigned in this case?

ICD-9-CM Diagnosis Code(s) with POA Indicator and MS-DRG:

_____

ICD-9-CM Procedure Code(s): _____

ICD-10-CM Code(s): _____

ICD-10-PCS Code(s): _____

4.19. The patient is a 44-year-old male who started having abdominal pain the day before yesterday. Subsequently he had diarrhea. He had 4 episodes of diarrhea last night and then 4 episodes in the morning. The stools have turned to fairly frank blood. Also the abdominal pain got worse, and he said he felt dizzy when he stood up. Patient admitted for treatment of dehydration. Patient has frank blood coming out from his bowels. Stool culture and sensitivity revealed *Salmonella*. Physician documented that the abdominal pain, diarrhea, and bleeding were due to Salmonella gastroenteritis. Patient put on Levaquin IV and also rehydrated. Patient responded well and was discharged. What codes are assigned?

ICD-9-CM Code(s):

a. 003.0, 276.51
b. 558.9, 003.0, 276.51
c. 003.0, 578.9, 276.51, 787.91
d. 276.51, 003.0

ICD-10-CM Code(s): _____

4.20. A patient with diabetes and osteoarthritis of the knee is admitted for bilateral direct inguinal hernia repair. The operative report states the repair is done laparoscopically with Marlex mesh. What is the correct code assignment?

ICD-9-CM Diagnosis Code(s) with POA Indicator and MS-DRG:

_____

ICD-9-CM Procedure Code(s): _____

ICD-10-CM Code(s): _____

ICD-10-PCS Code(s): _____

4.21. An 80-year-old patient with hypertension was admitted to the hospital for cholecystectomy. The patient underwent an attempted laparoscopic cholecystectomy, but due to extensive adhesions, it had to be converted to an open cholecystectomy with exploration of the common duct and choledocholithotomy. Final diagnostic statement: 1. Acute and chronic cholecystitis with choledocholithiasis and cholelithiasis. 2. Hypertension. Correct code assignment would be:

ICD-9-CM Diagnosis Code(s) with POA Indicator and MS-DRG:

_____

ICD-9-CM Procedure Code(s): _____

ICD-10-CM Code(s): _____

ICD-10-PCS Code(s): _____

4.22. A 5-month-old patient presents with vomiting, diarrhea, and growth failure. The discharge diagnosis was eosinophilic allergic gastroenteritis and colitis. What is the correct code assignment?

ICD-9-CM Diagnosis Code(s) with POA Indicator and MS-DRG:

_____

ICD-10-CM Code(s): _____

4.23. **Preoperative Diagnoses:** Extensive diverticulitis of sigmoid colon with perforation; obstruction of right colon and proximal transverse colon Crohn's disease

Postoperative Diagnosis: Same

Procedures: Exploratory laparotomy sigmoid colectomy; extended right hemicolectomy; permanent colostomy

Procedure Description: After consent was obtained for the procedure, risks and benefits were described at length. The patient was taken to the operating room and placed supine on the operating room table. Preoperatively the patient received 3 g of IV Unasyn. The patient was placed under general endotracheal anesthesia. PAS stockings were applied to both extremities. The patient's abdomen was then prepped and draped in the standard surgical fashion.

A midline laparotomy incision was made from just around the umbilicus to the pubic symphysis. The midline of the fascia was divided, and the abdomen was entered. With exploration of the abdomen, extensive diverticular disease of the distal sigmoid colon was noted.

First order of business was to mobilize the sigmoid colon for a sigmoid colectomy. The left ureter was identified and was far from the area of the sigmoid colon. The sigmoid colon was mobilized laterally to include the area of the diverticulitis. The sigmoid colon was mobilized down to the peritoneal reflection. The medial aspect of the sigmoid colon was also mobilized. The colon was then completely mobilized. A point of transaction was chosen at the proximal sigmoid colon. The mesentery was then taken down across the sacrum. The vessels were tied with 2-0 silk sutures. The sigmoid colon was mobilized down to the proximal rectum. Once the proximal rectum was identified, the sigmoid colon was again transected, this time using a contour Ethicon stapler with a blue load. Both the right and left ureters were identified prior to any transection of the sigmoid colon. A 3-0 Prolene suture was then tagged to either edge of the rectal staple line.

The right colon was then inspected. Multiple perforations with sites of deserosalization with exposed mucosa were identified in the right colon. The right colon was mobilized by taking down the white line of Toldt all the way up to and including the hepatic flexure. The omentum was taken off the transverse colon with electrocautery. Once the colon was completely mobilized and became a medial structure, the terminal ileum was transected this time also using a 45-mm GIA stapler with a blue load. A point of transaction was chosen in the mid transverse colon just proximal to the middle colic artery where the last site of deserosalization was identified. The mid transverse colon was divided with a GIA 45-mm stapler with a blue load. The mesentery to the right colon and transverse colon were then taken down with Pean clamps and tied with 2-0 silk sutures. The specimen was then passed off the field.

The abdomen was then irrigated. Hemostasis was assured. The ileocolic anastomosis was then created between the terminal ileum and the mid transverse colon. The bowel were positioned to lie along side each other, and a side-to-side functional end-to-end anastomosis was created using a 45-mm GIA stapler with a blue load. The enterostomes were then closed together with a running 3-0 PDS suture followed by interrupted 3-0 GI silks in a Lembert fashion. A stitch was placed at the crotch of each of the bowel connections. A finger was palpated at the anastomosis, and it was widely patent. Mesenteric defect was then closed using 3-0 Vicryl suture in a running fashion.

Attention then turned toward formation of the end-descending colostomy. The descending colon had already been mobilized enough to make it to the anterior abdominal wall without any difficulty. A point on the anterior abdominal wall on the left-hand side just below the umbilicus was chosen for the colostomy. A small 1.5- to 2-cm circular incision was made on the anterior abdominal wall midway through the rectus muscle. The anterior fascia was divided in a cruciate fashion. The rectus muscles were split, and two fingers were palpated through the defect into the abdominal cavity. The descending colon was then grasped with an Allis clamp and passed through the defect and exteriorized. There was no tension on the colon.

On the undersurface of the peritoneum, the colon was tagged with 3-0 GI silk sutures ×2.

The midline fascial incision was then closed with a running #1 looped PDS ×2. The surgical incision was then irrigated with copious saline. The skin was then closed with surgical staples. The ostomy was then matured by removing the staple line and sewing the ostomy in place with 3-0 Vicryl sutures. The sutures were sown in circumferentially. An ostomy appliance was applied.

Sterile dressings were applied, and the patient was awakened from general anesthesia and transported to the recovery room in stable condition.

ICD-9-CM Diagnosis Code(s) with POA Indicator and MS-DRG:

_____

ICD-9-CM Procedure Code(s): _____

ICD-10-CM Code(s): _____

ICD-10-PCS Code(s): _____

Endocrine, Nutritional, and Metabolic Diseases and Immunity Disorders

4.24.   This 75-year-old female admitted because of chronic diarrhea and dehydration. History of herpes zoster, right upper extremity, leading to monoparesis, right upper extremity, with postherpetic neuralgia on the right side of the chest. She has been treated with heavy doses of Neurontin with no significant relief. On admission her chest x-ray showed resolving lingular and left lower lobe pneumonia and pneumonia in the right perihilar region. The patient is being treated with Levaquin for the pneumonia. She had colonoscopy in the hospital to determine a cause of her iron deficiency anemia. Colonoscopy with biopsies taken of the small bowel as well as the rectosigmoid area showed no specific etiology. What codes are assigned?

ICD-9-CM Diagnosis Code(s) with POA Indicator and MS-DRG:

_____

ICD-9-CM Procedure Code(s): _____

ICD-10-CM Code(s): _____

ICD-10-PCS Code(s): _____

4.25.   A 55-year-old female was admitted with diabetic gastroparesis documented as due to steroid-induced diabetes. The patient is on long-term use of systemic corticosteroids, which are properly taken. What codes would be assigned?

ICD-9-CM Diagnosis Code(s) with POA Indicator and MS-DRG:

_____

ICD-10-CM Code(s): _____

4.26.   The following information is contained in the health record.

Chief Complaint: History of nausea with severe vomiting for the past 2 to 3 days. Diabetes mellitus diagnosed at the age of 12 years.

Hospital Course: This 31-year-old male patient has a history of type I diabetes mellitus and is on 15 units of NPH and 10 of Regular in the morning, and 10 units of NPH and 5 of Regular in the evening. The patient started having symptoms of nausea. The patient at the same time had increased frequency of urination and polydipsia with evidence of uncontrolled diabetes. The patient was severely dehydrated on admission. There was no evidence of thrombophlebitis, varicosities, or edema on examination of the extremities. The patient was hydrated and, as a result, his blood sugar decreased from more than 600 to normal levels. The patient was discharged with the diagnosis of diabetic ketoacidosis, type 1.

What code(s) are assigned for this admission?

ICD-9-CM Diagnosis Code(s) with POA Indicator and MS-DRG:

_____

ICD-10-CM Code(s): _____

4.27.   From the health record of a patient requiring thyroid surgery:

History: Patient is a 50-year-old female who noted a swelling in the neck. Outpatient workup was done. Thyroid scan and thyroid sonogram revealed moderate enlargement of the left lobe of the thyroid gland measuring 1.1 × 2.2 cm, a solid nodule at the anterior aspect of the mid of the left lobe of thyroid measuring approximately 1 × 1.9 cm, a small cyst in the middle of the left lobe of the thyroid measuring 2.4 cm, normal right lobe of the thyroid, and a small cyst in the mid of the right lobe measuring 2.3 mm. Thyroid scan showed hot nodule, which is usually negative for malignancy. The fine-needle aspiration was strongly suspicious for papillary carcinoma.

Impression: Papillary carcinoma of the thyroid

Report of Operation:

Preoperative Diagnosis: Steroid nodule left lobe, rule out papillary carcinoma

Postoperative Diagnosis: Papillary carcinoma of thyroid

Procedure: Left thyroid lobectomy with isthmectomy and frozen section. Subsequently, patient underwent total thyroid right lobectomy.

Anesthesia: General endotracheal

Estimated Blood Loss: 50 cc. Replacement: IV fluids, sponge count, needle count times two correct

Technique: After patient was well anesthetized with general endotracheal anesthesia, a sand bag was placed underneath the shoulder blades. The neck was extended and stabilized and placed on a foam head pillow. Entire neck and anterior chest was prepped and draped in the usual manner. The skin incision site was marked with -2-0 VICRYL suture with pressure. Preempt analgesia was obtained with infiltration of .25 percent

Marcaine. Transverse skin incision was made in the anterior part of the neck, which was deepened through the subcutaneous tissue and the platysma. Upper and lower flaps were raised, upper flap up to the thyroid cartilage, lower flap up to the sternal notch. Hemostasis obtained with cautery as well as -3-0 VICRYL sutures. Midline fascia was incised. Strap muscles on the left side were separated from the underlying thyroid gland. Strap muscles were retracted laterally with a Green retractor. Middle thyroid veins were identified, divided between the clamps, ligated with -3-0 VICRYL suture. Patient was noted to have palpable thyroid nodule on the left lower part of the thyroid gland. Superior thyroid vessels were identified. External of the superior laryngeal nerve was identified and protected. Superior thyroid vessels were divided close to the thyroid clamp between the Mixter clamp and ligated with -2-0 VICRYL suture. Recurrent laryngeal nerve was identified and protected throughout the procedure. Superior and inferior parathyroids were identified, protected with their vasculature. Inferior thyroid vessels were divided close to the thyroid capsule after its branching to preserve the blood supply to the parathyroid gland. Isthmus was divided between the clamps, and the entire thyroid lobe was removed and sent for frozen section, which was reported to be a papillary carcinoma. After the pathology report, the decision was made to proceed with the total thyroidectomy, which was carried out in the following manner:

Strap muscles on the right side were separated from the right thyroid gland. Middle thyroid vessels were divided between the clamps, ligated with -3-0 VICRYL suture. Superior and inferior thyroid poles were identified. Superior thyroid vessels were divided close to the upper pole. During the procedure, the external branch of the superior laryngeal nerve was identified and protected. The divided vessels were ligated with -2-0 VICRYL suture. Recurrent laryngeal nerve was identified and protected. Inferior and superior parathyroid glands were identified and protected with vasculature. Inferior thyroid vessel branches were divided between the clamps; thereby the blood supply to the parathyroid glands was preserved. Care was taken to protect the recurrent laryngeal nerve throughout the procedure. The right lobe of the thyroid was completely removed after satisfactory hemostasis. No drains were placed. The strap muscles were approximated with interrupted -3-0 VICRYL suture. Platysma and subcutaneous tissue was approximated with interrupted -4-0 VICRYL suture. Skin approximated with subcuticular -4-0 Dexon. Sterile dressings were applied. At the end of the procedure the vocal cords were inspected. They were moving equally well. The patient tolerated the entire procedure well and was discharged in stable condition to the recovery room.

Discharge Information: Patient discharged after 2 days, with no complications.

Diagnosis: Papillary carcinoma of the thyroid, left and right lobes, with follicular pattern. Papillary carcinoma positive in one cervical lymph node. Will follow up with me in the office.

What are the correct codes in this case?

ICD-9-CM Diagnosis Code(s) with POA Indicator and MS-DRG:

_____

ICD-9-CM Procedure Code(s): _____

ICD-10-CM Code(s): _____

ICD-10-PCS Code(s): _____

4.28.   This 51 year-old male is a Type I insulin-dependent diabetic admitted for treatment of a grade III foot ulcer which involved necrosis of the muscle on the left foot with gangrenous changes resulting from diabetic neuropathy, atherosclerosis, and chronic peripheral vascular insufficiency. Excisional debridement of the ulcer to the muscle is accomplished.

Which of the following answers would be correct?

ICD-9-CM Code(s):

a. 250.71, 440.23, 250.61, 357.2, 86.22
b. 250.71, 440.24, 250.61, 357.2, 707.15, 83.45
c. 250.01, 440.20, 785.4, 357.2, 707.15, 86.28
d. 250.71, 440.24, 250.61, 357.2, 707.15, 86.28

ICD-10-CM Code(s): _____

ICD-10-PCS Code(s): _____

Disorders of the Genitourinary System

4.29.   From the health record of a patient with urinary retention admitted through the emergency department:

Discharge Summary

Pertinent History: The patient is a 34-year-old female admitted through the ER with severe, stabbing, low back pain and inability to urinate. The patient has a long history of pelvic inflammatory disease, with three surgical episodes to remove implants. CT scan revealed a mass in the area of the kidneys.

Hospital Course: The patient was admitted, prepped, and taken to surgery. Exploratory laparotomy revealed an area of pelvic inflammatory disease involving both kidneys in dense adhesions. Cultures indicate chlamydia. Both ureters were almost totally blocked. Dense adhesions were painstakingly taken down. This was done very carefully and required several hours of surgery. Care was taken not to sever the kidneys or ureters. INTERCEED adhesion barrier was applied.

Postoperatively, the patient was pain free.

Discharge Instructions: The patient was discharged home to return to see me in the office in 1 week.

Diagnosis: Severe pelvic adhesions, chlamydia infection.

Which of the following code sets would be reported for this admission?

ICD-9-CM Code(s):

a. 614.9, 079.98, 59.02
b. 614.6, 079.98, 59.02, 99.77
c. 614.6, 079.88, 54.59, 99.77
d. 614.3, 079.98, 59.02, 99.77

ICD-10-CM Code(s): _____

ICD-10-PCS Code(s): _____

4.30. From the health record of a patient requiring radical surgery:

Discharge Summary

Pertinent History: The patient is a 68-year-old female admitted through the ER. The patient's abdomen is enlarged to about 18-week size; however, the patient states she has actually lost 22 pounds over the past few weeks. Patient says her appetite has disappeared. Patient is admitted for workup and definitive treatment.

Hospital Course: The patient's CT scan and MRI revealed a suspicious mass in the pelvis. Patient was taken to surgery, where exploration revealed and pathology report later confirmed right ovarian cancer. A radical abdominal hysterectomy was performed, which in this case included removal of the uterus and upper vagina. Also performed were regional pelvic lymph nodes dissection (entire lymph node chain was resected) and bilateral salpingo-oophorectomy. The patient tolerated the procedure well.

Discharge Instructions: The patient was discharged home to see me in the office in 1 week for removal of staples and scheduling for oncologist consultation.

Which of the following code sets should be reported for this admission?

ICD-9-CM Code(s):

a. 183.0, 68.41, 65.61, 40.3
b. 183.0, 68.69, 65.61, 40.3
c. 198.6, 68.61, 65.61, 40.3
d. 183.0, 68.69, 65.61, 40.59

ICD-10-CM Code(s): _____

ICD-10-PCS Code(s): _____

4.31. This 80-year-old female patient was admitted with fever, malaise, and left flank pain. A urinalysis was performed and showed bacteria more than 100,000/mL. This was followed by a culture, showing *Escherichia coli* growth documented as *E. coli* urinary tract infection (UTI). On day 2 the patient had an exacerbation of chronic obstructive pulmonary disease (COPD) and was treated with an inhaler. This resolved the same day. Patient is also on current medication therapy for hypertension and arteriosclerotic heart disease (ASHD) of the native vessels. What codes are assigned for this encounter?

ICD-9-CM Diagnosis Code(s) with POA Indicator and MS-DRG:

_____

ICD-10-CM Code(s): _____

4.32.   This is a 47-year-old female admitted to the hospital for a scheduled total abdominal hysterectomy and bilateral salpingo-oophorectomy due to submucous leiomyoma of the uterus. The patient also has extensive endometriosis of the uterus, ovaries, and pelvic peritoneum. On the day of admission the patient was taken to surgery and, in addition to the scheduled procedure, lysis of extensive pelvic adhesions was also carried out. In the process of removing the adhesions, the physician accidently punctured the small bowel. This small puncture was quickly repaired. The patient was diagnosed with acute blood-loss anemia with a documented loss of 1,500 ml of blood during surgery. The remainder of the postoperative course was uneventful and the patient was discharged on day 4. Assign the codes for the diagnoses only.

ICD-9-CM Diagnosis Code(s) with POA Indicator and MS-DRG:

_____

ICD-10-CM Code(s): _____

4.33.   This 38-year-old mother of four children has been treated for nearly 20 years for severe cystic breast disease. The patient has elected to have her breasts removed to relieve the pain. She is also very worried about developing breast cancer because her mother died from breast cancer at age 42 years. She has had numerous breast biopsies, and each time they are benign. She may consider plastic reconstruction later, but is not interested in it now. She is in good health. She was taken to surgery, and bilateral simple mastectomies were performed. The pathology report shows severe cystic disease of both breasts. What codes are assigned?

ICD-9-CM Diagnosis Code(s) with POA Indicator and MS-DRG:

_____

ICD-9-CM Procedure Code(s): _____

ICD-10-CM Code(s): _____

ICD-10-PCS Code(s): _____

4.34.   This elderly patient has been treated for hypertension for many years. Otherwise he is in relatively good condition considering his age. He was brought to the ER and admitted in acute renal failure due to severe dehydration with hyponatremia. What code(s) are assigned for this case?

ICD-9-CM Diagnosis Code(s) with POA Indicator and MS-DRG:

_____

ICD-10-CM Code(s): _____

4.35. The 56-year-old patient who has type I diabetes mellitus is admitted with acute renal failure. Past medical history includes: hypertension, diabetic nephropathy, and chronic kidney disease stage IV. What codes are assigned?

ICD-9-CM Diagnosis Code(s) with POA Indicator and MS-DRG:

_____

ICD-10-CM Code(s): _____

4.36. A 56-year-old patient with end-stage renal failure has a bloodstream infection due to the central dialysis catheter. He is admitted for replacement of the catheter. What diagnosis code(s) are assigned?

ICD-9-CM Diagnosis Code(s) with POA Indicator and MS-DRG:

_____

ICD-10-CM Code(s): _____

Infectious Diseases

4.37. This is a 35-year-old HIV-positive male with progressive lymphadenopathy and unexplained fevers, night sweats, and chills. Low osmolar CT scan of the chest, abdomen, pelvis, and neck showed extensive lymphadenopathy involving mediastinum and left hilum, paratracheal nodal chains, retroperitoneum, right iliac nodal chains, and right inguinal nodes. There were several areas of atelectasis evident in the right lung. Lymph node biopsy suspicious for tuberculosis and in fact was AFB-positive. The patient was placed on respiratory isolation and serial sputums were obtained. The patient's sputum contained positive AFB on concentrated specimen. Also during the course of hospitalization, the patient complained of swelling in the bilateral lower extremities. Dopplers were negative for DVT. The patient was diagnosed with tuberculosis of intrathoracic, retroperitoneum, and inguinal lymph nodes, tubercle bacilli found by microscopy. The patient will be referred to the clinic for management of his HIV disease and associated tuberculosis. What diagnosis codes are assigned?

ICD-9-CM Diagnosis Code(s) with POA Indicator and MS-DRG:

_____

ICD-10-CM Code(s): _____

4.38. The discharge diagnosis for a patient admitted with urosepsis due to streptococcus and white blood cell count of 15,000. Urine culture and blood cultures were positive for streptococcus. After query to the physician regarding the meaning of the term *urosepsis*, an addendum was added to the record: Sepsis with streptococcal septicemia and urinary tract infection (UTI), both due to streptococcus B. What codes are assigned?

ICD-9-CM Diagnosis Code(s) with POA Indicator and MS-DRG:

_____

ICD-10-CM Code(s): _____

4.39. This 25-year-old patient was admitted with difficulty breathing. She has AIDS and is in the 21st week of pregnancy. Workup shows *Pneumocystis carinii* pneumonia. What codes are assigned in this case?

ICD-9-CM Diagnosis Code(s) with POA Indicator and MS-DRG:

_____

ICD-10-CM Code(s): _____

4.40. This 53-year-old male with emphysema, previous lung transplant 2 years ago, was admitted with history of elevated temperature of 101 degrees with associated malaise, fatigue, and headache. The patient continued to have temperature elevations after admission. He was started on intravenous ganciclovir and intravenous Imipenem. Blood and urine cultures were basically nondiagnostic. He underwent a bronchoscopy for bronchoalveolar lavage from his left transplanted lung, which did not show any evidence of viral or bacterial pathogens. The BAL was performed by washing out the alveolar tissue in order to obtain alveolar tissue for diagnosis. Blood CMV antigen test was positive and hence he was diagnosed with CMV infection. He has had a persistent cough, and microscopy confirmed the presence of pulmonary tuberculosis. The physician documentation shows the infiltrating pulmonary tuberculosis and CMV are HIV-related. Patient was treated with ethambutol. What codes are assigned?

ICD-9-CM Diagnosis Code(s) with POA Indicator and MS-DRG:

_____

ICD-9-CM Procedure Code(s): _____

ICD-10-CM Code(s): _____

ICD-10-PCS Code(s): _____

4.41. This 23-year-old female is admitted with pneumonia. She also has multiple bilateral lesions of the vulva and vagina with fluid-filled blisters. The history includes fever, and pain for 2 days. Sputum cultures show group A streptococcus. History also includes pain, particularly with urination, and itching of the genitals. Physician documents group A streptococcus pneumonia, vulvovaginitis due to herpes. What codes are assigned?

ICD-9-CM Diagnosis Code(s) with POA Indicator and MS-DRG:

_____

ICD-10-CM Code(s): _____

Disorders of the Skin and Subcutaneous Tissue

4.42. An elderly nursing home patient was admitted for pneumonia. He has frequent aspiration because of difficulty swallowing due to a previous stroke. This pneumonia was documented as aspiration pneumonia. He was also found on admission to have stage 2 decubitus ulcer on the left buttock. The patient received skin care by the nursing staff for this ulcer. What codes are assigned in this case?

ICD-9-CM Diagnosis Code(s) with POA Indicator and MS-DRG:

_____

ICD-9-CM Procedure Code(s): _____

ICD-10-CM Code(s): _____

ICD-10-PCS Code(s): _____

4.43. This patient had surgery 2 weeks ago for appendicitis. She is admitted now because of fever, pain, and redness at the operative site. There is evidence of cellulitis of the operative wound, and cultures confirm *Staphylococcus aureus* as the cause. She received IV antibiotics. She also has type II diabetes mellitus and is on oral antidiabetic medication. What codes are assigned?

ICD-9-CM Diagnosis Code(s) with POA Indicator and MS-DRG:

_____

ICD-10-CM Code(s): _____

4.44. This nursing home patient was admitted to the hospital with severe cellulitis in the leg. The cultures grew streptococcus B, and this was documented by the physician as the cause of the cellulitis. Patient was given IV antibiotics. He also has dominant right-sided hemiplegia from an old cerebrovascular accident (CVA) and was found to have a stage 1 decubitus ulcer of the right lower back. What code(s) are assigned?

ICD-9-CM Diagnosis Code(s) with POA Indicator and MS-DRG:

_____

ICD-10-CM Code(s): _____

4.45. This 85-year-old patient, who is a resident at the skilled nursing facility, was admitted with a severe decubitus ulcer on the right buttock, stage II, and a small chronic ulcer on the left heel limited to the skin area. Patient also has Alzheimer's disease. The treatment was an excisional debridement of the skin of the heel and an open excisional debridement into the muscle of the buttock. What is the code assignment?

ICD-9-CM Diagnosis Code(s) with POA Indicator and MS-DRG:

_____

ICD-9-CM Procedure Code(s): _____

ICD-10-CM Code(s): _____

ICD-10-PCS Code(s): _____

4.46. This 29-year-old female patient is admitted for wide local excision of melanoma on the back. She also has a history of asthma. The melanoma is a 2-mm lesion so a margin of 2 cm of normal skin was removed as well. After surgery, she had an acute exacerbation of her asthma treated with two nebulizer treatments with Alupent. The wide excision was performed and a full-thickness skin graft from the left thigh was applied. The donor site was sutured closed directly. What codes are assigned?

ICD-9-CM Diagnosis Code(s) with POA Indicator and MS-DRG:

_____

ICD-9-CM Procedure Code(s): _____

ICD-10-CM Code(s): _____

ICD-10-PCS Code(s): _____

Behavioral Health Conditions

4.47. **Case Scenario:** A patient in a state of acute intoxication presented for care. The patient's 12-year alcohol dependence is consistent with a high level of daily alcohol consumption. The patient was admitted for alcohol detoxification and rehabilitation. On the second day of admission, he began experiencing withdrawal symptoms of sweating and nausea. On the third day, the sweating became more profuse, and he developed irregular tremors and tachycardia. The delirium tremors were managed medically. The patient did not experience any seizures. Hallucinations abated by day 4. By day 5, the patient was resting more comfortably, and plans for rehabilitation were initiated. The patient expressed a desire to reduce his alcohol abuse to a "controlled" level. A motivational treatment plan was developed and implemented, with the short-term goal of assisting the patient in reaching a stable level of use; that is, controlled drinking and a long-range goal of motivating the patient to accept a goal of total abstinence. Initially, the patient actively participated in the program, but his motivation waned, and he left the program after signing out AMA without meeting any of the rehabilitation goals.

Which of the following code sets most accurately reflects this case scenario?

ICD-9-CM Code(s):

a. 291.81, 303.01, 94.63, 94.39
b. 291.81, 303.90, 94.62, 94.39
c. 291.0, 303.01, 94.63, 94.39
d. 291.0, 303.90, 94.62, 94.39

ICD-10-CM Code(s): _____

ICD-10-PCS Code(s): _____

4.48. This 30-year-old male was admitted after being transferred from the outpatient therapy services because of severe major depressive disorder with psychotic features. After a complete neuropsychological, personality, and behavioral psychological evaluation, the risks and benefits of ECT were reviewed and explained to the patient and his family. Single seizure unilateral ECT was administered three times per week. The patient tolerated the therapy well and responded quickly with overall improvement in the acute phase of his depressive disorder. After establishing adequate therapeutic levels of lithium, the patient was discharged to be managed as an outpatient. What codes are assigned?

ICD-9-CM Diagnosis Code(s) with POA Indicator and MS-DRG:

_____

ICD-9-CM Procedure Code(s): _____

ICD-10-CM Code(s): _____

ICD-10-PCS Code(s): _____

4.49. This patient has been living at home, but his dementia has been getting progressively worse. He was diagnosed with Alzheimer's disease over 2 years ago. The family called the police because he was missing from home. A search was conducted and an observant passerby called in a report of an elderly man who seemed to be disoriented at a nearby public park. He was found after several hours and brought to the hospital. He had fallen in the park and had a laceration on his right knee that required suturing of the subcutaneous tissue and skin. What codes are reported in this case?

ICD-9-CM Diagnosis Code(s) with POA Indicator and MS-DRG:

_____

ICD-9-CM Procedure Code(s): _____

ICD-10-CM Code(s): _____

ICD-10-PCS Code(s): _____

4.50. The patient was brought to the ER and then admitted because of acute alcohol inebriation. The discharge diagnosis is acute and chronic alcoholism, continuous. The patient also has a history of hypertension, for which he is currently taking medication for. What codes are assigned?

ICD-9-CM Diagnosis Code(s) with POA Indicator and MS-DRG:

_____

ICD-10-CM Code(s): _____

4.51. This 65-year-old chronic cigarette smoker for the past 40 years was admitted to the hospital with acute exacerbation of her chronic obstructive pulmonary disease. She has a history of anxiety syndrome due to hypothyroidism, and is maintained on medications for both the anxiety and the hypothyroidism. No symptomatology at the time of admission. On hospital day 2, she developed extreme anxiety and a psychiatric consultation was ordered. What codes are assigned in this case?

ICD-9-CM Diagnosis Code(s) with POA Indicator and MS-DRG:

_____

ICD-10-CM Code(s): _____

Disorders of the Musculoskeletal System and Connective Tissue

4.52. This patient was admitted for treatment of a traumatic left second metatarsal fracture. The fracture site was opened and reduced, followed by placement of three internal Kirschner wires. Two pins were then placed, and an external fixator frame was connected to the pins to provide pressure and hold them in reduction. What codes are assigned in this case?

ICD-9-CM Diagnosis Code(s) with POA Indicator and MS-DRG:

_____

ICD-9-CM Procedure Code(s): _____

ICD-10-CM Code(s): _____

ICD-10-PCS Code(s): _____

4.53. A patient is admitted with an infected right partial hip prosthesis. The prosthesis was removed, and the patient underwent a total hip titanium-polyethylene arthroplasty. What are the correct code assignments?

ICD-9-CM Diagnosis Code(s) with POA Indicator and MS-DRG:

_____

ICD-9-CM Procedure Code(s): _____

ICD-10-CM Code(s): _____

ICD-10-PCS Code(s): _____

4.54.   A patient was admitted for recurrent dislocation of the left shoulder. The operation included an abrasion acromioplasty with Mitek suture placement. Which of the following is the correct code assignment?

ICD-9-CM Code(s):

a. 718.31, 81.82
b. 718.31, 81.83
c. 831.00, 81.82
d. 718.32, 81.82

ICD-10-CM Code(s): _____

ICD-10-PCS Code(s): _____

4.55.   This is a 65-year-old lady with complaints of low-back pain with radiation down her right leg to her foot. This pain has been progressively worse over the last several months. MRI scan of the lumbar spine showed degenerative disc disease at L2–3, L3–4, and L4–5; L3–L4 with mild central canal stenosis; and facet arthropathy at L3–L4 and L4–L5. Past medical history includes coronary artery disease, hypertension, and lumbar osteoarthritis. Her current medications include Lipitor, Avapro, Ecotrin, Imdur, Lasix, K-Dur, calcium, and Vioxx. She had a CABG two years ago and PTCA with cardiac stents placed three years ago. Patient admitted for lumbar epidural steroid injections for her lumbar radiculopathy due to degenerative disc disease as noted on MRI results. Which of the following answers would be correct?

ICD-9-CM Code(s):

a. 722.52, 721.3, 414.00, 401.9, V45.81, V45.82, 03.92, 99.23, 88.93
b. 722.52, 721.3, 724.02, 724.4, 414.00, 401.9, V45.81, V45.82, 03.92, 99.23, 88.93
c. 724.4, 414.00, 401.9, V45.81, V45.82, 03.92, 99.23, 88.93
d. 722.52, 721.3, 414.00, 401.9, V45.81, V45.82, 03.91, 88.93

ICD-10-CM Code(s): _____

ICD-10-PCS Code(s): _____

4.56.   This 70-year-old female has been treated for progressive increasing pain in her back. She is to the point that she is unable to move. She was brought to the ER and admitted after x-ray shows severe compression fractures of the lumbar vertebrae due to her senile osteoporosis. An injection of local anesthetic was done into the spinal canal. What codes are assigned?

ICD-9-CM Diagnosis Code(s) with POA Indicator and MS-DRG:

_____

ICD-9-CM Procedure Code(s): _____

ICD-10-CM Code(s): _____

ICD-10-PCS Code(s): _____

4.57. This 45-year-old male patient in whom conservative treatment for degenerative disk disease of the lumbar spine has failed came to the hospital. The discectomy was performed at L5 and total spinal disk prosthesis inserted to restore disk function and anatomy. What procedure code(s) are assigned?

ICD-9-CM Code(s):

a. 80.51
b. 80.51, 84.65
c. 84.65, 80.51
d. 84.65

ICD-10-PCS Code(s): _____

4.58. What procedure code(s) is/are assigned for open osteotomy of the capitates and lunate bones, right hand?

ICD-9-CM Procedure Code(s): _____

ICD-10-PCS Code(s): _____

4.59. ## Discharge Summary

Date of Admission: 06/28/XX

Date of Discharge: 07/07/XX

Diagnoses: 1. Status post fractured right femoral neck.
2. Chronic obstructive pulmonary disease.
3. Rheumatoid arthritis, steroid dependent.
4. Osteoporosis.

Pertinent History: The patient was admitted on the 28th of June after a fall. She did not pass out but just fell and fractured her hip. She fell off of a stool at home. She underwent surgery for this. She had a hemiarthroplasty. She tolerated the procedure well and was transferred to A Pavilion for continued physical therapy and rehabilitation.

Pertinent Laboratory: CBC initially showed a white count of 15,400, subsequently the white count is 10,900 with 78 neutrophils. H&H was stable at 12.2 and 36.9. Theophylline level was 10.3, therapeutic.

Hospital Course: The patient tolerated physical therapy well. She was able to give her own Lovenox shots. She was anxious to go home on Saturday. Orthopedics had planned for 14 more days of Lovenox, and that will be given by the patient and prescribed by Dr. Thomas's group. She will be back in about 3 weeks. She will continue with her current medications, which are proventil 2 puffs q.i.d., Fosamax 10 mg q.a.m., Soma 350 mg q.i.d., Lovenox 30 mg q. 12 hours, folic acid 1 mg q. day, Lasix 40 mg b.i.d., Atrovent 2 puffs q. 6 hours, synthroid

0.075 q day, potassium 20 mEq b.i.d., prednisone 20 mg a day, Theo-Dur 100 mg in the morning and 200 mg in the evening. She takes Sonata and she will continue with 5 mg q.h.S. She will continue with her laxative of choice. She will restart her Nasonex, Celebrex, Vicodin, and Vanceril when she gets home. She will stay on a regular diet. Activities per her primary care physician. She will see me back in 3 weeks.

History and Physical Examination

Admission Date: 6/28

Chief Complaint: Hip fracture.

Present Illness: The patient is a 79-year-old white female who slipped off of a stool in the apartment's kitchen while talking to her daughter. She was apparently trying to do too many things at one time, trying to clean some books or something like that and then just slipped and fell off and fractured her hip. She lives alone, had to call for help. She denies any type of passing out, no head injury, and no history of falling a lot before.

Past Medical History: The patient denies any kind of past history of chest pains, exertional chest pain. She stopped smoking some time ago but continues to be mildly short of breath and that has been stable.

She has no gastrointestinal (GI) symptoms, only occasionally some mild stress incontinence.

Medications:
1. Nasonex nasal spray
2. Soma 350 mg 1 q.i.d.
3. Potassium 10 mEq. 2 b.i.d.
4. Celebrex 200 mg q.d.
5. Synthroid 0.075 q.d.
6. Vicodin p.r.n.
7. Fosamax 10 mg q.a.m.
8. Theo-Dur 200 mg ~ in the morning and 1 in the evening
9. Folic acid 1 q.d.
10. Lasix 40 mg b.i.d.
11. Prednisone 10 mg. 2 g.d.
12. Vanceril inhaler
13. Atrovent inhaler
14. Albuterol inhaler

Allergies: Halcion, which causes her to hallucinate.

Medical History: Her medical history includes rheumatoid arthritis, chronic obstructive pulmonary disease (COPD), osteoporosis, and congestive heart failure (CHF).

Social History: She is a widow, stopped smoking 12 years ago. Does not use any alcohol.

Family History: Noncontributory.

Physical Examination: Finds her alert and oriented in no acute distress. Her blood pressure is 140/68, pulse 74, respirations 18. She was afebrile. HEENT: Examination was negative. Neck: Supple without any adenopathy, no bruit was heard. Chest: Clear to auscultation. Heart: Sounds regular without any murmur or gallop. Abdomen: Soft, positive bowel sounds, nontender, no bruits heard. Extremities: Showed normal vascular status.

Laboratory and X-Ray Data: She has a complete blood count (CBC) and urinalysis essentially normal. EKG shows no acute changes. Chest x-ray is pending at this time. If that is normal, she will be able to go on to surgery; that is decided on by Dr. Rowan.

Impression(s): 1. Fracture right femoral neck.
                    2. Chronic obstructive pulmonary disease and rheumatoid arthritis. She is steroid dependent so we are going to increase the amount of steroids that she is taking right now. Continue her on her inhalers and restart her oral medications as directed later.

Operative Report

Date: 06/28

Preoperative Diagnosis: Displaced right femoral neck hip fracture.

Postoperative Diagnosis: Displaced right femoral neck hip fracture.

Operation: Right hip hemiarthroplasty (Zimmer LD/Fx cemented monopolar metal prosthesis).

Anesthesia: Spinal.

Indications: This is a 79-year-old, previously ambulatory female with a history of rheumatoid arthritis, osteoporosis, steroid-dependent, and emphysema, with the above diagnosis. Risks, benefits, and alternatives of the above procedure were explained to the patient in detail, and she consented to proceed.

Operative Procedure: The patient was taken to the operating room and placed in the lateral position on the transfer bed, where spinal anesthesia was administered. She was transferred to the left lateral decubitus position on a beanbag on the operative table. Padded all bony prominences. Peritoneum was sealed off with Steri-Drape. The right hip was prepped and draped in the usual sterile fashion. Longitudinal incision over the greater trochanter and proximal femur was performed curving posteriorly proximally along the gluteus maximus. Sharp dissection to the skin, Bovie dissection to the subcutaneous tissues down to tensor fascia lata, identifying the greater trochanter. Besides the tensor fascia lata and along with the incision splitting the fibrous gluteus maximus, controlling bleeders with Bovie cautery. Piriformis was identified and short external rotators were tagged with a #5 Tycron suture. These are moved from their insertion. T capsulotomy was performed. Displaced hip fracture was identified, femoral head was removed and measured, copious irrigation was performed, acetabular was visibly and palpable normal appearing. Sagittal saw was used to make cut in the femoral neck. Box osteotome was used to gain lateral entrance to the canal. The canal finder was used, easily locating the femoral canal. Sequential broaching was performed up to a 14, which fit well. Stating the appropriate anteversion. Trawled with an endofemoral head. Had full range of motion without instability and grossly equal leg lengths. I could bring the hip and knee up to 90 degrees of flexion, neutral adduction, start to internally rotate to 30 degrees before it would become unstable. Hip was redislocated, trial components were removed. Measured the canal for a centralizer. I placed a distal cement restrictor 2 cm distal to the component. Copious lavage of the canal was performed and brushed. Acetabulum was irrigated clean; palpable and visibly free of loose fragments. It was packed off with lap sponge. Dried the femoral canal. Placed cement in the femoral canal with retrograde manor using proximal pressurizer. Placed the 14-mm Zimmer LD/Fx with a distal centralizer in the appropriate anteversion, held in place with a cement set. Copious irrigation was performed. After the cement set, placed the final endo head, tapped into position with Morris taper, reduced the head. Could take the hip through the same range of motion without any instability. The short external rotator is in the drill holes in the greater trochanter. The tensor fascia lata closed with interrupted -0-0 VICRYL suture. We copiously irrigated each layer. Subcutaneous tissue closed with interrupted -2-0 VICRYL sutures, skin was closed with staples. Sterile dressing was applied.

ICD-9-CM Diagnosis Code(s) with POA Indicator and MS-DRG:

_____

ICD-9-CM Procedure Code(s): _____

ICD-10-CM Code(s): _____

ICD-10-PCS Code(s): _____

Neoplasms

4.60. The following documentation is from the health record of a terminally ill oncology patient.

Discharge Summary

History of Present Illness: The patient is an 80-year-old white female with a known history of advanced metastatic carcinoma of the breast, widely metastatic. The patient was admitted because of increasing shortness of breath and severe pain. The pain, which was worse in her left chest, was associated with increasing shortness of breath. At the time of admission, the patient was in so much pain that she was unable to remember her history. The patient initially presented for congestive heart failure over 1 year ago. This was subsequently found to be secondary to metastatic breast cancer, post left mastectomy, 3 years ago. The patient had previously been on chemotherapy.

Laboratory Data and Hospital Course: The patient was treated initially with IV pain medication to control her pain. Subsequently, she became able to be stable on oral medication. By the time of discharge, the patient was stable on oral Vicodin, and she was able to eat. Blood sugars were improved, and her Tolinase was withheld. Laboratory results at time of discharge included BUN 17, creatinine 1, sodium 141, potassium 4.5, chloride 105, CO_2 25, alkaline phosphatase elevated at 170 with

GGT 267, SGOT 68. Admission BUN was up to 38 with creatinine 1.3 secondary to dehydration. By the time of discharge, these had improved. Admission glucose 225, down to 110 at discharge. Patient treated with Lanoxin and Lasix for CHF.

Medications at Discharge Include: Aldactone, 25 mg twice a day; Lanoxin, 0.125 mg daily; Metamucil, 5 cc in 4 ounces of juice twice a day; Tolinase, 250 mg half tablet b.i.d. (but hold if preceding Accu-Chek is less than 125); Reglan, 10 mg p.o. a.c.; Pepcid, 20 mg b.i.d.; Lasix, 40 mg daily (only if pedal edema is present); Vicodin tablets, 1 every 3 hours p.r.n. for pain.

Discharge Diagnoses: 1. Uncontrolled pain, secondary to widely metastatic breast carcinoma
2. Dehydration
3. Type II diabetes mellitus, uncontrolled
4. Congestive heart failure

Which of the following is the correct ICD-9-CM code assignment?

ICD-9-CM Code(s):

a. 338.3, 199.1, V10.3, 276.51, 250.02, 428.0
b. 174.9, 276.51, 250.02, 428.0
c. 199.1, V10.3, 276.51, 250.02, 428.0
d. 786.59, 199.1, 276.51, 250.02, 428.0

ICD-10-CM Code(s): _____

4.61. This 60-year-old male had bronchoscopy with brushings, washings, and fine-needle aspiration due to left lung tumor. The bronchoscope was advanced into the left upper lobe. Brushings were taken followed by transbronchial lavage to the area and then two fine-needle aspirations. The pathology report describes tissue from the fine-needle biopsy of the left upper lobe of the lung, bronchoalveolar lavage and bronchial brushings of the left upper lobe as well as bronchus brushing. Final diagnosis was oat cell carcinoma of the left upper lobe of the lung and emphysema. What are the code assignments for this patient?

ICD-9-CM Diagnosis Code(s) with POA Indicator and MS-DRG:

_____

ICD-9-CM Procedure Code(s): _____

ICD-10-CM Code(s): _____

ICD-10-PCS Code(s): _____

4.62. This female patient with terminal carcinoma of the breast, metastatic to the liver and brain, was admitted with dehydration. Patient rehydrated with IVs and discharged, with no treatment given to the cancer. What are the codes assigned?

ICD-9-CM Diagnosis Code(s) with POA Indicator and MS-DRG:

_____

ICD-10-CM Code(s): _____

4.63. This 45-year-old female patient was diagnosed with right breast carcinoma 3 years ago, at which time she had a mastectomy performed with chemotherapy administration. She has been well since that time with no further treatment but yearly checkups. She has metastasis in 3 axillary lymph nodes. She is admitted now with visual disturbances, dizziness, headaches, and blurred vision. Workup was done that revealed metastasis to the brain. What is the correct code assignment for this admission?

ICD-9-CM Diagnosis Code(s) with POA Indicator and MS-DRG:

_____

ICD-10-CM Code(s): _____

4.64. This patient was admitted for chemotherapy due to a primary hepatocellular carcinoma of the transplanted liver. What codes are assigned?

ICD-9-CM Code(s):

a. V58.11, 155.0
b. V58.11, 155.0, 199.2
c. V58.11, 996.82, 199.2, 155.0
d. 996.82, 199.2, 155.0

ICD-10-CM Code(s): _____

4.65. This patient was admitted with a large pelvic mass and underwent an exploratory laparotomy. Pathology confirmed carcinoma of the left ovary with extensive metastasis to the omentum. A total greater omentectomy, excision of left ovarian mass, and radical abdominal hysterectomy were performed, which in this case included removal of the uterus and upper vagina. Bilateral salpingo-oophorectomy was also performed. What codes are assigned?

ICD-9-CM Diagnosis Code(s) with POA Indicator and MS-DRG:

_____

ICD-9-CM Procedure Code(s): _____

ICD-10-CM Code(s): _____

ICD-10-PCS Code(s): _____

4.66. A patient with known carcinoma of the pancreatic head is admitted with an Hgb of 9.1. She has been receiving Docetaxel chemotherapy and the physician determines this new anemia as an adverse effect of the chemotherapy. The patient is treated with darbepoetin alpha and IV iron. The patient is discharged with an improvement in the Hgb to 11.3. Assign the correct diagnostic code(s).

ICD-9-CM Diagnosis Code(s) with POA Indicator and MS-DRG:

_____

ICD-10-CM Code(s): _____

Disorders of the Nervous System and Sense Organs

4.67. This is one of multiple hospital admissions for this 37-year-old white male with a history of meningoencephalitis 20 years ago. He developed obstructive hydrocephalus as a late effect/sequela and underwent ventriculoperitoneal shunting of the right lateral ventricle using a high-pressure valve. The patient is now complaining of numbness in his right leg, headaches, and diplopia. The patient had a low osmolar CT head scan which showed a slight increase in the hydrocephalus involving the fourth ventricle. Impression was shunt malfunction. He is admitted this time for VP shunt revision. Ventricular shunt was replaced via open approach and was functioning well at the time of discharge. Which of the following is the correct code assignment?

ICD-9-CM Code(s):

  a. 996.2, 331.4, 326, 02.42, 87.03
  b. 331.4, 326, 02.42, 87.03
  c. 996.63, 331.4, 02.42
  d. 996.2, 02.42, 87.03

ICD-10-CM Code(s): _____

ICD-10-PCS Code(s): _____

4.68. This 32-year-old female patient was admitted with intractable partial epilepsy. The patient was monitored and her epilepsy medications were adjusted. The rest of her hospital stay was uneventful. What codes are assigned?

ICD-9-CM Diagnosis Code(s) with POA Indicator and MS-DRG:

_____

ICD-10-CM Code(s): _____

4.69. This 19-year-old college student was brought to the ER and admitted with high fever, stiff neck, chest pain, cough, and nausea. A lumbar puncture was performed, and results were positive for meningitis. Chest x-ray revealed pneumonia. Sputum cultures grew *Pneumococcus*. Patient was treated with IV antibiotics and was discharged with the diagnosis of pneumococcal meningitis and pneumococcal pneumonia. What codes are assigned?

ICD-9-CM Diagnosis Code(s) with POA Indicator and MS-DRG:

_____

ICD-9-CM Procedure Code(s): _____

ICD-10-CM Code(s): _____

ICD-10-PCS Code(s): _____

4.70. This patient was admitted when MRI revealed cerebral aneurysm. After admission, a cerebral angiogram was performed and showed nonruptured arteriosclerotic aneurysm of the anterior cerebral artery. An aneurysmectomy by anastomosis was performed using Marlex graft replacement. What codes are assigned?

ICD-9-CM Diagnosis Code(s) with POA Indicator and MS-DRG:

_____

ICD-9-CM Procedure Code(s): _____

ICD-10-CM Code(s): _____

ICD-10-PCS Code(s): _____

4.71. This is a 71-year-old female admitted with a complaint of right-sided weakness. She denies any fever, shortness of breath, cough, headaches, or chest pain. Patient has NIDDM, controlled by diet. Patient currently smokes. Mild right-sided paralysis was found on physical examination. Patient is right-handed. Gadolinium-enhanced brain MRI demonstrated subacute middle cerebral artery infarct in the left basal ganglia. Discharge diagnosis was CVA—subacute infarct. Physical therapy and speech therapy for her hemiparalysis and dysphasia started and will continue at the rehabilitation facility where she was transferred.

Which of the following answers would be correct?

ICD-9-CM Code(s):

a. 434.91, 438.21, 438.12, 250.00, 305.1, 88.91, 93.39, 93.72
b. 434.91, 342.91, 784.59, 250.00, 305.1, 88.91, 93.39, 93.74
c. 436, 250.00, 305.1, 88.91, 93.39, 93.74
d. 434.91, 342.91, 784.59, 250.00, 305.1, 88.91, 93.39, 93.72

ICD-10-CM Code(s): _____

ICD-10-PCS Code(s): _____

Newborn/Congenital Disorders

4.72. A 6-month-old baby with a left-sided, incomplete upper cleft lip and cleft soft palate is admitted and undergoes surgical repair of both deformities.

Which of the following codes would be correct?

ICD-9-CM Code(s):

a. 749.02, 749.12, 27.62, 27.54
b. 749.22, 27.54, 27.63
c. 749.02, 749.12, 27.69
d. 749.22, 27.62, 27.54

ICD-10-CM Code(s): _____

ICD-10-PCS Code(s): _____

4.73. The patient is an 18-day-old baby girl admitted after it was noticed she was developing drainage from the umbilical cord. Upon admission she was placed on intravenous Cefotaxime and Ampicillin, later changed to Cefotaxime and Clindamycin. A culture taken from the umbilical stump grew Staphylococcus aureus and Group H streptococcus. After the first day, there was great improvement, and the baby continued to improve. She remained afebrile, has continued to eat very well, and she shows no sign of abdominal tenderness or peritonitis. The mother was instructed to watch the child closely and to notify the office if there is any redevelopment of the redness, swelling, or discharge. Recheck in 2 weeks for 1 month check-up. Discharge diagnosis: *Staphylococcus aureus* and Group H streptococcus omphalitis of the newborn. What codes are assigned?

ICD-9-CM Diagnosis Code(s) with POA Indicator and MS-DRG:

_____

ICD-10-CM Code(s): _____

4.74. An infant is born by cesarean section at 27 weeks' gestation. The baby weighs 945 g. The baby's lungs are immature, and the baby develops respiratory distress syndrome, requiring a 25-day hospital stay in the NICU. Discharge diagnosis: Extreme immaturity, with 27-week gestation, with respiratory distress syndrome, delivered by cesarean section.

Which of the following diagnosis codes would be correct?

ICD-9-CM Code(s):

a. V30.01, 765.03, 765.24
b. 765.03, 769
c. V30.01, 765.03, 765.24, 769
d. V30.01, 769

ICD-10-CM Code(s): _____

4.75. **Hospital Summary:** A male newborn, born at this hospital with pre-axial polydactyly of the thumbs and cleft deformities of both hands and feet, had a harsh murmur heard posteriorly and faint femoral pulses on initial newborn exam. The newborn was 39 weeks gestation and was born vaginally. Cardiology was consulted and determined a diagnosis of coarctation of the aorta and a very small conoventricular ventricular septal defect. The newborn had surgical repair of the coarctation but the VSD could not be repaired at this young age due to closeness to the aortic valve. Cardiology will follow to manage the VSD. Orthopedics was consulted for the hand and feet deformities and will schedule serial repairs after the age of about 1 year. The family will be seen by Medical Genetics as an outpatient for possible determination of a syndrome that encompasses this combination of defects. Assign the correct diagnostic code(s).

ICD-9-CM Diagnosis Code(s) with POA Indicator and MS-DRG:

_____

ICD-10-CM Code(s): _____

4.76. This full-term female infant was born in this hospital by vaginal delivery. Her mother has been an alcoholic for many years and would not stop drinking during her pregnancy. The baby was born with fetal alcohol syndrome and was placed in the NICU. What codes are assigned?

ICD-9-CM Diagnosis Code(s) with POA Indicator and MS-DRG:

_____

ICD-10-CM Code(s): _____

Pediatric Conditions

4.77. A child has second- and third-degree burns of the left lower leg and second- and third-degree burns of the lower back with a total of 16% total body surface area (TBSA), 9% third-degree. What is the correct code assignment?

ICD-9-CM Diagnosis Code(s) with POA Indicator and MS-DRG:

_____

ICD-10-CM Code(s): _____

4.78. Patient admitted with cervical lymphadenopathy. Left lymph node excisional biopsy confirmed Hodgkin's sarcoma disease. Megavoltage electron radiotherapy was begun postoperatively.

Which of the following is the correct code set?

ICD-9-CM Code(s):

a. 201.21, 40.40, 92.29
b. 201.91, 40.40, 92.29
c. 201.21, 40.11, 92.24
d. 201.91, 40.11, 92.24

ICD-10-CM Code(s): _____

ICD-10-PCS Code(s): _____

4.79. This 7-year-old child was brought to the hospital with congenital heart problems. During her stay a cardiac catheterization with a non-drug-eluting stent implantation to the left lower pulmonary vein is performed. The stent is implanted via the catheter. What is the correct code assignment for the percutaneous dilation of left pulmonary vein with insertion of stent?

ICD-9-CM Procedure Code(s): _____

ICD-10-PCS Code(s): _____

4.80.   The 2-year-old female was admitted to the hospital after being seen in the ER because of vomiting and diarrhea. She received Phenergan suppositories but the vomiting and diarrhea persisted. She was given an intravenous bolus of normal saline followed by intravenous D5 one-quarter, with potassium added, to correct the 5% dehydration. At the time of admission, mucous membranes were tacky. The abdominal examination revealed markedly increased bowel sounds; abdomen was mildly distended, but nontender. There were no masses and no organomegaly. Laboratory evaluation at the time of admission included a Chem-7 profile, which was remarkable for a BUN of 22 and a CO_2 of 19.5. On repeat the following day, the Chem-7 revealed values that were essentially within normal limits. The CBC on admission revealed a white blood cell count of 13,500 with hemoglobin increased at 54.1%, and there was a left shift. On repeat evaluation, the white cell count was down to 5,100, and the indices were within normal limits. Throat culture revealed normal flora; Rotavirus antigen was positive and found to be the cause of the gastroenteritis.

Which of the following answers would be correct?

ICD-9-CM Code(s):

a. 008.61, 276.51
b. 276.51, 558.9
c. 276.51, 008.61
d. 008.8

ICD-10-CM Code(s): _____

ICD-10-PCS Code(s): _____

4.81.   This 3-month-old infant was brought to the ER by the babysitter after she did not wake up from a nap. The babysitter admits to shaking the baby because she would not stop crying earlier in the day. She was admitted to ICU and was unconscious for 8 hours. Diagnosis at discharge: Shaken infant syndrome, subdural hematoma, loss of consciousness for 8 hours, and total retinal detachment, right eye. What codes are assigned?

ICD-9-CM Diagnosis Code(s) with POA Indicator and MS-DRG:

_____

ICD-10-CM Code(s): _____

Conditions of Pregnancy, Childbirth, and the Puerperium

4.82. The patient presented through the ED with severe abdominal pain, amenorrhea. Serum human chorionic gonadotropin (hCG) was lower than normal. There were also endometrial and uterine changes. Patient diagnosed with right tubal pregnancy. A laparoscopic salpingectomy with removal of tubal pregnancy was performed. Which of the following is the correct code assignment?

ICD-9-CM Code(s):

a. 633.80, 66.62
b. 633.10, 66.62
c. 633.10, 66.4
d. 633.10, 66.02

ICD-10-CM Code(s): _____

ICD-10-PCS Code(s): _____

4.83. From the health record of a patient experiencing a spontaneous abortion:

Diagnosis: Incomplete spontaneous abortion

Postoperative Diagnosis: Same

Operation: Dilatation and curettage

History: This 22-year-old female, gravida IV, para II, AB I, comes in today because of crampy abdominal pain and passing fetal tissue at home. Apparently her last menstrual period was 9 weeks ago, and she had been doing well, and this problem just started today.

Procedure: The patient was placed on the operating table in the lithotomy position, prepped, and draped in the usual manner. Under satisfactory intravenous sedation, the cervix was visualized by means of weighted speculum, grasped in the anterior lip with a sponge forceps. Cord was prolapsed through the cervix and vagina, and a considerable amount of placental tissue was in the vagina and cervix. This was removed. A sharp curet was used to explore the endometrial cavity, and a minimal amount of curettings was obtained. The patient tolerated the procedure well. What codes are assigned?

ICD-9-CM Code(s):

a. 635.91, 69.09
b. 634.91, 69.09
c. 634.91, 69.02
d. 635.91, 69.02

ICD-10-CM Code(s): _____

ICD-10-PCS Code(s): _____

4.84. This 25-year-old female was admitted at 38 weeks gestation for induction of labor due to mild pre-eclampsia. The patient failed to dilate during medical induction. The decision was made to perform a cesarean section due to the failed induction. What is the principal diagnosis?

ICD-9-CM Code(s):

a. 642.41
b. 659.11
c. 659.01
d. 652.51

ICD-10-CM Code(s): _____

4.85. This is a 26-year-old patient who had previous cesarean section for delivery for fetal distress. She had normal antepartum care and has had no complications. We are going to attempt a VBAC for this delivery. She is admitted in her 39th week in labor. The fetus is in cephalic position and no rotation is necessary. The labor continues to progress and 5 hours later she is taken to delivery. During the delivery she was fatigued, so low outlet forceps were required over a midline episiotomy which was subsequently repaired by an episiorrhaphy. A single liveborn infant was delivered. What codes are reported?

ICD-9-CM Diagnosis Code(s) with POA Indicator and MS-DRG:

_____

ICD-9-CM Procedure Code(s): _____

ICD-10-CM Code(s): _____

ICD-10-PCS Code(s): _____

4.86. The following documentation is from the OB record of a 33-year-old female patient.

Admit Note: 2/27

This is a 33-year-old G2 P0, with an estimated delivery date of 2/28, and estimated gestational age of 40 weeks. She presents for induction secondary to gestational diabetes mellitus. The diabetes has been managed by diet throughout the pregnancy. The patient also has diastasis recti that occurred three weeks ago, which has kept her at bedrest since that time. PNL: 0 positive, rubella immune. PE: AVSS, Abdomen FH 40 cm, EFW 3800–4000 grams. Cervix is closed/50%/-3/post/ceph. Plan is for Pitocin induction with epidural at the beginning of active labor.

Progress Note: 2/28 09:15

Patient is having uterine contractions every 3–8 minutes. Cervix is 1 cm/100%/floating. Patient desires not to start Pitocin yet. Feels that she is in labor. FHR reactive, baseline 120's with accelerations.

Progress Note: 2/28 19:25

Patient's uterine contractions have resolved. Cervix unchanged. Discussed options, would like to go home to sleep and return in a.m. for Pitocin induction. Discharged home for tonight to sleep. Admit in a.m., start IV Pitocin as per protocol and clear liquid diet. Assign the correct diagnostic code(s).

ICD-9-CM Diagnosis Code(s) with POA Indicator and MS-DRG:

_____

ICD-10-CM Code(s): _____

Disorders of the Respiratory System

4.87. The patient was admitted with increasing shortness of breath, weakness, and nonproductive cough. Treatment included oxygen therapy. Final diagnoses listed as acute respiratory insufficiency and acute exacerbation of chronic obstructive pulmonary disease (COPD). Which of the following is the correct diagnostic code assignment?

ICD-9-CM Code(s):

a. 491.21
b. 491.21, 518.82
c. 518.81, 491.21
d. 518.82, 491.21

ICD-10-CM Code(s): _____

4.88. A ventilator-dependent patient (due to emphysema) is admitted to the hospital at 10 a.m. on January 1. He is admitted for dehydration and is placed on the hospital's ventilator upon admission. The patient is discharged January 6 at 1 p.m. What is the appropriate code assignment?

ICD-9-CM Code(s):

a. 492.8, 276.51, 96.72
b. 276.51, 492.8, V46.11, 96.72
c. 276.51, 496, V46.11, 96.71
d. 492.8, 276.51, V46.11, 96.72

ICD-10-CM Code(s): _____

ICD-10-PCS Code(s): _____

4.89. The patient is a 59-year-old female who is quadriplegic after C5–6 fracture and C5–6 spinal cord injury from motor vehicle accident 1 year ago. Admitted because of a 2-day history of shortness of breath, fevers, and productive cough of green yellow sputum. She has not had much of an appetite and has not been eating or drinking much for the past 2 days. The patient is allergic to Penicillin. An x-ray revealed left-sided pneumonia. She was admitted to the hospital and given intravenous antibiotics for her pneumonia, IV fluids for dehydration, and oxygen. Her pO$_2$ in the Emergency Room was 50 on room air. She was started on hand-held nebulizer treatment, and her hypoxemia rapidly improved. Serum electrolytes were normal except for potassium of 3.3. This was corrected with additional potassium. At the time of discharge, she was breathing easy on room air and was discharged home. What codes are assigned?

ICD-9-CM Diagnosis Code(s) with POA Indicator and MS-DRG:

_____

ICD-10-CM Code(s): _____

4.90. **Discharge diagnosis:**

Moderate persistent asthma with status asthmaticus
Acute exacerbation of chronic obstructive pulmonary disease

Hospital Course: The patient presented with gradual increase in shortness of breath, which was unresponsive to home nebulizer treatments. In the emergency room, he received more respiratory treatments; however, he failed to improve. Therefore, the patient was admitted to the hospital. At the time of admission, the theophylline level was 5.9. Chest x-ray showed no evidence of active infiltrates. The patient was bolused with intravenous steroids and started on frequent respiratory therapy treatments. IV aminophylline boluses and drip were used to increase his theophylline level to therapeutic range. The patient gradually cleared and by the next day was much better. His IV aminophylline was changed to p.o. The Ventolin treatments were decreased to q 4 hr. and his steroids were rapidly tapered back to 10 mg. of Prednisone. What diagnosis codes are assigned?

ICD-9-CM Diagnosis Code(s) with POA Indicator and MS-DRG:

_____

ICD-10-CM Code(s): _____

4.91. A 75-year-old male was admitted to the hospital in acute respiratory failure. He has emphysema due to his continuous cigarette smoking for over 50 years. Sputum cultures showed streptococcus A pneumonia. He was intubated in the ER and started on mechanical ventilation. Thirty-six hours later he was extubated and was able to breathe on his own. He was started on Chantix™ to treat his dependence on nicotine. Diagnosis: Acute respiratory failure, pneumonia due to streptococcus A, and emphysema. What codes are assigned?

ICD-9-CM Diagnosis Code(s) with POA Indicator and MS-DRG:

_____

ICD-9-CM Procedure Code(s): _____

ICD-10-CM Code(s): _____

ICD-10-PCS Code(s): _____

Trauma and Poisoning

4.92. From the health record of a high-school athlete:

Discharge Summary: The patient is a 16-year-old male who received a hard tackle while playing football. He was unconscious at the playing field and was brought by ambulance to the emergency department. MRI brain showed a right subdural hematoma. Repeat MRI brain 1 hour later showed the hematoma to be growing. The patient remained unconscious. Vital signs were continuously monitored and remained within normal limits. The patient was taken to the OR, where the hematoma was evacuated via craniotomy. Postoperative course has been uneventful. The patient awakened and stated he was hungry. He has no memory of the event or the period of the football game. The patient is now discharged on the seventh postoperative day.

Which of the following code sets would be correct for this scenario?

ICD-9-CM Code(s):

a. 852.23, E886.0, E849.4, E007.0, E000.8, 01.31, 88.91, 88.91
b. 852.26, E886.0, E849.4, E007.0, E000.8, 01.31, 88.91, 88.91
c. 852.33, E886.0, E849.4, E007.0, E000.8, 01.39, 88.91, 88.91
d. 852.26, E886.0, E849.4, E007.0, E000.8, 01.39, 88.91, 88.91

ICD-10-CM Code(s): _____

ICD-10-PCS Code(s): _____

4.93. The patient is being seen due to right knee pain and decreased mobility. Previously the patient had a right total knee replacement for osteoarthritis. The patient also has extensive medical problems which were all monitored and treated while he was in the hospital: Parkinson's disease, hypertensive heart disease, congestive heart failure, bilateral capsular glaucoma, old MI six months ago, and recent abnormal cardiac stress test. Evaluation of the right knee indicated that patient had aseptic loosening of the tibial component of the knee. The orthopedic consultant indicated that the patient would need to be scheduled for a revision arthroplasty once he was cleared by cardiology for surgery. The cardiac clearance will be done as an outpatient and the procedure will then be scheduled. Assign the correct diagnostic code(s).

ICD-9-CM Diagnosis Code(s) with POA Indicator and MS-DRG:

_____

ICD-10-CM Code(s): _____

4.94. This 35-year-old female patient was a driver involved in an automobile accident when she was rear-ended by another driver in a car. She was seen in the emergency room complaining of pain in the arm and neck. She was brought into the hospital by the EMTs on a backboard and after proper splinting to the right arm. It was evident that compound fractures were present. After a CT scan of the head and neck, the patient was removed from the backboard.

She was admitted to the hospital for an open reduction, internal fixation of the type II fractures of the radius and ulna. The surgery was completed without problems. Postoperative x-rays show the radial and ulnar shafts in good alignment. Patient was advised to wear a collar for her cervical strain.

Final Diagnoses, in Order of Significance:
        Compound radius and ulna shaft fractures
        Whiplash injury, cervical spine

What are the correct codes to report for this service?

ICD-9-CM Diagnosis Code(s) with POA Indicator and MS-DRG:

_____

ICD-9-CM Procedure Code(s): _____

ICD-10-CM Code(s): _____

ICD-10-PCS Code(s): _____

4.95. This 32-year-old patient was brought to the emergency department after a gas leak caused an explosion at his home. He was admitted with third-degree burns of the upper back involving 9 percent of the body surface. What codes are assigned?

ICD-9-CM Diagnosis Code(s) with POA Indicator and MS-DRG:

_____

ICD-10-CM Code(s): _____

4.96. This nursing home patient is admitted with extensive cellulitis of the abdominal wall. The examination performed reveals that his existing gastrostomy site is infected. He had a feeding tube inserted 4 months ago because of carcinoma of the middle esophagus. The physician confirms that the responsible organism is *Staphylococcus aureus*.

ICD-9-CM Diagnosis Code(s) with POA Indicator and MS-DRG:

_____

ICD-10-CM Code(s): _____

4.97. This patient was walking along the railroad tracks when a train hit him. He was taken to the Medical Center by ambulance. Surprisingly, there were no internal injuries, and the only injury sustained was significant trauma to both lower legs. Discharge diagnosis was bilateral traumatic amputation. A revision by further amputation of the traumatic amputations of the mid tibia and fibula to the high tibia and fibula was performed on both legs.

ICD-9-CM Diagnosis Code(s) with POA Indicator and MS-DRG:

_____

ICD-9-CM Procedure Code(s): _____

ICD-10-CM Code(s): _____

ICD-10-PCS Code(s): _____

4.98. From the health record of a patient who is status post joint replacement:

Discharge Summary: The patient is an active 61-year-old male, who underwent right total hip arthroplasty approximately 3 years ago. The patient is very active and walks several miles every day and enjoys playing golf. He has recently experienced several instances of failure of the right hip prosthesis. This is well documented in several ED visits for dislocation of the prosthetic hip. The patient was now admitted for scheduled replacement of the right hip arthroplasty. The patient was taken to surgery, where the old prosthesis was found to be eroded and bent, causing the repeated dislocations. The prosthesis was removed and replaced with a titanium/polyethylene prosthesis without incident. The patient was begun on physical therapy for prosthetic gait training while in the hospital to help regain mobility. The patient was discharged on the fifth day postop to continue the physical therapy as an outpatient.

Which of the following codes would be used to report the above scenario?

ICD-9-CM Diagnosis Code(s) with POA Indicator and MS-DRG:

_____

ICD-9-CM Procedure Code(s): _____

ICD-10-CM Code(s): _____

ICD-10-PCS Code(s): _____

4.99.   **Discharge Summary:** The patient is a 45-year-old female who fell while walking her dog. She was walking on the sidewalk in her neighborhood and accidently tripped and subsequently fell. She sustained a comminuted fracture of the shaft of her right tibia confirmed by x-ray done in the emergency room. She also hit her head on a fire hydrant and suffered a slight concussion but no loss of consciousness. The patient was admitted and taken to surgery, where an open reduction with internal fixation was accomplished with good alignment of fracture fragments. Postop course was uneventful and the patient was discharged home with daily physical therapy.

ICD-9-CM Diagnosis Code(s) with POA Indicator and MS-DRG:

_____

ICD-9-CM Procedure Code(s): _____

ICD-10-CM Code(s): _____

ICD-10-PCS Code(s): _____

Chapter 5

Case Studies from Ambulatory Health Records

Note: Even though the specific cases are divided by setting, most of the information pertaining to the diagnosis is applicable to most settings. Even the CPT codes in the ambulatory and physician sections may be reported in the same manner. The differences in coding in these two settings may involve modifier reporting, evaluation and management CPT code reporting, and other health plan reporting guidelines unique to settings. If you practice or apply codes in a particular type of setting, you may find additional information in other sections of this publication that may be pertinent to you.

Every effort has been made to follow current recognized coding guidelines and principles, as well as nationally recognized reporting guidelines. The material presented may differ from some health plan requirements for reporting. The ICD-9-CM codes used are effective October 1, 2012, through September 30, 2013, and the HCPCS (CPT and HCPCS Level II) codes are in effect January 1, 2013, through December 31, 2013. The current standard transactions and code sets named in HIPAA have been utilized. The 2013 draft edition of ICD-10-CM was utilized.

Instructions: Assign all applicable ICD-9-CM diagnosis codes including V codes and E codes. Assign all applicable ICD-10-CM diagnosis codes including Z codes and external cause codes. Assign all CPT Level I procedure codes and HCPCS Level II codes. Assign Level I (CPT) and Level II (HCPCS) modifiers as appropriate. Outpatient healthcare settings represented in the case examples include emergency room (ER), urgent care, outpatient surgery, observation, ancillary outpatient, wound care, interventional radiology, radiation therapy, or other outpatient department. Final codes for billing occur after codes are passed through payer edits. Medicare utilizes the National Correct Coding Initiative (NCCI) edits. CMS developed the NCCI edit list to promote national correct coding methodologies and to control improper coding leading to improper payments for Medicare Part B. The purpose of the NCCI edits is to ensure the most comprehensive code is assigned and billed rather than the component codes. In addition, NCCI edits check for mutually exclusive pairs.

Cases are presented as either multiple choice or fill in the blank.

- For multiple-choice cases:
  - Select the letter of the appropriate code set.

- For the fill-in-the-blank cases:
  - Assign up to three reasons for visit ICD-9-CM codes to describe the reason for unscheduled visits such as emergency room. Reason for visit coding is required on the claim submission for all "unscheduled" outpatient visits.
  - ICD-9-CM and ICD-10-CM: Sequence the first-listed diagnosis first followed by the secondary diagnoses including any appropriate Classification of Factors Influencing Health Status and Contact with Health Service codes, External Causes of Injury and Poisoning (ICD-9-CM) codes, and External Causes of Morbidity (ICD-10-CM) codes.
  - Sequence the CPT procedure code first followed by additional procedure codes including modifiers as appropriate (both CPT Level I and HCPCS Level II modifiers).
  - Assign HCPCS Level II codes only if instructed (case specific).
  - Assign evaluation and management (E/M) codes only if instructed (case specific).
    - Medicare Type A Emergency Department visits are reported with CPT Level I codes 99281–99285 and critical care codes 99291 and 99292.
    - Medicare Type B Emergency Department visits are reported with Level II HCPCS codes G0380–G0384.

The scenarios are based on selected excerpts from health records. In practice, the coding professional should have access to and refer to the entire health record. Health records are analyzed and codes assigned based on physician documentation. Documentation for coding purposes must be assigned based on medical record documentation. A physician may be queried when documentation is ambiguous, incomplete, or conflicting. The queried documentation must be a permanent part of the medical record.

The objective of the cases and scenarios reproduced in this publication is to provide practice in assigning correct codes, not necessarily to emulate complete coding that can be achieved only with the complete medical record. For example, the reader may be asked to assign codes based on only an operative report; in real practice, a coder has access to documentation in the entire medical record.

The *ICD-9-CM Official Guidelines for Coding and Reporting of Outpatient Services*, published by the National Center for Health Statistics (NCHS), supplements the official conventions and instructions provided within ICD-9-CM. Adherence to these guidelines when assigning ICD-9-CM diagnosis codes is required under the Health Insurance Portability and Accountability Act (HIPAA) of 1996. Additional official coding guidance can be found in the American Hospital Association (AHA)'s *Coding Clinic* publication.

Disorders of the Blood and Blood-Forming Organs

5.1.   This 35-year-old patient was brought to the ER for GI bleeding. He was given 3 units of packed red cells. He was taken to the same-day surgery suite, and the colonoscopy showed angiodysplasia of the transverse colon, which was controlled with laser. What codes are assigned for this case?

ICD-9-CM and CPT Code(s):

a. 569.85, 45382, 36430-59
b. 578.9, 569.84, 45382, 36430, 36430, 36430
c. 578.9, 45382, 36430-59
d. 569.84, 578.9, 45382

ICD-10-CM Code(s): _____

5.2. This 20-year-old female came to the outpatient procedure area with a diagnosis of anemia. A bone marrow aspiration was performed in the following manner.

Manubrial area was prepped with Betadine. Skin and periosteum anesthetized with 2 percent Xylocaine. Skin incision was made with #11 Bard Parker blade, and marrow aspirations performed with U of IL sternal needle. Patient tolerated the procedure with no complaints or complications. Advised to resume normal activity.

Diagnosis: Iron deficiency anemia

Pathology Report

Specimen Received: Bone marrow aspiration and biopsy

Pathologic Diagnosis: Slightly hypercellular marrow with diminished iron consistent with iron deficiency anemia

Microscopic Description: The bone marrow specimen is adequate. The marrow appears to be slightly hypercellular with a cell-to-fat ratio of 60/40. Megakaryocytes are easily found. Most of them are of normal morphology. There is nothing to suggest a primary or metastatic neoplastic proliferation. Granuloma is not found. The maturation of myeloid cells is complete. A Prussian blue stain obtained on both specimens shows diminished stainable iron. The specimen appears to be marrow aspiration. Bone trabecula are not seen in any of it. A reticulin stain was obtained. There is no evidence of significant increase in reticulin in the marrow stroma.

The marrow smears show adequate number of spicules. The complete maturation of myeloid cells is confirmed. Hemoglobinization of erythroid cells is slightly deficient. There is no evidence of excessive number of blasts. The myeloid/erythroid ratio is within normal limits. Plasma cells amount to less than 1 percent of the cells counted.

A review of the peripheral blood smear received shows no abnormal morphological changes in any of the cell lines.

What would be the correct codes assigned in this case?

ICD-9-CM and CPT Code(s):

a. 285.9, 38220
b. 280.9, 38220
c. 285.9, 38220, 38221-59
d. 280.8, 38230

ICD-10-CM Code(s): _____

5.3. This 18-year-old patient with an abnormal blood test underwent bone marrow aspiration from the sternum. The area was cleaned with antiseptic solution, and a local anesthetic was injected. The needle was inserted beneath the skin and rotated into the cortex and the sample taken. The needle was repositioned slightly, and a new syringe attached, and a second sample was obtained. These were sent to the laboratory for analysis. The results show acute lymphoblastic leukemia. How is this coded?

ICD-9-CM and CPT Code(s): _____

ICD-10-CM Code(s): _____

5.4.   A 40-year-old female had recent surgery for melanoma of the left arm, documented as Clark level IV. She has no obvious signs of metastasis or adenopathy, but staging needs to be done. Under general anesthesia, a sentinel node biopsy of the deep axillary nodes is performed with a gamma counter probe. An injection of isosulfan blue dye was performed, and the nodes followed carefully to the single bright blue node. This node was excised and sent for frozen section, which proved to be positive for melanoma.

Assign the correct codes and modifier for this encounter.

ICD-9-CM and CPT Code(s): _____

ICD-10-CM Code(s): _____

5.5.   This 12-year-old male African-American patient is admitted to the ER with chest pain and pulmonary infiltrates. He has sickle cell disease. Treatment was aimed at reducing the chest pain to improve breathing. He was transferred to a larger children's hospital for admission for his sickle cell crisis and acute chest syndrome. What code(s) would be assigned for the diagnosis in this case?

ICD-9-CM Reason for Visit Code(s): _____

ICD-9-CM and CPT Code(s): _____

ICD-10-CM Reason for Visit Code(s): _____

ICD-10-CM Code(s): _____

Disorders of the Cardiovascular System

5.6.   The following documentation is from the health record of a 67-year-old male.

Procedure: Placement of a dual chamber implantable pacing cardioverter-defibrillator

Indications: Patient has moderate ischemic cardiomyopathy, prior infarct and stent

Description of Procedure: After informed consent was obtained, the patient was brought to the cardiac lab. The procedure was done under conscious sedation with fluoroscopic guidance. 1% Lidocaine was used to anesthetize the skin under the left clavicle, and a skin incision was made. A pocket was made for the ICD generator and leads, securing good hemostasis. The left subclavian vein was easily cannulated twice using a pediatric set, which was upsized to regular 037 wires, the position of which was checked under fluoro.

I then dilated the access volts with 9-French dilators and used 7-French access sheaths through which a 7-French ventricular lead was advanced and placed under fluoroscopic guidance. It was an active fixation lead. The numbers looked good, and the lead was sutured down. There was no diaphragmatic stimulation.

A 7-French lead was then advanced under fluoroscopic guidance and placed in the right atrial appendage. The numbers looked good. There was no diaphragmatic stimulation and the lead was sutured down. The leads were then attached to the generator, which was tested and sutured down in the pocket. The wound was irrigated several times with antibiotics during and at the end of the case. Wound was closed in layers. The patient tolerated the procedure well without any complications.

The ICD is Model Virtuoso DRD 154AWG. Atrial and ventricular leads are Medtronic. Battery voltage is 3.17 volts. Sensed P waves of 2.5 millivolts through the PSA, slew rate of 0.6 volts per second, impedance of 539 ohms, threshold of 17 volts at 0.5 milliseconds, current of 3.9 milliamperes, sensed R waves of 21 millivolts, slew rate of greater than 4 volts per second, impedance of 965 ohms, threshold of 0.8 volts at 0.5 milliseconds, and current of 0.8 milliamperes.

Through the device, sensed P waves of 2.3 millivolts, impedance of 472 ohms, threshold of 1 volt at 0.5 milliseconds, sensed R waves of 12.1 millivolts, impedance of 752 ohms, threshold of 1 volt at 0.1 milliseconds, HVB impedance of 38 ohms, HVA impedance of 44 ohms.

Defibrillator threshold testing was done. Battery was B2AX, rhythm induced was ventricular fibrillation with T shock, impedance of 43 ohms, energy delivered was 20 joules, charge time was 3.8 seconds, sensitivity was 1.2, and it was successful.

Tachy parameters are VF zone of 300 milliseconds at 200 beats. Therapies are 30 joules and then 35 times 5 with 80 P during charging for VT. Monitor zone is between 150 and 200 beats per minute. Brady parameters are AAI with backup DDD. Managed ventricular pacing at 50 to 120. PAV of 180. SAV of 150. Mode switch at 171.

Impression: Successful dual chamber ICD implantation as noted above. ESP testing of leads and generator. The patient will be monitored in observation, will get further doses of antibiotics, and be sent home when stable.

What CPT code(s) describe(s) this cardiac lab service?

a. 33240
b. 33225, 33240
c. 33249, 93641
d. 33249, 93640, 93641

5.7. A pediatric patient requires a transesophageal echocardiogram to evaluate an atrioventricular canal defect present since birth. Which codes are reported for this outpatient service?

ICD-9-CM and CPT Code(s):

a. 745.4, 93315
b. 745.69, 93315
c. 745.69, 93312
d. 429.71, 93312

ICD-10-CM Code(s): _____

5.8.   This 45-year-old patient is scheduled for the ambulatory surgical center to have an INFUSAID pump installed. He has primary liver cancer, and the pump is being inserted for continuous administration of 5-FU.

The right subclavian vein was cannulated without difficulty and the guidewire passed centrally. The subcutaneous tunnel and pocket were then created and the catheter passed through the tunnel. The central venous catheter was placed and connected to the secured pump. The pump was filled with the chemotherapy agent provided by the hospital, and the patient is observed for adverse reaction and then is discharged home.

What codes are assigned for this episode?

ICD-9-CM and CPT Code(s): _____

ICD-10-CM Code(s): _____

5.9.   This 55-year-old patient has a history of unstable angina, hypertension, and chronic systolic heart failure. He is seen in the ER after prolonged chest pain that was not relieved by medication. Cardiac enzymes are elevated, and EKG shows anterior infarct. A decision was made to admit patient to observation and perform a cardiac catheterization and coronary angiography. Left heart catheterization was performed in order to perform a left ventriculogram. He tolerated the procedure well and will be discharged. Diagnosis: Acute anterior myocardial infarction (STEMI), chronic systolic heart failure, hypertension. What are the correct codes?

ICD-9-CM Reason for Visit Code(s): _____

ICD-9-CM and CPT Code(s): _____

ICD-10-CM Reason for Visit Code(s): _____

ICD-10-CM Code(s): _____

5.10.   This 82-year-old male patient was shoveling snow and collapsed in his driveway. He arrived in the emergency department unresponsive and in asystole. A "code blue" was called, and CPR was administered without a return to consciousness. The final diagnosis on the ER record was "Cardiopulmonary arrest, probably secondary to an acute myocardial infarction induced by exertion." Which diagnosis codes are reported?

ICD-9-CM Reason for Visit Code(s): _____

ICD-9-CM Code(s): _____

ICD-10-CM Reason for Visit Code(s): _____

ICD-10-CM Code(s): _____

5.11.   Under local anesthesia and ultrasound guidance, a patient underwent radiofrequency ablation of an incompetent greater saphenous vein in the right lower extremity. Assign the appropriate CPT code(s).

a. 36475-RT
b. 36475-RT, 36000
c. 36478-RT
d. 36475-RT, 76942

5.12. The elderly patient was seen in the same-day surgery unit for insertion of a subclavian venous catheter for treatment of his prostate carcinoma.

Operative Report: The patient's right upper chest was prepped and draped in the usual manner. Local anesthesia was obtained using Xylocaine. A percutaneous subclavian venous catheter was inserted and secured at the skin level with 4-0 nylon. A sterile dressing was applied. The catheter was irrigated with Heparin and the patient was sent to recovery.

What codes are assigned for this ambulatory surgery?

ICD-9-CM and CPT Code(s): _____

ICD-10-CM Code(s): _____

Disorders of the Digestive System

5.13. The following documentation is from the health record of a female patient.

Outpatient Operative Report

This patient with hiatal hernia is admitted to same-day surgery for repair.

Description of Procedure: The patient was placed under satisfactory general endotracheal anesthesia. She was then placed in the lithotomy position. Foley was placed. Orogastric tube was inserted. The abdomen was prepped and draped in normal sterile fashion. A supraumbilical incision was made to the midline, and the fascia was incised to enter the abdomen. Under direct visualization, a 0 VICRYL stitch was placed on each side of the fascia, and a blunt Hasson trocar was inserted. The abdomen was insufflated with CO_2. Under direct visualization, two 11-mm ports were placed in the left subcostal region, and 11-mm and 12-mm ports were placed in the right subcostal region.

The liver bed was then lifted up off the gastrohepatic ligament. The gastrohepatic ligament was taken down with harmonic scalpel. The right crus of the diaphragm was identified and dissected out with harmonic scalpel and blunt dissection. I dissected out the phrenicoesophageal ligament anteriorly and came around identifying the left crus. I then took down the short gastrics from the midportion of the greater curvature of the stomach up to the GE junction, using harmonic scalpel and taking care to not damage the spleen. Once we had adequately taken down the short gastrics, the posterior ligament was then mobilized behind the esophagus, and the stomach easily pulled through with no tension and no twist on the esophagus and easily laid in place.

The hiatal hernia was then repaired with a posterior cruropexy stitch of 0 ETHIBOND. The wrap was then brought around and was placed approximately 2 cm into the esophagus with a horizontal mattress pledgeted 0 ETHIBOND stitch. A second interrupted stitch was placed just through-and-through on the stomach below this. At the end of the procedure, there was no tension or twist on the esophagus and no bleeding apparent. All ports were removed under direct visualization and there appeared to be hemostasis. The fascia at the supraumbilical incision was closed with 0 VICRYL. The skin was anesthetized with local anesthetic and then closed with 4-0 subcuticular MONOCRYL.

Which codes are reported for this case?

ICD-9-CM and CPT Code(s):

a. 553.3, 43327
b. 553.3, 43280
c. 551.3, 43280
d. 553.3, 43328

ICD-10-CM Code(s): _____

5.14.   This 59-year-old female patient came into the emergency room because of passing melanotic stools. The emergency room physician initially saw her. The gastroenterologist was called into consultation. Because of the massive amounts of bleeding, it was decided to proceed with endoscopy. The endoscope was passed into the esophagus, stomach, and duodenum. Blood and clots were noted. This patient could possibly have a duodenal ulcer, but because of the amount of blood, it was difficult to delineate an ulcer crater. Diagnosis: Melanotic stools, and possibly duodenal ulcer. What codes are assigned in this case?

ICD-9-CM Reason for Visit Code(s): _____

ICD-9-CM and CPT Code(s): _____

ICD-10-CM Reason for Visit Code(s): _____

ICD-10-CM Code(s): _____

5.15.   This 77-year-old patient admitted to the special procedures room is having an endoscopic-directed percutaneous endoscopic gastrostomy tube placed because of moderate malnutrition. The patient has had a stroke, with residual right dominant-sided hemiparesis. Assign the codes that the hospital would use to bill this service.

ICD-9-CM and CPT Code(s): _____

ICD-10-CM Code(s): _____

5.16.   A 39-year-old male has been treated for symptomatic cholelithiasis without improvement. Patient comes to outpatient surgery for a laparoscopic cholecystectomy. Due to previous abdominal surgery, adhesions were encountered. During the course of the laparoscopic cholecystectomy procedure, the adhesions were lysed, but this did not prolong the procedure.

What codes are assigned?

ICD-9-CM and CPT Code(s): _____

ICD-10-CM Code(s): _____

5.17. The following documentation is from the health record of an outpatient surgical patient.

Preoperative Diagnosis:	Rectal mass Change in bowel habits
Postoperative Diagnosis:	Rectal prolapse Colonic polyps. Biopsies × 2 Significant sigmoid diverticulosis with nonspecific colitis
Procedure:	Colonoscopy performed to the level of the cecum, 110 cm

Procedure: The 62-year-old male patient was prepped in the usual fashion, followed by placement in the left lateral decubitus position. I administered 3 mg of Versed. Monitoring of sedation was assisted by a trained registered nurse. Next, the Pentax Video Endoscope was passed through the rectal verge after a negative digital examination and advanced to the level of the cecum. The scope was then slowly retracted with a circular tip motion. There was mild nonspecific colitis noted. She did have significant sigmoid diverticulosis and several small polyps just inside the rectum, as well as a large prolapsing mass of mucosa approximately 5 cm inside the rectum. This appears to have prolapsed previously. Two of the small polyps were biopsied using the cold biopsy forceps and sent to pathology for examination. The remainder of the examination was unremarkable. The patient tolerated the procedure well.

Pathology Report

Clinical Information: Change in bowel habits. Colonoscopy performed.

Gross Examination: The specimen is labeled polyps × 2 at 3 cm. Submitted are 2 fragments of tan tissue measuring up to 0.3 cm in greatest dimension.

Microscopic Examination: Sections examined at multiple levels show 2 fragments of rectal mucosa in which the surfaces and subjacent crypts show no evidence of adenomatous or neoplastic changes.

Diagnosis: Rectum, biopsies at 3 cm: rectal polyps

What codes are assigned in this case?

ICD-9-CM and CPT Code(s): _____

ICD-10-CM Code(s): _____

5.18. The following documentation is from the health record of an outpatient surgical patient.

Preoperative Diagnosis:	Right inguinal hernia
Postoperative Diagnosis:	Right inguinal hernia, direct and indirect
Procedures:	Repair of right inguinal hernia with mesh

Procedure: This 45-year-old male was prepped in the usual manner for an initial hernia repair. After satisfactory spinal anesthesia, the inguinal area was draped in the usual sterile manner. A transverse incision was made above the inguinal ligament and carried down to the fascia of the external oblique, which was then opened, and the cord was mobilized. The ilioinguinal nerve was identified and protected. A relatively large indirect hernia was found. However, there was an extension of the hernia, such that one could definitely tell there had been a long-standing hernia here that probably had enlarged fairly recently. The posterior wall, however, was quite dilated and without a great deal of tone and bulging, and probably fit the criteria for a hernia by itself. Nonetheless, the hernia sac was separated from the cord structures, and a high ligation was done with a purse-string suture of 2-0 silk and a suture ligature of the same material prior to amputating the sac. The posterior wall was repaired with Marlex mesh, which was sewn in place in the usual manner, anchoring two sutures at the pubic tubercle tissue, taking one lateral up the rectus sheath and one lateral along the shelving border of Poupart's ligament past the internal ring. The mesh had been incised laterally to accommodate the internal ring. Several sutures were used to tack the mesh down superiorly and laterally to the transversalis fascia. Then the two limbs of the mesh were brought together lateral to the internal ring and secured to the shelving border of Poupart's ligament. The mesh was irrigated with gentamicin solution. The subcutaneous tissue was closed with fine VICRYL, as was the internal oblique. Marcaine was infiltrated in the subcutaneous tissue and skin. The wound was closed with fine nylon. The patient tolerated the procedure well.

Pathology Report

Gross Description

Specimen: Right inguinal hernia sac

The specimen consists of a pink to blue-gray membranous piece of tissue measuring 5.5 cm in maximum dimension. Blocks are made.

Clinical: Right inguinal hernia

Assign the correct codes and modifier for this encounter.

ICD-9-CM and CPT Code(s): _____

ICD-10-CM Code(s): _____

5.19.   The following documentation is from the health record of an outpatient surgical patient.

Preoperative Diagnosis:	Chronic cholelithiasis
Postoperative Diagnosis:	Chronic cholelithiasis Subacute cholecystitis
Operation:	Laparoscopic cholecystectomy Intraoperative cholangiogram

Procedure: The patient is a 44-year-old female brought to the operating room, placed in supine position, and who underwent general endotracheal anesthesia. After adequate induction of anesthesia, the abdomen was prepped and draped in the usual fashion. The patient had several previous lower midline incisions and right flank incision; therefore, the pneumoperitoneum was created via epigastric incision to the left of the midline with a Verres needle. After adequate pneumoperitoneum was created, the 11-mm trocar was placed through the extended incision in the left epigastrium just to the left of the midline. The trocar was placed, and the laparoscope and camera were in place. Inspection of the peritoneal cavity revealed it to be free of adhesions, and an 11-mm trocar was then placed under direct vision through a small infraumbilical incision. The scope and camera were then moved to this position, and the gallbladder was easily visualized. The gallbladder was elevated, and Hartmann's pouch was grasped. Using a combination of sharp and blunt dissection, the cystic artery was identified. The gallbladder was somewhat tense and subacutely inflamed. Therefore, a needle was passed through the abdominal wall into the gallbladder, and the gallbladder was aspirated free until it collapsed. One of the graspers was held over this region to prevent any further leakage of bile. Again, direction was turned to the area of the triangle of Calot. The cystic duct was dissected free with sharp and blunt dissection. A small opening was made in the duct, and the cholangiogram catheter was passed. The cholangiogram revealed no stones or filling defects in the bile duct system. The biliary tree was normal. There was good flow into the duodenum, and the catheter was definitely in the cystic duct. The catheter was removed, and the cystic duct was ligated between clips, as was the cystic artery. The gallbladder was then dissected free from the hepatic bed using electrocautery dissection, and it was removed from the abdomen through the umbilical port. Inspection of the hepatic bed noted that hemostasis was meticulous. The region of dissection was irrigated and aspirated dry. The trocars were removed, and the pneumoperitoneum was released. The incisions were closed with Steri-Strips, and the umbilical fascial incision was closed with 2-0 Maxon. The patient tolerated the procedure well; there were no complications. She was returned to the recovery room awake and alert.

What codes would be assigned?

ICD-9-CM and CPT Code(s): _____

ICD-10-CM Code(s): _____

5.20. A 61-year-old male patient is being assessed for possible colon cancer and treated in the special procedure unit of the hospital. He undergoes a colonoscopy into the ascending colon with biopsy of a suspicious area in the transverse colon using the cold biopsy forceps. In addition, a colonic ultrasound of the area is performed, with transmural biopsy of an area of the mesentery adjacent to the transverse colon. Assign the appropriate CPT codes.

   a. 45384, 45342
   b. 45380, 45391
   c. 45384, 45392
   d. 45380, 45392

5.21. The following documentation is from the health record of an outpatient.

Preoperative Diagnosis:	Aspiration pneumonitis
Postoperative Diagnosis:	Aspiration pneumonitis
Operative Procedure:	NJ Tube Placement

Description of Procedure: The identity of the patient was confirmed. The planned procedure was confirmed with staff. Consent was verified. The patient was prepared with IV sedation.

An 8 Fr CorPak tube was lubricated and inserted into stomach. Fluoroscopic guidance was provided by radiology. This allowed passage of the tube through the pylorus, through the duodenum, and into the jejunum. Position of the tube was confirmed by contrast instillation. Water flushed well through the tube. The tube was taped securely to the face. The patient was sent to the recovery room in good condition.

Impression: 1. Successful NJ tube placement

ICD-9-CM Reason for Visit Code(s): _____

ICD-9-CM and CPT Code(s): _____

ICD-10-CM Code(s): _____

5.22. The patient was seen in the ER after accidentally swallowing a crown from a tooth. A rigid esophagoscopy for foreign body removal was ordered.

Procedure: The 33-year-old was taken to OP surgery where conscious sedation was induced. An esophageal speculum was introduced and a small crown was grasped and removed using the speculum. Compression on the trachea was released. The esophagus was evaluated using a 6 × 30 esophagoscope and there appeared to be no remaining fragments or injuries to the esophagus. The esophagoscope was removed and the patient was sent to the PACU in good condition.

What code(s) are assigned for this outpatient encounter?

ICD-9-CM and CPT Code(s): _____

ICD-10-CM Code(s): _____

5.23. The patient was seen in the endoscopy suite for evaluation of previously diagnosed guaiac-positive stools. The EGD revealed no abnormalities except for a suspicious area in the duodenum which was biopsied. The scope was removed and a colonoscope introduced. The rectum, sigmoid colon, and descending colon were examined. After some difficulty, the scope was passed through the splenic flexure; the transverse colon had multiple polyps. Two large adenomatous polyps were removed by snare technique and two additional polyps were biopsied.

What code(s) are used to report this encounter?

ICD-9-CM and CPT Code(s): _____

ICD-10-CM Code(s): _____

5.24. The following documentation is from a health record from an OP surgery.

> **Preoperative Diagnosis:**   Ventral hernia.
>
> **Postoperative Diagnosis:**   Ventral hernia.
>
> **Operation Performed:**   Ventral hernia repair via laparoscopy.

Description of Procedure: The patient was prepped and draped in the usual fashion after being placed in a supine position. A 1-cm incision was made and a Veress needle was introduced into the abdominal cavity. A ten mm trocar was inserted and the laparoscope introduced. Additional trocars were inserted. Direct observation of the abdomen revealed a 2- to 3-cm hernia defect just below the umbilicus. Following plication of the rectus abdominal muscle, mesh Marlex was fashioned to an appropriate size, applied around the area, and sutured using 2.0 Prolene suture. Two Jackson-Pratt drains were placed in the subcutaneous area and attached using 2-0 thread.

The scope and trocars were removed and incisions sutured. The patient tolerated the procedure well and left the OR in good condition.

What code(s) are assigned in this case?

ICD-9-CM and CPT Code(s): _____

ICD-10-CM Code(s): _____

Endocrine, Nutritional, and Metabolic Diseases and Immunity Disorders

5.25. This 17-year-old patient presents to the emergency room with a chief complaint of severe right lower quadrant abdominal pain. The patient describes the pain as tightness and an intense cramping feeling. She has had increased bowel movements that provide some relief from the cramping. The pain seems much more intense after milk or ice cream. The patient is also currently menstruating but describes these cramps as different and worse. She is on no medication, no birth control, and is not sexually active.

Emergency Department diagnoses: Lactose intolerance, uterine menstrual cramps

ICD-9-CM Reason for Visit Code(s): _____

ICD-9-CM: _____

ICD-10-CM Reason for Visit Code(s): _____

ICD-10-CM Code(s): _____

5.26. The patient is diagnosed with a recurrent thyroglossal duct cyst. The surgeon locates the cyst using palpation, and an incision is created. The cyst is then excised. What is the correct CPT code assignment for this service?

    a. 60200
    b. 60210
    c. 60280
    d. 60281

5.27.   A 45-year-old female presents to the outpatient surgery unit of the hospital with a complaint of neck swelling. The physician noted diffuse swelling of the neck with enlargement of the thyroid gland. The patient exhibits no clinical signs of hyperthyroidism. The physician suspects lymphoma, and a biopsy is performed. A large, hollow core needle is passed through the skin into the thyroid. Tissue is sent for histopathology. A diagnosis of thyroid gland follicular lymphoma is confirmed and chemotherapy is planned.

What is the correct code assignment?

ICD-9-CM and CPT Code(s): _____

ICD-10-CM Code(s): _____

Disorders of the Genitourinary System

5.28.   A 55-year-old female patient presents to the same-day surgical unit with stress incontinence and requires repair for midline cystocele and incomplete vaginal prolapse. The physician elects to perform a paravaginal defect repair on both sides. An abdominal incision is made and entry into the space of Retzius is gained. Six sutures are placed through the anterior lateral edge of the vaginal wall and then through the fascia condensation over the obturator internus muscle from the inferior aspect of the pubic bone along the arcus tendinous to the ischial spine. Additional anchors were placed at the level of the urethrovesical junction on both sides to correct the cystocele.

Which of the following code sets is reported for this service?

ICD-9-CM and CPT Code(s):

a. 625.6, 618.01, 618.2, 57284, 51840
b. 625.6, 57284-50
c. 618.02, 57240
d. 618.01, 625.6, 57284

ICD-10-CM Code(s): _____

5.29.   This 77-year-old male patient is a nursing home patient who is admitted to the special procedure unit at the hospital. Patient is stress incontinent and continually leaks urine. To treat this, the urologist introduces a mechanical obstruction in the urethra that prevents leakage. Using an endoscope, the physician injects a solution of polytetrafluoroethylene into the region of the distal sphincter of the urethra, then inserts an inflatable bladder neck sphincter with pump, reservoir, and cuff. Which of the following code sets is reported for this surgery?

ICD-9-CM and CPT Code(s):

a. 788.37, 788.32, 53445, 51715
b. 788.39, 51715
c. 788.37, 53440
d. 788.37, 788.32, 53445

ICD-10-CM Code(s): _____

5.30. This 68-year-old male patient presents to the clinic with a chief complaint of inability to void. He has a history of several urinary tract infections in the past. The physician orders a urinalysis with a diagnosis of acute urinary retention. Urine is obtained by the nursing staff using a straight catheter. What codes would be submitted by the facility for the nursing services provided that day?

ICD-9-CM and CPT Code(s):

a. 788.20, V13.02, 51701
b. 788.20, 51702, P9612
c. 788.20, V13.02, P9612
d. 599.0, 51701

ICD-10-CM Code(s): _____

5.31. This patient, a 47-year-old male with adenoma of the prostate, is being treated in the outpatient surgery suite. The urologist inserts an endoscope in the penile urethra and dilates the structure to allow instrument passage. After endoscope placement, a radiofrequency stylet is inserted, and the diseased prostate is excised with radiant energy. Bleeding is controlled with electrocoagulation. Following instrument removal, a catheter is inserted and left in place. Which of the following code sets will be reported for this service?

ICD-9-CM and CPT Code(s):

a. 600.20, 53852
b. 600.20, 52601
c. 600.00, 53852
d. 222.2, 53850

ICD-10-CM Code(s): _____

5.32. The patient is a 22-year-old male with left testicular pain and scrotal swelling over the past 3 hours. No dysuria, no penile discharge, no fever and is able to void well. No trauma to groin. Pain 5/10. The physician orders an ultra-sound which demonstrates a testicle that is free-floating in the scrotum with the spermatic cord looped once around the middle of the testicle. The patient was against surgical intervention and opted to try manual detorsion. The patient was warmed with hot packs to loosen the scrotal skin, and the physician manipulated the testicle until the spermatic cord felt loosened. Reultrasound confirmed proper position, and the patient's pain was substantially relieved. The patient was sent home with a list of precautions and instructions to return with any increase in pain.

What codes are reported by the facility? Do not include an E/M code for this case.

ICD-9-CM Reason for Visit Code(s): _____

ICD-9-CM and CPT Code(s): _____

ICD-10-CM Reason for Visit Code(s): _____

ICD-10-CM Code(s): _____

5.33. A 90-year-old female nursing home patient with a long history of chronic urinary tract infections is brought to the emergency room after developing a fever of 102°F with generalized abdominal pain. The patient has senile dementia with delirium and is unable to communicate. The history was obtained from nursing home transfer records. Nonautomated urinalysis with microscopy was performed but was not remarkable. The physician's assessment stated "fever of unknown origin." The patient was treated with Tylenol and started on a broad-spectrum antibiotic and referred to her primary care physician for follow-up first thing in the morning.

What codes are reported by the ER facility coding? Do not include E/M codes in this example, but do include laboratory codes, even though they would be reported by the chargemaster.

ICD-9-CM Reason for Visit Code(s): _____

ICD-9-CM and CPT Code(s): _____

ICD-10-CM Reason for Visit Code(s): _____

ICD-10-CM Code(s): _____

5.34. Patient is a 59-year-old admitted to the same-day surgery suite. Patient is a type I diabetic with diabetic nephropathy and end-stage renal disease now requiring dialysis. A Cimino-type direct arteriovenous anastomosis is performed by incising the skin of the left antecubital fossa. Vessel clamps are placed on the vein and adjacent artery. The vein is dissected free and the downstream portion of the vein is sutured to an opening in the artery using an end-to-side technique. The skin incision is closed in layers.

What codes are reported for this service?

ICD-9-CM and CPT Code(s): _____

ICD-10-CM Code(s): _____

5.35. A 28-year-old patient admitted for same-day surgery with a history of abdominal surgery and is experiencing sharp pain in the pelvic area. Diagnostic workup has presented no etiology. An exploratory laparoscopy was performed and revealed adhesions around the fallopian tubes and ovaries. The adhesions were taken down during the procedure. What codes will be reported?

ICD-9-CM and CPT Code(s): _____

ICD-10-CM Code(s): _____

5.36. An 80 year-old male patient was taken to the special procedure unit for cystoscopy after developing gross hematuria. The cystoscopy revealed a 2.5 cm tumor in the trigone and a 2.1 cm tumor of the posterior wall. Both tumors were fulgurated. The patient was diagnosed with urothelial cell carcinoma.

What codes are reported?

ICD-9-CM and CPT Code(s): _____

ICD-10-CM Code(s): _____

5.37. A patient with advanced renal cell carcinoma is admitted to the interventional radiology department to undergo percutaneous radiofrequency ablation of four tumors of the right kidney. Assign the appropriate CPT code for this procedure.

Code(s): _____

Infectious Diseases

5.38. A 22-year-old male patient presents to the emergency room with symptoms of right upper quadrant pain, fever, profound malaise, and bloody diarrhea. An infectious consultation was obtained and diagnosis was made of acute *Entamoeba histolytica* dysentery. What code(s) are assigned?

ICD-9-CM Reason for Visit Code(s): _____

ICD-9-CM Code(s): _____

ICD-10-CM Reason for Visit Code(s): _____

ICD-10-CM Code(s): _____

5.39. A 29-year-old male patient presents to the hospital emergency room with a vesicular eruption and severe itching on the penis, scrotum, buttocks, and groin. Itching is severe at night. Assessment: Infestation with *Sarcoptes scabiei*. Plan: Permethrin 5% cream is applied to the affected area and a prescription provided for whole-body treatment of the entire household. What diagnosis code is reported for this encounter?

ICD-9-CM Reason for Visit Code(s): _____

ICD-9-CM Code(s): _____

ICD-10-CM Reason for Visit Code(s): _____

ICD-10-CM Code(s): _____

5.40. This 3-year-old patient presents to the emergency department with history of sudden bloody diarrhea. The stool culture demonstrated *Escherichia coli*. The patient went swimming with his child-care-center class the previous day at a nearby water park. The physician documented: acute enteritis, due to enterotoxigenic *E. coli*. What is the correct ICD-9-CM diagnostic code for this encounter?

ICD-9-CM Reason for Visit Code(s): _____

ICD-9-CM Code(s): _____

ICD-10-CM Reason for Visit Code(s): _____

ICD-10-CM Code(s): _____

5.41. The patient is seen for latent TB infection. He had a positive TB skin test last week and presents today for counseling on the start of INH 300 mg/day, orally. The patient also has moderate Bipolar I disorder and is currently depressed. Because of this, the physician spends considerable time discussing the need to take the INH daily, along with all other prescribed medication.

What diagnosis code(s) describe this case?

ICD-9-CM Reason for Visit Code(s): _____

ICD-9-CM Code(s): _____

ICD-10-CM Reason for Visit Code(s): _____

ICD-10-CM Code(s): _____

Disorders of the Skin and Subcutaneous Tissue

5.42. This is a record from a same-day surgery.

Preoperative Diagnosis:	Basal cell carcinoma of right nasal tip; lesion on right cheek.
Postoperative Diagnosis:	Pathology pending. Probable sebaceous hyperplasia.
Procedures:	Excision of lesion of the right nasal tip; placement of full thickness skin graft; excision of cheek lesion.

Description of Procedure: Under satisfactory premedication, the patient was brought to the Operating Room and using a loupe magnification, the area of excision was mapped out. 1% Xylocaine with Epinephrine was then utilized to anesthetize the nasal tip and also the keratosis on the right cheek. The 1.0-cm lesion in the right cheek was excised. The 0.9-cm nasal specimen was then excised after prepping and draping. The excision went down to the alar cartilage. Specimen was sent for frozen section. The specimen showed no basal cell cancer. The pathologist commented that it might be sebaceous hyperplasia. It appeared to be completely excised. Full thickness skin graft was then harvested from the right post auricular region. The area here was then closed after some cauterization of small bleeders with the battery-operated cautery. Closure was with interrupted 4-0 Vicryl and then a running 4-0 Prolene mattress suture. The graft was defatted and then sewn into position. The length of the graft was 1.1×1 cm. 5-0 Nylon was utilized to secure the graft. Xeroform and 2×2 gauze were then placed over the operative area. A Band-Aid was placed over the keratosis site. The patient tolerated the procedure quite well and was sent to the ASU.

Pathology Report

Tissue(s) Submitted:	Specimen A: Lesion—right nasal tip.
	Specimen B: Lesion—right cheek.

Gross Description:

A. Specimen is received in fixative and consists of a 1.3×0.7 cm ellipse of skin with a longitudinal cut. There is a suture along one long axis. This axis is marked with black ink and a central section through the ellipse is made. Frozen section diagnosis: sebaceous lobules, and a small follicular cyst.

B. Specimen is received in fixative and consists of an oval, gray, friable 0.6-cm piece of skin.

Microscopic Description:

Five microscopic slide(s) examined.

Diagnosis:

A. Basal cell carcinoma, skin of right nasal tip.

Comment: Surgical resection margins are free of neoplastic cells. Although initial frozen section did not reveal basal cell carcinoma, deeper sections of the frozen piece reveal basal cell carcinoma.

B. Seborrheic keratosis, skin of right cheek.

Assign the correct codes for this same-day surgery encounter.

ICD-9-CM and CPT Code(s): _____

ICD-10-CM Code(s): _____

5.43. A 45-year-old female patient presents for wide exision of a 2.0 cm malignant melanoma of the right posterior calf. The area excised resulted in a 4.3 cm × 2.5 cm defect requiring rotational advancement flap closure. The pathology report shows clear margins.

What are the correct codes to report? The procedure is performed in the outpatient surgery suite at the hospital.

ICD-9-CM and CPT Code(s):

a. 173.70, 14001
b. 172.7, 14001
c. 172.7, 14001, 11606
d. V76.43, 14000

ICD-10-CM Code(s): _____

5.44. An ambulatory surgery operative report for a 75-year-old male patient states that the patient received a full-thickness graft of the cheek following lesion removal of a basal carcinoma. The lesion plus margins are documented to be 3.2 cm in diameter. A 10-sq-cm graft is applied with donor skin from his thigh, closed by suture.

Which of the following code sets is correct for this surgery?

ICD-9-CM and CPT Code(s):

a. 173.31, 15240, 11646
b. 173.31, 15240, 15004
c. 173.31, 15275, 15004, 11644
d. 173.31, 15240, 11644

ICD-10-CM Code(s): _____

5.45. From the health record of a patient undergoing foot surgery in the outpatient surgical unit:

Indication for Procedure: The patient is a 60-year-old female who has a persistently ingrowing great toenail on the right foot that has had two past infections. The infection is now clear and the patient presents for wedge resection of the toenail. She also has pernicious anemia, Friedreich's ataxia, and heart disease. Because of these conditions, a digital block will be used for the procedure.

Procedure: Wedge resection of toenail

Procedure Description: The patient is placed in the supine position, with the knees flexed, and the right foot is flat on the table. The toe is prepped and cleansed. A standard digit block is performed with 1% lidocaine using a 10-ml syringe and a 30 gauge needle. Approximately 3 ml is instilled on each side of the toe.

After waiting 10 minutes, a sterilized rubber band is placed around the base of the toe. The toe is resterilized and draped with the toe protruding. A nail elevator is slid under the cuticle to separate the nail plate from the overlying proximal nail fold. The lateral one fourth of the nail plate is identified as the site for the partial lateral nail removal. A bandage scissors is used to cut from the distal end of the nail straight back beneath the proximal nail fold. A straight, smooth, new lateral edge to the nail plate is created. The lateral piece of nail is grasped with a hemostat and removed in one piece, pulling straight out.

Electrocautery ablation is used to destroy the nail matrix where the nail was removed. The matrix is treated twice. Antibiotic ointment is applied and a bulky gauze dressing is placed. The foot is placed in a surgical boot. Post-op instructions are given for daily cleansing with warm water, and strenuous exercise is to be avoided completely for at least 1 week. The patient tolerated the procedure well and understands the discharge instructions.

What codes would be assigned for reporting the facility services?

ICD-9-CM Reason for Visit Code(s): _____

ICD-9-CM and CPT Code(s): _____

ICD-10-CM Reason for Visit Code(s): _____

ICD-10-CM Code(s): _____

5.46. A 17-year-old male patient presents to the hospital outpatient surgery center for surgery. Destruction was performed on 8 viral warts on the left arm. Destruction was done using cryosurgery and curettage. What codes are reported?

ICD-9-CM and CPT Code(s): _____

ICD-10-CM Code(s): _____

5.47. This 14-year-old boy is seen in the emergency room today. He was helping his father outside, who was installing a new bedroom window in their single family home, and the window fell. The glass broke, cutting the boy on his hand, forearm, and leg. He received a 2-cm laceration on his left hand, a 3-cm laceration on his left forearm, and a 2.5-cm laceration on his lower right leg. The lacerations on the hand and forearm were repaired with a simple repair. The laceration on the leg was deeper and required a layered repair. Assign the correct codes for this encounter.

ICD-9-CM Reason for Visit Code(s): _____

ICD-9-CM and CPT Code(s): _____

ICD-10-CM Reason for Visit Code(s): _____

ICD-10-CM Code(s): _____

5.48.

Preoperative Diagnosis:	Burn scar contracture with hypertrophic and keloid scarring anterior neck.
Postoperative Diagnosis:	Burn scar contracture with hypertrophic and keloid scarring anterior neck.
Procedure Performed:	Excision of keloid and release of anterior neck (20 × 8 cm).
Anesthesia:	General.
Estimated Blood Loss:	Minimal.

Indications for Procedure: This 18-year-old male had very severe hypertrophic burn scar to his anterior neck region. He is a keloid former by his previous history. He has been successfully treated with an acellular dermal replacement in the past. Our plan today after release of his neck and excision of the keloid is application of Integra to the defect on the anterior neck.

Description of Procedure: The patient was brought to the operating room and placed in the supine position on the OR table where general anesthesia and endotracheal intubation were accomplished without difficulty. After this was done, the patient was placed in a slightly hyper-extended position on the neck with a roll behind his shoulders and with sterile towels in the usual manner. A line was then drawn across the site of maximal contracture on the anterior neck and this was incised, carried down to scar into the platysma muscle. A large amount of hypertrophic and keloid scar was excised from the upper part of the flap. After this was released, the face was not distorted any longer and the contracture had been alleviated. The size of the defect with this was 20 × 8 cm. After bleeding was controlled with electrocautery, Integra was prepared, and one sheet was meshed 1:1 and applied on to the wound and secured with staples. Following this, stretched burn netting was applied over the Integra for support by Reston foam wet, irrigation catheters, and wet burn dressings. Spandex was used to complete the dressing.

The patient was then awakened, extubated, and transferred to the recovery room in good condition.

Assign the correct codes for this encounter.

ICD-9-CM and CPT Code(s): _____

ICD-10-CM Code(s): _____

5.49.   A 38-year-old female patient underwent a left lumpectomy and placement of an afterloading balloon catheter into the left breast in the special procedure room. Assign the appropriate CPT code(s).

a. 19297-LT
b. 19301-LT, 19297-LT
c. 19301-RT
d. 19120-LT

5.50.   A 75-year-old female patient is treated in the wound care clinic. She presents with a large sacral decubitus and a small decubitus on her buttock. The large sacral ulcer was a Stage II. Procedure performed by the surgeon: Full-thickness excisional debridement to the sacral decubitus. Scalpel was used to remove devitalized tissue down to bleeding. Patient tolerated the procedure well. Assign the diagnosis code(s).

ICD-9-CM Code(s):

a. 707.03, 707.05
b. 707.03, 707.05, 707.22
c. 707.03, 707.22
d. 707.03, 707.05, 707.22, 707.20

ICD-10-CM Code(s): _____

Behavioral Health Conditions

5.51.   A 35-year-old female patient presents to the Community Mental Health Center for group therapy with the diagnosis of obsessive-compulsive disorder. A psychiatrist provides group therapy for obsessive-compulsive disorder. Which of the following code sets would be reported for the facility code?

ICD-9-CM and CPT Code(s):
a. 301.4, 90853
b. 300.3, 90785, 90853
c. 300.3, 90853
d. 300.3, 90847

ICD-10-CM Code(s): _____

5.52.   A 66-year-old patient is seen as an outpatient in the community mental health center and participates in multiple-family group psychotherapy for 45 minutes. Diagnosis: Agoraphobia with panic attacks. List the diagnosis and CPT procedure codes for facility reporting.

ICD-9-CM and CPT Code(s): _____

ICD-10-CM Code(s): _____

5.53.   A 15-year-old depressed male is seen in the emergency department after a failed suicide attempt. Right wrist with a 3-cm laceration with no injury to the tendon. Left wrist with a 2.0-cm laceration with no injury to the tendon. Both wrists required simple suture repair. Patient used a razor to cut himself in a suicide attempt while at home in the bathroom today. He stated he has become increasingly depressed and has not experienced these types of symptoms before. He denies psychotic symptoms. Assessment: Laceration to both wrists, repaired. Major depression, severe. Plan: A 24-hour hold was instituted and the patient was transferred for psychiatric care. Stitches removed in 10 days. List the diagnosis and CPT procedure codes for facility reporting.

ICD-9-CM Reason for Visit Code(s): _____

ICD-9-CM and CPT Code(s): _____

ICD-10-CM Reason for Visit Code(s): _____

ICD-10-CM Code(s): _____

5.54.   This 25-year-old female was brought to the ER because of an overdose of prescription drugs. Her roommate found her in her bedroom at their apartment and called 911. She has been treated recently for depression, and her bottle of amitriptyline was empty. The roommate also reports that her bottle of diazepam was empty. Roommate estimates that there may have been about 20 pills in each bottle. According to the evidence, it appears as if she used alcohol to take the pills, and this was confirmed during drug screening. She left a suicide note stating that she could not go on living. Aggressive measures included stomach pumping to remove pill fragments and cardiopulmonary resuscitation. She could not be revived and was pronounced dead at 2305. List the diagnosis and procedure codes for facility reporting.

ICD-9-CM Reason for Visit Code(s): _____

ICD-9-CM and CPT Code(s): _____

ICD-10-CM Reason for Visit Code(s): _____

ICD-10-CM Code(s): _____

Disorders of the Musculoskeletal System and Connective Tissue

5.55.   **Preoperative Diagnosis:**   Lipoma of the left posterior thigh.

   Postoperative Diagnosis: Same.

   Procedures: Excision of the above.

   Description of Procedure: The patient was taken to the Operating Room where good anesthesia was obtained with 40 cc of 1% Carbocaine. The transverse incision was made centered over the visible and palpable mass, carried down through the skin and into the deep subcutaneous tissue. The mass was noted and shelled out. It had no major neurovascular attachments. This was removed in its entirety. Copiously irrigated and aspirated. The fat layer was closed using 0 plain catgut. The skin was closed with 2-0 dermalon.

Estimated Blood Loss: Minimal. Dressings were applied and the leg wrapped with an ACE wrap for compression. She tolerated the procedure well and left the Operating Room in good condition.

Pathology Report

Clinical Diagnosis and History:

Operation: Excision soft tissue mass left thigh.

Tissue(s) Submitted: Specimen: soft tissue mass left lateral posterior thigh.

Gross Description: The specimen consists of several lobular portions of fatty tissue which together measure $4.5 \times 3 \times 2$ cm in greatest dimension. Multiple sections through the specimen reveal no areas of softening or of unusual consistency.

Microscopic Description: Sections show mature fat with a scant amount of intervening fibrous stroma.

Diagnosis: "Soft tissue mass left lateral posterior thigh": The appearance is compatible with a lipoma.

What code(s) are used to report this encounter?

ICD-9-CM and CPT Code(s): _____

ICD-10-CM Code(s): _____

5.56.   This 3-year-old male fell from a park bench at the playground and was unable to bear weight on the left leg. X-rays today determined that he sustained a midshaft fracture of the femur, which was reduced and placed in a spica cast under conscious sedation in the outpatient surgical suite. Total conscious sedation time was 1 hour and 40 minutes.

Which CPT codes are appropriate for reporting?

a. 27500, 99148, 99150
b. 27502
c. 27506, 99148 x4
d. 27506

5.57.   From the health record of a 16-year-old male patient requiring fracture care in the outpatient surgical unit:

Operative Report

Preoperative Diagnosis:	Displaced comminuted fracture of the lateral condyle, right elbow
Postoperative Diagnosis:	Same
Procedure:	Open reduction, internal fixation

Description: The patient was anesthetized and prepped with Betadine. Sterile drapes were applied, and the pneumatic tourniquet was inflated around the arm. An incision was made in the area of the lateral epicondyle through a Steri-Drape, and this was carried through subcutaneous tissue, and the fracture site was easily exposed. Inspection revealed the fragment to be rotated in two planes about 90 degrees. It was possible to manually reduce this quite easily, and the judicious manipulation resulted in an almost anatomic reduction. This was fixed with two pins driven across the humerus. These pins were cut off below skin level. The wound was closed with some plain catgut suture subcutaneously and 5-0 nylon in the skin. Dressings were applied to the patient and tourniquet released. A long arm cast was applied.

Which of the following is the correct code assignment?

ICD-9-CM and CPT Code(s):

a. 812.52, 24577, 29065
b. 812.42, 24579, 29065
c. 812.42, 24579-RT
d. 812.52, 24579-RT

ICD-10-CM Code(s): _____

5.58.   The patient was hit in the face by a soccer ball on the neighborhood soccer field, when playing soccer with her friends, sustaining a 2.3-cm superficial laceration to the right medial cheek. X-rays revealed a nasal fracture that required stabilization. The emergency room physician stabilizes the fracture with a splint and tape and repairs the laceration with simple suture of the skin.

ICD-9-CM Reason for Visit Code(s): _____

ICD-9-CM and CPT Code(s): _____

ICD-10-CM Reason for Visit Code(s): _____

ICD-10-CM Code(s): _____

5.59.   This 52-year-old male was brought to the same-day surgery area for treatment of an open fracture of the distal phalanx of his index finger on the right hand. Patient is right-handed and this injury occurred when the food-processing machine at work tipped over and his hand got caught. He works in the local food factory here in town. The patient had open treatment performed to remove the fracture fragments without any internal or external fixation hardware used. What diagnosis and procedure codes are reported?

ICD-9-CM and CPT Code(s): _____

ICD-10-CM Code(s): _____

5.60.   This 70-year-old male presents to outpatient surgery for correction of his hallux valgus of the left great toe. In the operating room, the surgeon resects the base of the proximal phalanx as well as removes the medial eminence of the associated metatarsal. The repair is completed with insertion of Kirshner wire to hold the joint in place. The surgeon documents the repair as a Keller bunionectomy.

Assign the correct codes and modifier for this encounter.

ICD-9-CM and CPT Code(s): _____

ICD-10-CM Code(s): _____

5.61. The procedure that involves transplantation of a piece of articular cartilage and attached subchondral bone from a cadaver donor to a damaged region of the articular surface of the knee joint is called a(n):

    a. Osteochondral autograft
    b. Osteochondral allograft
    c. Autologous chondrocyte implantation
    d. Anterior cruciate ligament repair

5.62. From the health record of a 47-year-old patient admitted for outpatient surgery on his knee:

Operative Report

Preoperative Diagnosis:	Severe chondromalacia patellar, right knee.
Postoperative Diagnosis:	Severe chondromalacia patella and medial femoral condylar, right knee.
Procedure Performed:	1. Arthroscopy. 2. Chondroplasty/debridement of patella and medial femoral condyle. 3. Lateral retinacular release, right knee.
Anesthesia:	General.

Indications: This 47-year-old man has a history of severe patellofemoral and anteromedial joint line pain. This has been treated with anti-inflammatory medications and physical therapy with persistent symptoms. He has tightness of his lateral retinaculum associated with lateral patellar compression syndrome and patellofemoral pain. He presents now for surgical treatment after failed conservative management.

Details of Operation: Patient was brought to the operating room and placed on the operating table in a supine position. After instillation of successful general anesthesia, the right knee was examined. Range of motion was full; no laxity to stress testing was noted. Marked patellofemoral crepitus was noted. The leg was then placed in the arthroscopic leg holder and the knee sterilely prepped and draped. The knee was injected with a total of 30 cc of 0.25 percent Marcaine with epinephrine. Standard arthroscopic portals were established. There were grade III changes over the superior aspect and medial aspect of the patella. The trochlear groove of the femur was softened and minimally fissured. The medial compartment was entered and showed grade III chondromalacia over the majority of the weight-bearing surface of the medial femoral condyle. The tibial plateau was mildly softened, as was the medial meniscus. Intercondylar notch revealed a normal anterior cruciate ligament. The lateral compartment also revealed mild degeneration of the posterior horn of the lateral meniscus and minimal chondromalacia of the tibial plateau. At that point, a full radius resector was placed, and a chondroplasty debridement was carried out of the patella and medial femoral condyle. An internal lateral retinacular release was then carried out using arthroscopic electrocautery to help decompress the patellofemoral area. The patient returned to the recovery room without complications.

What are the correct code assignments for this outpatient surgical case?

ICD-9-CM and CPT Code(s):

a. 719.46, 717.7, 29873-RT, 29877-RT-59
b. 719.46, 717.7, 27425-RT
c. 717.7, 29877-RT
d. 719.46, 717.7, 29999-RT, 29877-RT

ICD-10-CM Code(s): _____

5.63. **Operative Report:** Palmar Fasciectomy

Indications: This is a 93-year-old lady who presents with a Dupuytren contracture of the left palm, which has progressively involved the base of the middle and ring fingers with inability to straighten the fingers.

Preoperative Diagnosis:	Dupuytren contracture, left palm, involving the middle and ring fingers.
Postoperative Diagnosis:	Dupuytren contracture, left palm, involving the middle and ring fingers.
Procedure:	Palmar fasciectomy. Release of the contracture around the left middle and ring fingers.
Anesthesia:	IV Bier block.

Description of Procedure: With the patient under IV Bier block and in the supine position, the left hand was prepped and draped in a sterile fashion. A Z-shaped incision was made in the left hand and carried down to the median crease. The skin flap was dissected free from the palmar fascia. The thickened palmar ligament into the metocarpophalangeal joint of the ring and middle fingers was resected. The tourniquet was let down after about ½ hour and hemostasis was maintained in the operative field. There was good capillary refill to the fingers. The wound was copiously irrigated with saline. A Penrose drain was inserted and the wound was closed with interrupted 4-0 nylon. Pressure dressing was applied to the hand and a volar splint was applied.

The patient tolerated the procedure well. Blood loss during the procedure was less than 50 cc. The patient was sent home in good condition.

What CPT code(s) are assigned to this case?

Code(s): _____

5.64.   **Preoperative Diagnosis:**   Status post trauma with tri-malleolar fracture dislocation, left ankle, now completely healed

Postoperative Diagnosis: Same.

Procedure: Removal of deep internal fixation devices from specified bone.

Description of Procedure: With the patient under general anesthesia, the right lower extremity was prepped and draped in the usual sterile manner. Pneumatic tourniquet was in place and inflated. There was a palpable lateral screw in the distal third of the fibula. An incision was made over the screw head through a previous area of incision, carried down through the skin and subcutaneous tissue and superficial fascia. The screw was identified and was removed. The tip of the medial malleolus and screw heads were identified and the incision carried down though the previous incision and carried down through the skin and a small split in the fascia and deltoid. The screw heads were each identified and removed. There was no evidence of infection. Irrigation was carried out throughout. The wounds were closed using 3-0 nylon.

The patient had a dry bulky dressing applied. There was good circulation in the foot. She tolerated the procedure well and went to the recovery room in good condition.

Pathology Report

Gross Description: The specimen is received fresh, labeled with the patient's name and consists of two metallic, partially threaded screws each measuring 5 cm in length and each measuring 0.2 cm in diameter. Additional material consists of a metallic, entirely threaded screw which is 6 cm in length and 0.3 cm in diameter. Gross only. No sections submitted.

Microscopic Description: None.

Assign the correct code(s) and modifier for this encounter.

ICD-9-CM and CPT Code(s): _____

ICD-10-CM Code(s): _____

Neoplasms

5.65.   A patient has squamous cell carcinoma of the posterior pharyngeal wall and metastasis to the cervical lymph nodes. Following consultation with the oncology team, the patient refused surgical intervention and elected to begin radiation therapy daily on a 6-MV linear accelerator. The radiation was delivered by hyperfractionation technique. Each field was treated twice each day, through a pair of large opposing lateral head and neck fields covering the primary cancer, the suspected areas of extension, and the lymph nodes in the neck. (Three separate treatment areas are involved, and customized shielding blocks are employed to shield normal tissue and shape the field to follow the anatomic boundaries.) Prior to the encounter under consideration, the clinical treatment parameters and dosimetry calculations have been completed, and the simulation-aided field settings have been accomplished.

Which of the following codes will be reported by the hospital for the encounters for radiation therapy, keeping in mind the number of treatments that will be reported in the unit's field on the UB-04?

ICD-9-CM and CPT Code(s):

a. V58.0, 77413
b. 149.0, 77408
c. V58.0, 149.0, 196.0, 77413
d. 149.0, 196.0, 77412

ICD-10-CM Code(s): _____

5.66. A patient with a lung mass discovered on prior x-ray presents to the outpatient surgery area for a diagnostic bronchoscopy. Following anesthetic to the airway, a fiberoptic bronchoscope is introduced into the bronchial tree. A needle is advanced through a channel in the scope, and tissue is aspirated from the lung mass for pathologic evaluation under fluoroscopic guidance. Pathology report confirmed parenchymal tissue of the lung was obtained and reported a diagnosis of oat cell carcinoma.

Which of the following is the correct code assignment?

ICD-9-CM and CPT Code(s):

a. 162.9, 31629
b. 162.9, 31629, 77002
c. 162.9, 31625
d. 235.7, 31629, 77002

ICD-10-CM Code(s): _____

5.67. A Medicare patient is scheduled for breast biopsy of a palpable lump in the right breast. A much smaller lesion in the left breast is identified by a radiological marker shown on mammography. An excisional biopsy is performed on both sides. The specimen on the right is diagnostic for breast malignancy with clear margins, whereas the small lesion in the left breast is found to be only fibrocystic disease, without evidence of malignancy. Which of the following is reported?

ICD-9-CM and CPT Code(s):

a. 174.9, 610.1, 19120-RT, 19125-LT, 19290-LT
b. 611.72, 610.1, 19120-50
c. 174.9, 610.1, 19120-50, 19125-50, 19290-50
d. 174.9, 610.2, 19120, 19125-59, 19290

ICD-10-CM Code(s): _____

5.68. A 50-year-old male patient with a personal history of colonic polyps presents to the outpatient surgery department for a colonoscopy to rule out colon cancer. The patient has been experiencing rectal bleeding for approximately 6 weeks and has lost a significant amount of weight. A colonoscopy to the terminal ileum is performed. Just beyond the rectal vault, two polyps are found and excised by hot biopsy forceps. Further up into the sigmoid colon, a lesion was biopsied. The pathology report confirms a diagnosis of colon cancer in the lesion found, and the polyps were found to be villous adenoma.

What codes are assigned in this case?

ICD-9-CM and CPT Code(s): _____

ICD-10-CM Code(s): _____

5.69.   A patient presents to the hospital outpatient department for chemotherapy treatment. She is a 15-year-old female with acute lymphoblastic leukemia. The chemotherapy agent is listed as an injection of lyophilized cyclophosphamide, 200 mg IV push. What codes, including the medication, would be reported?

ICD-9-CM, CPT, and HCPCS Code(s): _____

ICD-10-CM Code(s): _____

Disorders of the Nervous System and Sense Organs

5.70.   A 36-year-old female patient presents to the ED with a severe headache, listlessness, light sensitivity, nausea, and vomiting. The headache has been growing in intensity over the last 3 days. The patient does not have a fever. The patient has a programmable cerebrospinal fluid shunt in place and after MRI of both the head and the abdomen, it is determined that there is fluid accumulation in the intracranial portion of the shunt, indicating malfunction. The neurosurgeon takes the patient to the outpatient surgical suite and performs a magnetic adjustment of the valve pressure. The diagnoses are documented as headache and idiopathic normal pressure hydrocephalus, blocked ventricular shunt.

Excluding the E/M code and the MRI codes assigned by the chargemaster, what codes would be assigned for the facility in this case?

ICD-9-CM and CPT Code(s): _____

ICD-10-CM Code(s): _____

5.71.   A patient with Lou Gehrig's disease presents to the hospital-based outpatient neurology department for EMG testing. A needle electromyography of the legs and both of the eyes was conducted. Which of the following code set combinations would be reported?

ICD-9-CM and CPT Code(s):

a. 335.20, 92265-50, 95861
b. 335.24, 95868, 95861
c. 335.20, 95861, 92265
d. 335.29, 95861

ICD-10-CM Code(s): _____

5.72. From the health record of a patient requiring outpatient eye surgery:

Operative Report

Preoperative Diagnosis:	Type I diabetes patient with severe retinal microaneurysmal diabetic retinopathy, OU
Postoperative Diagnosis:	Same
Operation:	Vitrectomy followed by laser photocoagulation, OU

Description of Procedure: An Ocutome is used to go behind the iris and cut and suction the vitreous mechanically. After vitreous removal, a laser is used to treat the remaining retinal disorders in all four retinal quadrants and prevent further retinal hemorrhage. Procedure repeated.

Which of the following code sets is reported for this service?

ICD-9-CM and CPT Code(s):

a. 250.51, 362.01, 67040-50
b. 362.01, 362.81, 67040-50
c. 250.50, 362.02, 67039-LT-RT
d. 250.51, 362.02, 67105, 67145

ICD-10-CM Code(s): _____

5.73. From the health record of a patient with cataracts treated in outpatient surgery at the Eye Center:

Operative Report

Procedure:	Extracapsular cataract extraction with intraocular lens implantation, left eye
Diagnosis:	Bilateral cataracts

Technique: The patient was given a retrobulbar injection of 2.5 to 3.0 cc of a mixture of equal parts of 2 percent lidocaine with epinephrine and 0.75 percent Marcaine with Wydase. The area about the left eye was infiltrated with an additional 6 to 7 cc of this mixture in a modified Van Lint technique. A self-maintaining pressure device was applied to the eye, and a short time later, the patient was taken to the OR.

The patient was properly positioned on the operating table, and the area around the left eye was prepped and draped in the usual fashion. A self-retaining eyelid speculum was positioned and 4-0 silk suture passed through the tendon of the superior rectus muscle, thereby deviating the eye inferiorly. A 160° fornix-based conjunctival flap was created, followed by a 150° corneoscleral groove with a #64 Beaver blade. Hemostasis was maintained throughout with gentle cautery. A 6-0 silk suture was introduced to cross this groove at the 12 o'clock position and looped out of the operative field. The anterior chamber was then entered superiorly temporally, and after injecting Occucoat, an anterior capsulotomy was performed without difficulty. The nucleus was easily brought forward into the anterior chamber. The corneoscleral section was opened with scissors to the left and the nucleus delivered with irrigation and gentle lens loop manipulation. Interrupted 10-0 nylon sutures were placed at both the nasal and lateral extent of the incision. A manual irrigating-aspirating setup then was used to remove remaining cortical material from both the anterior and posterior chambers.

At this point, a modified C-loop posterior chamber lens was removed from its package and irrigated and inspected. It then was positioned into the inferior capsular bag without difficulty, and the superior haptic was placed behind the iris at the 12 o'clock location. The lens was rotated to a horizontal orientation in an attempt to better enhance capsular fixation. Miochol was used to constrict the pupil, and a peripheral iridectomy was performed in the superior nasal quadrant. In addition, three or four interrupted 10-0 nylon sutures were used to close the corneal scleral section. The silk sutures were removed, and the conjunctiva was advanced back into its normal location and secured with cautery burns at the 3 o'clock and 9 o'clock positions. Approximately 20 to 30 mg of both gentamicin and Kenalog were injected into the inferior cul-de-sac in a subconjunctival and sub-Tenon fashion. After instillation of 2 percent pilocarpine and Maxitrol ophthalmic solution, the eyelid speculum was removed and the eye dressed in a sterile fashion. The patient was discharged to the recovery room in good condition.

Assign the correct codes and modifier for this encounter.

ICD-9-CM and CPT Code(s): _____

ICD-10-CM Code(s): _____

5.74. The following documentation is from the health record of a 10-year-old female.

Indication for Procedure: The patient is a 10-year-old girl who has a history of refractory seizure disorder, now in almost a continual seizing state.

Description of Procedure: This is a digital electroencephalogram recorded using the 10-20 Electrode Placement System. The recording was performed after sleep deprivation. The patient was both awake and asleep during the recording.

During the EEG hookup the patient began having a seizure. At the beginning of the recording, well into the seizure, there were generalized polyspikes overlying 1–2 hertz diffuse delta waves that evolved in frequency. The patient was given diastat to stop the seizure. Post-ictally, there was diffusely increased beta range activity and intermittent vertex waves. The patient fell asleep and there was a buildup of diffuse delta activity with overlying beta activity. This appeared to be a buildup to another seizure. The recording was stopped before another seizure began.

Impression: Very abnormal EEG with a generalized idiopathic epileptic seizure, with status epilepticus. Refractory seizure disorder, per history.

Assign the correct codes and modifier for this encounter.

ICD-9-CM Reason for Visit Code(s): _____

ICD-9-CM and CPT Code(s): _____

ICD-10-CM Reason for Visit Code(s): _____

ICD-10-CM Code(s): _____

5.75. The patient has known chronic glaucoma, more severe in the left eye. She is brought to the outpatient procedure suite and anesthetized with a periocular anesthetic. The left eye is prepared and sterilely draped, followed by insertion of a lid speculum. A clear corneal incision is made temporally with the diamond blade approximately 3.4 mm in width. Viscoelastic material is injected into the anterior chamber over the pupil and lens to increase and maintain anterior chamber depth. Viscoelastic is then injected under the iris for 180° to visualize the ciliary body processes with the endoscope. The endoscope is inserted through the temporal incision, viewing the nasal ciliary processes. The ciliary processes are coagulated through the endoscope with the endpoint of shrinkage and whitening.

Assign the appropriate CPT code for the described procedure.

a. 66710-LT
b. 66711-LT
c. 66720-LT
d. 66700-LT

5.76. From the health record of a patient scheduled for eye surgery:

Surgery Date: 04/10/XX

Preoperative Diagnosis: Endophthalmitis, left eye.

Postoperative Diagnosis: Endophthalmitis, left eye.

Operative Procedure:
1. Pars plana vitrectomy, left eye.
2. Intravitreal vancomycin (1 mg left eye).
3. Intravitreal ceftazidime (2 mg left eye).
4. Intravitreal triamcinolone (4 mg left eye).

Anesthesia: Retrobulbar anesthesia with 5 cc of a 50/50 mixture of 2 percent lidocaine and 0.75 percent Marcaine.

Indications: This patient is status post tap and injection on April 1, 20XX. She presents with vitreous debris, poor vision, and a history of endophthalmitis.

Description of Procedure: After informed written consent was obtained, the patient was brought to the operating room and was prepped and draped in the usual sterile fashion. Retrobulbar anesthesia was performed with 5 cc of a 50/50 mixture of 2 percent lidocaine and 0.75 percent Marcaine in the retrobulbar space of the left eye without any complications. She was then prepped and draped in the usual sterile fashion. A speculum was placed in the left eye.

A standard 20-gauge pars plana vitrectomy was carried out with the pars placed 3 mm posterior to the limbus. A full vitrectomy was performed. Posterior vitreous detachment was induced and then further vitrectomy was carried out. The sclerotomy was closed with 7-0 VICRYL, as was the conjunctiva. Then, 0.1 mL of vancomycin (1 mg), 0.1 mL of ceftazidime (2 mg), and 0.1 mL of triamcinolone (4 mg) were injected into the vitreous cavity at the end of the case.

The patient was patched after atropine and Maxitrol were applied to the eye. The patient will follow up tomorrow at 8 a.m.

No qualified resident was available for the case.

What are the correct codes for this ambulatory surgery?

ICD-9-CM and CPT Code(s):

a. 360.00, 67036-LT, 66030-59-LT
b. 360.03, 67036-LT, 66030-59-LT
c. 360.00, 67036-RT
d. 998.59, 360.00, 67036-LT, 66030-LT

ICD-10-CM Code(s): _____

Newborn/Congenital Disorders

5.77.   A baby was born in the hospital to a woman who lacked prenatal care and contracted rubella during pregnancy, passing it on to her fetus. The baby was born with multiple deformities, including a congenital cortical and zonular cataract of the left eye. The baby is now 7 months old and ready for extracapsular phacoemulsification with intraocular lens replacement.

Which of the following code sets and modifier, if needed, would be reported for the surgery?

ICD-9-CM and CPT Code(s):

a. 743.30, 760.2, 66984-50
b. 366.03, 66984-LT
c. V30.00, 771.0, 743.32
d. 743.32, 66984-LT

ICD-10-CM Code(s): _____

5.78.   A newborn female is born with accessory digits of the right hand with a total of 5 normal fingers and 2 extra digits that do not contain bony structures. Which of the following code sets would be reported by the ASC facility tying off and removing these digits at the age of 2 weeks?

ICD-9-CM and CPT Code(s):

a. 755.01, 11200
b. 755.01, 28344-RT
c. 755.00, 28899
d. 755.01, 26587

ICD-10-CM Code(s): _____

5.79.   A baby boy is born with hypospadias. At 7 months of age, the first stage of surgical correction is undertaken, which requires transplantation of the prepuce, but no skin flaps. What are the correct codes for this ambulatory surgery, as reported by the hospital?

ICD-9-CM and CPT Code(s): _____

ICD-10-CM Code(s): _____

5.80. This child was born with a bilateral hydrocele. He also has reducible inguinal hernias on both sides. The condition has become troublesome, and the parents and pediatrician have decided that surgical correction is warranted for this 3-year-old. Surgeon performed a bilateral hernia repair with hydrocelectomy.

Postoperative Diagnosis: Bilateral hernia repair with hydrocelectomy

Report diagnosis and CPT procedure codes.

ICD-9-CM and CPT Code(s): _____

ICD-10-CM Code(s): _____

Pediatric Conditions

5.81. The following documentation is from the health record of a 6-year-old female patient.

Preoperative Diagnosis: Unilateral incomplete cleft of lip

Postoperative Diagnosis: Unilateral incomplete cleft of lip

Operation: Secondary correction with complete take-down of unilateral cleft lip

Description of Procedure: After the proper operative consent was obtained from the parents, the patient was brought to the operating room. She was comfortably placed on the operating room table and induced with general endotracheal anesthesia. The patient's oral facial region was then prepped with Betadine and draped sterilely. Normal anatomical landmarks were then carefully marked out on the patient's lip. This was tattooed with methylene blue. 2% Xyocaine with 1:100,000 epinephrine was infiltrated into the lip. A revision rotation advancement flap was carefully marked out. This included cutting out an area at the nasal base where there was a significant depression. The rotation flap was cut first. This was done with a 15-blade. The dissection was carried down through skin. There was significant scar on the lip, and it was completely cut through. The advancement flap was then cut. Tissue was left on the advancement flap to be rotated up when the flap was thin at the nasal base. Hemostasis was again secured. The orbicularis muscle was dissected from the skin and from the mucosa. Hemostasis was again verified. Muscle was then brought together. This was done with interrupted 4-0 Vicryl suture. Vermillion was closed with 5-0 Chromic. The lip itself was closed with 5-0 Rapid Catgut. The patient tolerated the procedure well. Sponge, instrument, and needle count were correct.

ICD-9-CM Reason for Visit Code(s): _____

ICD-9-CM and CPT Code(s): _____

ICD-10-CM Reason for Visit Code(s): _____

ICD-10-CM Code(s): _____

5.82.   Tonsillectomy and Adenoidectomy: Chronic Adenoiditis and Tonsillitis

Preoperative Diagnosis: Chronic adenoiditis and tonsillitis.

Postoperative Diagnosis: Chronic adenoiditis and tonsillitis.

Anesthesia: General.

Complications: None.

Descriptions: The 6-year-old female was brought to the operating room where general anesthesia was induced and maintained through an endotracheal tube. A Crowe-Davis mouthgag was inserted and red rubber Robinson placed through the nose and retrieved through the oropharynx for retraction of the palate. An adenoid curette was used to remove the adenoid tissue from the nasopharynx. Hemostasis was obtained with electrocautery. The left tonsil was grasped, and using electrocautery it was dissected from the fossa and transected at the base. The right tonsil was removed in a similar manner. The patient was awakened, extubated, and then taken to the recovery room in satisfactory condition.

Which CPT codes would be used to report this encounter?

a. 42825, 42830
b. 42820, 42820
c. 42821
d. 42820

5.83.   **Emergency Room Service**

Chief Complaint: Coughing, history of asthma, on Albuterol MDI, no allergies.

S: Patient is an 11-year-old male, who is seen today with cough that started 3 days ago, growing progressively worse. He states that he coughs when walking short distances. Peak flows have been around 200 at home but hard to measure due to coughing. Personal best is 300. Has been using Albuterol MDI with little success today. He had some loose stools yesterday, and Mom says that his activity level is severely reduced. Appetite moderate to minimal, totally unlike him. Some nasal allergy symptoms due to tree season. No chest pain. No nausea or vomiting.

O: Young white male in moderate respiratory distress. W: 81 lbs P: 64 RR: 24 T: 100.4 HEENT: PERRLA. TMs bilaterally are clear. Nose: congested with rhinorrhea. Oropharynx: mild erythema. Neck: supple. Full ROM. Thyroid normal. Lungs have bilateral wheeze in the left lower lobe. Heart RRR w/o gallop or murmur. Abdomen: positive bowel sounds, soft, nontender. No organomegaly is noted.

Data: Peak flows here are 200, 210, 200 with coughing. Pulse Ox is 97. Albuterol 0.5 cc aerosol via nebulizer is given with resulting peak flows of 230, 240, and 220 and repeat nebulizer at .05 cc in 15 minutes with improvement to 250.

A: Cough, acute asthma exacerbation due to seasonal allergies.

P: Albuterol 2 puffs QID. Prednisone 40 mg qd × 3 days, rest at least today, until appetite and energy improve. Follow up with PMD in 3 days for adjustment in asthma care plan or sooner if symptoms don't improve.

Excluding the E/M code, assign the correct codes for this encounter.

ICD-9-CM, CPT, and HCPCS Level II Code(s): _____

ICD-10-CM Code(s): _____

5.84.   A 6 year-old boy was brought to the Emergency Department after he fell from the jungle gym he was climbing at the city park. He fell about 10 feet from the top of the equipment to the sandy surface below. EMS reports there with loss of consciousness and a generalized seizure.

Upon exam, the patient had a decreased level of consciousness and head injury. The patient was hemodynamically stable with oxygen saturations greater than 95%. His Glasgow Coma Scale was depressed at 10. X-rays revealed a hairline occipital skull fracture. No spinal fracture was appreciated. No other injuries were identified except for a minor abrasion of the left forearm. The patient's level of consciousness improved but the child developed recurrent vomiting. The child was transferred via helicopter to University Hospital for further observation.

Transfer diagnosis: (1) Occipital skull fracture; (2) Concussion with loss of consciousness lasting about 45 minutes; (3) Generalized seizure; (4) Vomiting

ICD-9-CM Reason for Visit Code(s): _____

ICD-9-CM Code(s): _____

ICD-10-CM Reason for Visit Code(s): _____

ICD-10-CM Code(s): _____

5.85.   This 4-year-old child was brought to the ER because of cough and fever. The mother was worried about pneumonia, and the physician's office was closed for the weekend. X-ray was negative. Diagnosis: upper respiratory infection with bilateral acute conjunctivitis. What diagnosis code(s) are assigned?

ICD-9-CM Reason for Visit Code(s): _____

ICD-9-CM Code(s): _____

ICD-10-CM Reason for Visit Code(s): _____

ICD-10-CM Code(s): _____

Conditions of Pregnancy, Childbirth, and the Puerperium

5.86.   A patient in the 26th week of pregnancy had a 1-hour glucose screening test. Results of this test showed a blood sugar level of 160 mg/dL. Subsequently, the patient presents to the outpatient laboratory department with a physician order for a 3-hour glucose tolerance test. The reason for the test as documented on the order is: abnormal glucose on screening, rule out gestational diabetes. What is the correct code set for this outpatient ancillary services encounter?

ICD-9-CM and CPT Code(s):

a. 790.22, V22.2, 82951
b. 648.83, 82951
c. 648.83, 82950
d. 648.80, 82951, 82952

ICD-10-CM Code(s): _____

5.87.   This 26-year-old gravida 1, para 0 female has been having spotting and has been on bedrest. She awoke this morning with severe cramping and bleeding. Her husband brought her to the hospital. After examination it was determined that she has had an incomplete early spontaneous abortion. She is in the 10th week of her pregnancy. She was taken to outpatient surgery, and a dilatation and curettage was performed. There were no complications from the procedure. She is discharged home with instructions to follow up with the physician in the office.

Which of the following is the correct code set?

ICD-9-CM and CPT Code(s):

a. 637.91, 58120
b. 634.91, 59812
c. 634.91, 58120
d. 634.92, 59812

ICD-10-CM Code(s): _____

5.88.   This 23-year-old female is expecting her first child. She comes into the radiology department for an outpatient antenatal ultrasound to confirm the gestational age of the fetus and rule out fetal growth retardation. A real-time image was taken of the fetus estimated to be at 16 weeks. What diagnosis codes and associated procedure codes (even though they may be chargemaster-assigned codes) are assigned?

ICD-9-CM and CPT Code(s): _____

ICD-10-CM Code(s): _____

5.89.   This patient has a history of infertility and has been seeing her OB/GYN physician for more than 2 years. It was elected to perform a hysterosalpingogram at the outpatient surgery center to assess the patency of the fallopian tubes.

Procedure Report

The patient was prepped and draped in the usual manner. The cervical os was cannulated and Sinografin injected in retrograde fashion under fluoroscopic control. The body of the uterus appears normal. No filling defects are seen. There is no evidence of synechiae. The right fallopian tube is occluded approximately 1 cm from the body of the uterus. The left fallopian tube is patent and demonstrates free spill of contrast into the peritoneal cavity.

Assign the codes for this encounter.

ICD-9-CM and CPT Code(s): _____

ICD-10-CM Code(s): _____

Disorders of the Genitourinary System

5.90. Operative Report

Preoperative Diagnosis:	A 5-mm stone in the right lower pole.
Postoperative Diagnosis:	A 5-mm stone in the right lower pole.
Operation Performed:	Right extracorporeal shockwave lithotripsy.
Anesthesia:	Intravenous sedation.

Indications for Procedure: This is a 32-year-old young man who recently presented with right renal colic. An x-ray showed a stone in the proximal ureter. On June 1, 20XX, he underwent cystourethroscopy, the stone was successfully flushed into the kidney, and a double-J stent was placed in the ureter. Today, he presents for ESWL. An x-ray confirmed location of the stone in the right lower pole.

Description of Procedure: The patient was placed onto the treatment table and sedated. He was positioned over the shockwave electrode. Biaxial Fluoroscopy was utilized to position the stone at the focal point of the shockwave generator. The stone was treated with a total of 3,000 shocks. At the conclusion of the procedure, the stone appeared to have fragmented nicely, and the patient was discharged to the PACU.

Which of the following CPT code(s) are reported for thise service?

a. 52332, 50590
b. 50590
c. 52353
d. 50590, 52353

5.91. Operative Report

Indications: The patient is a 50-year-old gentleman with 4 children. He desires a permanent form of birth control via vasectomy.

Preoperative Diagnosis:	Elective vasectomy.
Postoperative Diagnosis:	Elective vasectomy.
Procedure:	Bilateral trans-scrotal segmental vasectomy.
Anesthesia:	Local with 1% Xylocaine infiltration.

Estimated Blood Loss:	Minimal.
Drains:	None.
Complications:	None.
Findings:	Normal testes and normal vas deferens.

Description of Procedure: The patient was taken to the procedure room where, in the supine position, he was prepped and draped in routine fashion. The left vas deferens was identified and isolated. Local anesthesia was obtained using infiltration of 1% Xylocaine without epinephrine. An incision was made overlying the vas deferens. The vas deferens was identified and delivered to the operative field. A 2.5-cm segment of vas deferens was then excised between hemostats. The ends of the vasa were then cauterized with electrocautery. The distal end was sutured and folded back upon itself with 3-0 chromic. The proximal end was sutured and folded back upon itself. Hemostasis was obtained. Next, attention was directed to the right side where the procedure was performed in mirror-image fashion. After confirming adequate hemostasis, the vasa were returned to the normal location within the scrotum. The skin was closed using interrupted sutures of 3-0 chromic. The patient was returned to the recovery room in good condition.

What code(s) are assigned for this encounter?

ICD-9-CM and CPT Code(s): _____

ICD-10-CM Code(s): _____

5.92.   This is a record of an emergency room visit:

Admission Date:	1/1/20XX
Discharge Date:	1/1/20XX
Discharge Diagnosis:	Torsion, right appendix testis.
Operation:	Right scrotal exploration; excision appendix testis
Surgeon:	
Complications:	None.
Allergies:	None.
Disposition/Medications:	Follow-up in 2 weeks. No medications.
Special Instructions:	Parents instructed to keep incision clean.

Summary: HPI - patient is a 4-year-old white male patient who has a moderate intellectual disability as well as obesity; otherwise he gets along reasonably well. However, the patient presented to his pediatrician this morning with a 1 hour history of sudden onset of testicular pain. Physical exam at that time was suggestive for testicular torsion, and he was admitted for surgical repair. Physical exam showed an obese white male, who was crying. Lungs clear. Heart regular, without murmur or gallop. Abdomen obese; no masses appreciated; bowel sounds normal active. Genital exam showed a small penis which was engulfed in the suprapubic fat; testes down bilaterally; the right side was exquisitely tender.

Laboratory values on admission: WBC 8.7, with 33 segs, 58 lymphs; hgb 14.3.

Patient was admitted and taken to the Operating Room immediately, and right scrotal exploration was undertaken. The appendix testis was found to be hemorrhagic and cyanotic. It was excised. The testicle otherwise appeared fine. The right testicle was fixed in the scrotum. It was not felt necessary to explore the left side for fixation. Postoperatively the patient did well. He was discharged later that evening in good condition.

Pathology Report

Gross Description: The specimen consists of a dark reddish-brown polyp-like tissue fragment, 8 × 4 × 4 mm. The entire specimen is submitted.

Microscopic Description: The specimen consists of histologic sections of a papillomatous tissue fragment lined by what appears to be mesothelium. The core of the specimen is composed of extremely loose connective tissue showing vascular congestion and hemorrhage.

Diagnosis: Appendix—testis: Edema and hemorrhage.

What code(s) are assigned to this case?

ICD-9-CM and CPT Code(s): _____

ICD-10-CM Code(s): _____

Disorders of the Respiratory System

5.93.   A patient with chronic obstructive asthma and an acute exacerbation of chronic bronchitis presents to the ED in respiratory distress.

Which answer represents the correct diagnosis coding for this case?

ICD-9-CM Code(s):

a. 493.22
b. 493.21, 491.21
c. 493.20
d. 491.21

ICD-10-CM Code(s): _____

5.94.   This 65-year-old smoker with hemoptysis and chronic cough is scheduled for an outpatient bronchoscopy with an endobronchial biopsy of the lesion in the bronchus. The pathology report states "well-differentiated oat cell carcinoma of the upper bronchus." What codes would be reported?

ICD-9-CM and CPT Code(s): _____

ICD-10-CM Code(s): _____

5.95.   This 59-year-old male patient has recovered from an extended period of time on a ventilator with a tracheostomy and is now ready for closure. The physician repairs the tracheal defect with good result, not requiring plastic repair. What codes are reported?

ICD-9-CM Reason for Visit Code(s): _____

ICD-9-CM and CPT Code(s): _____

ICD-10-CM Reason for Visit Code(s): _____

ICD-10-CM Code(s): _____

Trauma and Poisoning

5.96.   While running, a 10-year-old boy began choking on a small latex balloon and was rushed from the amusement park to the emergency department. The balloon is lodged in the trachea just past the larynx and threatening to obstruct his breathing. The piece of latex balloon is carefully removed from the trachea by use of biopsy forceps through flexible fiberoptic laryngoscope following administration of topical anesthesia.

Which codes are reported for this service in addition to the ED visit code?

ICD-9-CM Code(s):

a. 934.0, E912, E000.8, E849.4, 31577
b. 934.0, E912, E849.4, 31511
c. 784.99, E912, E000.8, E849.4, 31530
d. 933.1, 31577

ICD-10-CM Code(s): _____

5.97.   This 23-year-old female is brought to the emergency department after being found by her college roommate. Sometime within the last hour and a half after the roommate left, the patient ingested her entire bottle of verapamil (estimated at over 20 pills) as a suicide attempt, evidenced by a note. The physician ordered a high-dose glucagon HCl administration as an antidote, consisting of 10 mg/100 ml of D5W in an IV over 2 minutes, followed by a 5 mg/100 ml of D5W per hour for 2 more hours. A gastric lavage and aspiration were also performed. The patient's vital signs stabilized and lab work returned to normal over the next several hours. The patient was transferred to an inpatient psychiatric facility for follow-up treatment on her suicide attempt.

Assign the correct codes for this encounter.

ICD-9-CM, CPT, and HCPCS Level II Code(s): 972.9; 43753

ICD-10-CM Code(s): _____

5.98. This 32-year-old female was burned by hot grease in her kitchen 1 week ago. She is seen in the hospital-based wound clinic for large dressing changes on both upper extremities following second-degree burns to both arms. This is accomplished without requiring anesthesia.

What codes are assigned for this service?

ICD-9-CM and CPT Code(s): _____

ICD-10-CM Code(s): _____

5.99. A physician performed an aspiration via thoracentesis on a patient in observation status in the hospital. The patient has advanced lung cancer with malignant pleural effusion. Later the same day, due to continued accumulation of fluid, the patient was returned to the procedure room and the same physician performed a repeat thoracentesis.

Report diagnosis and procedure codes. Do not report observation codes.

Assign the correct codes and modifier for this encounter.

ICD-9-CM and CPT Code(s): _____

ICD-10-CM Code(s): _____

5.100. A 12-year-old boy presents with his father to the ER due to open wounds to his arm, hand, and upper leg. The injury occurred when the boy fell on a barbed-wire fence at the farm while running in the field. Diagnosis: Multiple lacerations to the right forearm, right hand, and left thigh. Procedure: Suture repair of the following: single-layer closure, 4.0 cm, forearm; layered closure, 3.0 cm, hand; 6.0 simple repair, thigh.

ICD-9-CM Reason for Visit Code(s): _____

ICD-9-CM and CPT Code(s): _____

ICD-10-CM Reason for Visit Code(s): _____

ICD-10-CM Code(s): _____

5.101. From the health record of a patient seen in the emergency room/observation area for an allergic reaction:

Discharge Summary

Date of Discharge: 01/08/XX

Chief Complaint: Allergic reaction to Bactrim, resulting in angioedema and mild respiratory distress.

Hospital Course: Fifty-six-year-old male admitted for angioedema after taking Bactrim for an ear infection. The patient had mild respiratory distress and marked swelling of his hands, face, and his oropharynx. The patient was given IV steroids in the Emergency Room and was admitted overnight for observation. The patient's swelling rapidly improved and by the morning after his admission he was back to baseline. He had no complaints of shortness of breath and desired to go home.

Condition on Discharge: Good. Activity: As tolerated. Diet: As tolerated.

Medications: Home medications only including:

1. Celebrex 200 mg one b.i.d.

2. Isosorbide 30 mg once a day.

3. Atenolol 25 mg per day.

4. Lipitor 10 mg per day.

Follow-Up: Will be as needed with primary care physician if ear problem returns and/or if he has any evidence of recurrent swelling and/or respiratory distress.

Emergency Assessment

Chief Complaint: Swelling, itching, and change in voice.

Present Illness: This is a 56-year-old white male with a history of allergic reaction to an antibiotic in the past, who presents today after taking his second dose of Bactrim this morning at home. He then had acute onset of swelling, redness, itching, and change in voice; also states that he was slightly short of breath but no wheezing. He denies any nausea, vomiting, fevers, chills.

Past Medical History: Coronary artery disease, MI 2 years ago, is currently taking Celebrex, Isosorbide, Atenolol, Lipitor, and Bactrim that he just started on this morning.

Physical Examination: Appears very red, swollen diffusely with erythematous rash, macular type rash. Blood pressure is 146/77, heart rate of 120, respiration rate 18 and 02; saturation is 96%. On room air. HEENT: He does have swollen eyelids, both upper and lower eyelids, with also some facial swelling and some uvular swelling as well as some lateral pharyngeal and uvular swelling, which appears to be allergic in nature. His tongue appears also slightly swollen, does not have any neck swelling, also has an erythematous rash. Lungs: Clear to auscultation with no wheezing noted. Abdomen: Soft, nontender.

Ed Course: Received Benadryl 25 mg IV, Pepcid 20 mg IV, Solu-Medrol 125 mg IV. At this point, his voice was still changing, and decision was made to admit the patient to the hospital for observation and then to observe and given a second dose of Solu-Medrol and Benadryl. Consultation between patient's private physician.

Select the correct codes for this observation patient.

ICD-9-CM Code(s):

a. 961.0, 786.09, 995.1, 693.0, E857, E849.0
b. 995.20, E931.0, E849.0
c. 995.1, 786.09, E931.0, E849.0
d. 995.1, 786.09, 693.0, E930.9, E849.0

ICD-10-CM Code(s): _____

5.102. Operative Report

Preoperative Diagnosis: Circular saw injury with complex laceration of left index finger with laceration of extensor tendon and joint capsule; laceration collateral ligament, radial side; displaced fracture at base of the middle phalanx, articular involvement.

Postoperative Diagnosis: Circular saw injury with complex laceration of left index finger with laceration of extensor tendon and joint capsule; laceration collateral ligament, radial side; compound fracture, base of the middle phalanx, articular involvement.

Operation Performed

Debridement and repair extensor tendon and joint capsule. Repair radial collateral ligament and wound closure.

Anesthesia: Digital block

This is a 42-year-old white male who accidentally injured his left index finger on a circular saw while working on broken shutters at home in his garage. The patient sustained a jagged laceration over the dorsal radial aspect of the index finger at the proximal interphalangeal joint. The wound was deep, involving the joint capsule, extensor tendon, and collateral ligament. The bone was also involved, especially at the base of the middle phalanx into the apical surface. The sensation to the tip of the finger was intact, especially all of the radial side. The wound measured about 3 cm in length.

Procedure: 0.5 percent Marcaine was used as local anesthetic digital block. After anesthesia had been obtained, the hand was prepped and draped in the usual manner. Tourniquet then was placed at the base of the fingers. The wound was then debrided. The minute loose bone and articular surface had to be removed. Some skin debrided also was removed. After satisfactory debridement, the joint capsule and extensor tendon then were repaired with 5-0 PDS suture material. The radial collateral ligament also was repaired with the same suture material. The skin then was carefully approximated with 5-0 nylon. After completion, a dressing was applied. The tourniquet was released and there was good perfusion throughout the fingers. An aluminum splint was placed.

The patient received 1 g of Ancef in the emergency room. He will continue to take Keftab 500 mg twice daily for 4 days and Vicodin 1 tablet q.4h. p.r.n. for pain. The postoperative instructions were given. Also the patient was informed about his injury and complications, especially wound infection and some stiffness of the finger. The patient will be followed up in my office.

Assign the correct codes and modifier for this encounter.

ICD-9-CM and CPT Code(s): _____

ICD-10-CM Code(s): _____

Chapter 6

Case Studies from Physician-Based Health Records

Note: Although the specific cases are divided by setting, much of the information pertaining to the diagnosis is applicable in most settings. Even the CPT codes in the ambulatory and physician sections may be reported in the same manner. The differences in coding in these two settings may involve modifier reporting, evaluation and management CPT code reporting, and other health plan reporting guidelines unique to settings. If you practice or apply codes in a particular type of setting, you may find additional information in other sections of this publication that may be pertinent to you.

Every effort has been made to follow current recognized coding guidelines and principles, as well as nationally recognized reporting guidelines. The material presented may differ from some health plan requirements for reporting. The ICD-9-CM codes used are effective October 1, 2012, through September 30, 2013, and the HCPCS (CPT and HCPCS Level II) codes are in effect January 1, 2013, through December 31, 2013. The current standard transactions and code sets named in HIPAA have been utilized. The 2013 draft edition of ICD-10-CM was utilized.

Instructions: Assign all applicable ICD-9-CM diagnosis codes including V codes and E codes. Assign all CPT Level I procedure codes and HCPCS Level II codes. Assign Level I (CPT) and Level II (HCPCS) modifiers as appropriate. Final codes for billing occur after codes are passed through payer edits. Medicare utilizes the National Correct Coding Initiative (NCCI) edits. CMS developed the NCCI edit list to promote national correct coding methodologies and to control improper coding leading to improper payments for Medicare Part B. The purpose of the NCCI edits is to ensure the most comprehensive code is assigned and billed rather than the component codes. In addition, NCCI edits check for mutually exclusive pairs.

Cases in this workbook are presented as either multiple choice or fill in the blank.

- For multiple-choice cases:
  - Select the letter of the appropriate code set.
- For fill-in-the-blank cases:
  - Sequence the primary diagnosis first followed by the secondary diagnoses including appropriate V codes and E codes (both cause of injury and place of occurrence).
  - Sequence the primary CPT procedure code first followed by additional procedure codes including modifiers as appropriate (both CPT Level I and HCPCS Level II modifiers).

○ Assign HCPCS Level II codes only if instructed (case specific).

○ Assign evaluation and management (E/M) codes only if instructed (case specific).

The scenarios are based on selected excerpts from health records. In practice, the coding professional should have access to and refer to the entire health record. Health records are analyzed and codes assigned based on physician documentation. In physician practice, valuable information for coding purposes is available on the superbill; however, documentation for coding purposes must be assigned based on medical record documentation. A physician may be queried when documentation is ambiguous, incomplete, or conflicting. The queried documentation must be a permanent part of the medical record.

The objective of the cases and scenarios reproduced in this publication is to provide practice in assigning correct codes, not necessarily to emulate complete coding, which can only be achieved with the complete medical record. For example, the reader may be asked to assign codes based on only an operative report; in real practice, a coder has access to documentation in the entire medical record.

The *ICD-9-CM Official Guidelines for Coding and Reporting of Outpatient Services*, published by the National Center for Health Statistics (NCHS), supplements the official conventions and instructions provided within ICD-9-CM. Adherence to these guidelines when assigning ICD-9-CM diagnosis codes is required under the Health Insurance Portability and Accountability Act (HIPAA) of 1996. Additional official coding guidance can be found in the American Hospital Association (AHA)'s *Coding Clinic* publication.

Anesthesia Services

Note: The reporting of the anesthesia section code versus the CPT code is a payer-specific policy. For these exercises, the anesthesia section code is to be reported for practice in assigning these codes. The exercises in this section are not based on payer-specific requirements.

6.1.   Correctly apply the anesthesia code for 19367, a breast reconstruction with TRAM flap. Do not assign modifiers in this example.

CPT Code(s):

a. 00404
b. 00406
c. 00402
d. 00400

6.2.   An epidural was given during labor. Subsequently, it was determined that the patient would require a C-section for cephalopelvic disproportion because of obstructed labor. Assign the correct codes. Modifiers are not used in this example.

ICD-9-CM and CPT Code(s):

a. 660.11, 653.41, 64493
b. 660.11, 653.01, 01961

    c. 660.11, 653.41, 01967, 01968

    d. 660.11, 653.91, 01996

ICD-10-CM Code(s): _____

6.3.   A 3-year-old child came to the outpatient surgery center to have dental caries filled and caps placed on his teeth due to nursing bottle decay syndrome. Anesthesia was provided by an anesthesiologist. Assign the correct codes for the anesthesia services. Modifiers are included in this example.

ICD-9-CM and CPT Code(s):

    a. 521.00, 00170-AA-23

    b. 521.00, 00170-AA

    c. 520.7, 00170-P1-23-AA

    d. 521.30, 00170

ICD-10-CM Code(s): _____

6.4.   A 5-year-old patient was brought into the emergency room with a deep 2-cm laceration of his scalp. The child was combative and would not allow staff to cleanse the wound. The mother held the child in her lap while the ED physician administered 10 mg of Versed intranasally. When the child was sufficiently sedated, one of the ED nurses monitored the patient's vital signs, and the physician performed a layered repair of the laceration. The intra-service time for the procedure did not exceed 30 minutes.

Assign the correct CPT code(s) for the procedure and sedation for this case:

    a. 12031, 99143

    b. 12031, 99144

    c. 12031-47

    d. 12031-QS

6.5.   A 2-month-old infant is brought to the operating room for repair of coarctation of the aorta with a pump oxygenator. Anesthesia is provided by an anesthesiologist. The infant is in critical condition and may not survive. Assign the correct diagnosis and anesthesia codes, including physical status, Level I and II modifiers, and qualifying conditions for this procedure.

ICD-9-CM and CPT Code(s): _____

ICD-10-CM Code(s): _____

6.6.   A patient is brought to the emergency department with a ruptured aortic aneurysm and is taken immediately into surgery for operative repair. Which qualifying circumstance code is assigned to indicate that anesthesia for the surgery will be affected by the emergency status of this patient?

    a. 99140

    b. 99100

    c. 99116

    d. 99135

Disorders of the Blood and Blood-Forming Organs

6.7. The physician diagnoses acquired coagulopathy due to vitamin K deficiency. How is this coded?

ICD-9-CM Code(s): _____

ICD-10-CM Code(s): _____

6.8. A patient is admitted with cervical lymphadenopathy. A needle biopsy of a cervical lymph node is performed, and Hodgkin's sarcoma disease is confirmed. Which of the following is the correct code assignment?

ICD-9-CM and CPT Code(s):

a. 201.21, 38505
b. 201.91, 38505
c. 201.21, 38500
d. 785.6, 38510

ICD-10-CM Code(s): _____

6.9. From the physician services documentation of a 39-year-old male:

History of Present Illness: The patient is a 39-year-old African-American male who has a known history of sickle cell anemia. He was admitted to the hospital with diffuse extremity pains with minor complaints of pain along the right inguinal area. They started on Friday, became a little bit better on Saturday, then improved, and started again in the past 24 hours. He denies any problems with cough or sputum or production. He denies any problems with fever.

Past Medical History: See recent medical records in charts. He does have a new onset of diabetes, probably related to his hemochromatosis. He does have evidence of iron overload with high ferritins.

Review of Systems: Otherwise unremarkable except for those related to his pain. He denies any problems with fever or night sweats. No cough or sputum production. Denies any changes in gastrointestinal or genitourinary habits. No blood from the rectum or urine.

Physical Examination: This is a 39-year-old, African-American male who is conscious and cooperative. He is oriented × 3 and appears in no acute distress. Vital signs are stable. HEENT is remarkable for icterus present in oral mucosa and conjunctivae, which is a chronic event for him. The neck is supple. No evidence of any gross lymphadenopathy of the cervical, supraclavicular, or axillary areas. The heart is abnormally irregular in rate without any murmurs heard. Lungs are clear to auscultation and percussion. The abdomen is soft and benign without any gross organomegaly. Extremities reveal no edema. No palpable cords. He does have some tenderness along the inner aspects of his right lower extremity near the inguinal area; however, no masses were palpable and no point tenderness is noted.

The patient was treated for his painful sickle cell crisis with IV fluids and pain medications. He had a problem with his right inguinal area. He had evidence of pain. There was some pain on abduction of his right lower extremity. The examination really was unremarkable. There was no evidence of any Holman; no palpable cords, no masses were palpable.

Because of his sickle cell anemia, rule out the possibility of osteonecrosis of the femur. Complete x-rays of his femur and hip were carried out. However, these were both negative. Patient is being discharged after improvement. To follow up with me in 1 week.

Diagnoses: 1. Painful -sickle cell crisis
2. Type II diabetes mellitus
3. Chronic atrial fibrillation

Condition on Discharge: Stable

What diagnosis code(s) would the physician report on this case?

ICD-9-CM Code(s):

a. 282.61, 789.09, 427.31, 250.00
b. 282.62, 733.42, 427.31, 250.00
c. 282.62
d. 282.62, 427.31, 250.00

ICD-10-CM Code(s): _____

6.10. This established patient comes to the physician's office and after evaluation requires a glucose tolerance test. The physician drew the three specimens and performed the test at the office. List the correct CPT procedure code(s).

Code(s): _____

6.11. The physician documents that the patient has blood-loss anemia. Which diagnosis code is supported by this documentation?

ICD-9-CM Code(s):

a. 280.0
b. 285.1
c. 285.8
d. 285.9

ICD-10-CM Code(s): _____

Disorders of the Cardiovascular System

6.12. **Chief Complaint:** Left knee pain

Reason for Admission: Hypotension, bradycardia, and possible GI bleed

This 83-year-old patient presented to my office this morning complaining of knee pain and wanting to see an orthopedic surgeon for a knee replacement. My first impression of the patient was that he appeared lethargic and extremely tired-looking. Upon questioning, he stated that he was far more tired than normal and "just didn't feel good," attributing this to the chronic pain in the knee. I reviewed his meds and completed a 10-point review of systems, which revealed increasing bouts of periodic diarrhea with dark stool. He has overall poor health with multiple previous surgeries and hypertension that has been difficult to control. Other systems are negative for new complaints today. At the completion of our office visit, I arranged for a direct admission to the hospital. I saw him again at the hospital and continued the diagnostic workup.

No known allergies. Takes Lisinopril 40 mg daily, Coreg, half of a 25 mg pill twice per day, and Protonix daily. He is married and lives with his second wife. The first wife died in 1996. His mother lived to 93 and father lived to 96. He reports that they died of "old age."

Vital Signs: Blood pressure is 96/62. RR 18, P 54, T 97.3, Wt 197, down 6 pounds from last month with BMI of 28.67. General: Elderly male in no acute distress. Skin: Laminectomy scar on his lower back. No clubbing or cyanosis of his fingers and no suspicious lesions. Neurologic: He is alert and oriented but his timeline is unclear, especially relating to the diarrhea. Is far more concerned about his knee than anything else. Cranial nerves grossly intact and motor strength is 5/5. HEENT: Atraumatic, normocephalic. Anicteric sclera. No sinus tenderness. Posterior oropharynx is very irritated. Lips without cyanosis. NECK: Supple without adenopathy. No thyromegaly, nodules, or carotid bruits. CHEST: Normal symmetry. CARDIOVASCULAR: Rate is somewhat bradycardiac and very difficult tones to auscultate. Regular rhythm. LUNGS: Clear. ABDOMEN: Soft, nontender, nondistended, decreased bowel sounds, no hepatosplenomegaly, rebound, or rigidity. No inguinal adenopathy, 2+ inguinal pulses bilaterally. MUSCULOSKELETAL: Left leg shows some atrophy in the muscles and left knee looks larger than the right knee. No real swelling appreciated. Not warm. GU: Normal scrotal exam. No hernia. RECTAL: Perianal area is somewhat irritated. There is a large external hemorrhoid. Prostate is slightly enlarged. Stool is dark brown but heme negative.

Labs are pending. EKG shows a significant sinus bradycardia around 50–55 beats per minute. This does not appear to be atrial fibrillation. He has a somewhat widened QRS complex or intraventricular conduction delay. He does not peak T waves or have any other significant issues regarding arrhythmia.

Assessment:

1. Hypotension, potentially due to antihypertensive medication or based on decreased volume due to diarrhea and potential GI bleed.
2. Sinus bradycardia. Cause unclear but could also be due to volume depletion.
3. Diarrhea. Has had problems with anemia in the past but not currently. Potentially upper GI source since stool is dark.
4. Localized osteoarthrosis of left knee.

Plan: IV fluids, 2L over 8 hours and then will switch to 100 ml/hour of D5 normal saline. Blood was drawn in the office. Recheck comprehensive metabolic panel after IV hydration. Hold Lisinopril and Coreg until blood pressure stabilizes. Cardiology consult requested. GI consult requested. Will hold on evaluating any orthopedic issues until seen in follow-up in the office.

Assign the correct codes for this encounter.

ICD-9-CM and CPT Code(s): _____

ICD-10-CM Code(s): _____

6.13. The following documentation is from the health record of a 63-year-old female patient.

Admission Date:	11/19/XX
Discharge Date:	11/24/XX
Final Diagnoses:	1. Coronary artery disease
	2. Sick sinus syndrome
Procedures:	1. Permanent dual-chamber pacemaker insertion with atrial and ventricular leads
	2. Percutaneous transluminal coronary angioplasty (PTCA) of right coronary artery (RCA) with insertion of drug-eluting stent

History of Present Illness: The patient is a 63-year-old female who was admitted to another hospital on 11/19 after experiencing tachycardia. At that hospital, she underwent a cardiac catheterization, showing the presence of severe single-vessel coronary artery disease of the right coronary artery (RCA). The patient has a history of sick sinus syndrome. She was transferred to our hospital to undergo a percutaneous transluminal angioplasty.

Physical Examination: No physical abnormalities were found on the cardiovascular examination. Pulse 50, blood pressure 100/66. HEENT: PERRLA, faint carotid bruits. Lungs: Clear to percussion and auscultation. Heart: Normal sinus rhythm with a 2.6 systolic ejection murmur. Extremities and abdomen were negative. Laboratory data: Unremarkable.

Hospital Course: To manage the patient's sick sinus syndrome, a permanent AV sequential pacemaker was implanted by transvenous technique on 11/19. On 11/20, the patient underwent a PTCA without complications and good results were obtained. Postoperatively, the patient was stable and was subsequently discharged. Patient was discharged on the following medications: Cardizem, 30 mg p.o. q. 6 hours; ASA, 5 grains q. a.m.; Metamucil and Colace p.r.n; Nitro paste 1/2 inch q. 6 hours.

Which of the following is the correct code assignment for the procedures performed?

ICD-9-CM and CPT Code(s):

a. 427.0, 414.01, 92980, 33206
b. 414.01, 427.81, 92995, 33208
c. 414.01, 427.81, 92980, 33208
d. 427.81, 414.01, 92982, 33206

ICD-10-CM Code(s): _____

6.14. A patient is admitted with an acute exacerbation of congestive heart failure due to hypertensive heart disease. This patient has chronic systolic heart failure. The patient responds positively to Lasix therapy. The patient also has chronic kidney disease stage V and is a type I diabetic. Assign the correct diagnostic codes.

ICD-9-CM Code(s): _____

ICD-10-CM Code(s): _____

6.15. This 55-year-old male was brought to the ER with chest pain. The final diagnostic statement on the patient's record stated "preinfarction syndrome." What is the correct diagnostic code?

ICD-9-CM Code(s): _____

ICD-10-CM Code(s): _____

6.16. A patient had an implantable vascular access device placed 7 weeks ago for chemotherapy. This is administered each week in the ambulatory surgery department of the hospital. The full cycle is now complete and the vascular access device is no longer needed. The physician surgically removed the centrally tunneled central venous catheter. No services for the carcinoma of the sigmoid colon are provided. The cancer has not been resected yet because the chemotherapy was utilized in an attempt to shrink the tumor before surgery was initiated. The correct codes for reporting by the physician will be:

ICD-9-CM and CPT Code(s): _____

ICD-10-CM Code(s): _____

Disorders of the Digestive System

6.17. This 30-year-old male patient has exhausted all types of conservative treatment for his morbid obesity due to his excess calories intake. He has been treated by me in this clinic for 3 years. He has also been treated for hypertension and hypercholesterolemia. With these risk factors and with careful review of his condition and symptoms and with multiple consultations with him regarding the risks and benefits of the surgery, it is decided to perform a vertical-banded gastroplasty.

What diagnosis and CPT procedure codes are used in this surgical case?

ICD-9-CM and CPT Code(s):

a. 278.00, 401.9, 272.0, 43842, 43846–51
b. 278.01, 401.9, 272.0, 43842
c. 278.01, 401.9, 272.0, 43842, 43843–59
d. 278.01, 401.9, 272.0, 43848

ICD-10-CM Code(s): _____

6.18. This 25-year-old woman has been treated for Crohn's disease of the small intestine since 18 years of age. She has had several exacerbations but has been maintained on drug therapy. She is being seen now for extreme pain, which on x-ray shows small bowel obstruction. Patient is taken to surgery immediately. During the surgery, a partial excision of the terminal ileum is performed to release the obstruction. There is also a section of the jejunum that is very inflamed. This section is also resected. An end-to-end anastomosis is completed on all segments. The patient tolerates the procedure well. Which of the following is the correct code assignment?

ICD-9-CM and CPT Code(s):

a. 560.89, 555.0, 44120, 44121-51
b. 555.0, 560.89, 44120, 44121-51
c. 555.0, 560.89, 44120, 44121
d. 555.2, 560.89, 44020

ICD-10-CM Code(s): _____

6.19. During a colonoscopy, the surgeon biopsies an inflamed area in the ascending colon and removes a polyp in the descending colon with use of hot biopsy forceps. What is the correct CPT and modifier code assignment?

CPT Code(s): _____

6.20. The patient has a history of abdominal pain and blood in the stool. A colonoscopy was done earlier today and did not identify a bleed. As a further evaluation, the patient is undergoing a capsule endoscopy of the entire GI tract. The physician documentation states:

The patient was able to swallow the capsule orally without difficulty. Images were downloaded. The capsule was seen traversing the small bowel all of the way down to the cecum. Gastric images demonstrated no ulceration. Gastric passage time was 1 hour and 37 minutes. Careful review of small bowel images, which were of good quality, did not demonstrate any significant mucosal lesion. There was one single site suggestive of possible erosion seen in the ileum. The capsule was seen entering the ileocecal valve into the cecum.

Assign the correct codes for this encounter.

ICD-9-CM and CPT Code(s): _____

ICD-10-CM Code(s): _____

6.21. This 50-year-old male patient had an open cholecystectomy done with exploration of the common duct for stones. During the procedure an incidental appendectomy was performed. How are the CPT procedure codes reported if the third-party payer requires that both procedures be reported?

CPT Code(s): _____

6.22. The patient has both internal and external thrombosed hemorrhoids in a single group, excised in the outpatient surgical suite. What codes would be assigned by the surgeon?

ICD-9-CM and CPT Code(s):

a. 455.4, 455.1, 46255
b. 455.5, 455.2, 46260

    c. 455.4, 455.1, 46945, 46320

    d. 455.7, 46083, 46320

ICD-10-CM Code(s): _____

6.23. A laparoscopic cholecystectomy with cholangiography was performed on a 35-year-old female patient due to symptomatic cholelithiasis. The pathology report showed acute and chronic cholecystitis with cholelithiasis and was also documented by the physician. What codes would be assigned?

Assign the correct codes for this encounter.

ICD-9-CM and CPT Code(s): _____

ICD-10-CM Code(s): _____

6.24. The patient's gastric band has been adjusted so many times that it is losing its elasticity and starting to slip on her stomach and migrate up around her esophagus. She enters to undergo removal of her current gastric band and placement of a new adjustable band. Her weight loss has been steady and appropriate. Assign the CPT code(s) for the procedure of laparoscopic removal and replacement of an adjustable gastric band.

    a. 43773

    b. 43771, 43770

    c. 43774, 43770

    d. 43888

6.25. This is the health record of a patient treated in the ambulatory surgery center.

Preoperative Diagnosis:	Ankyloglossia
Postoperative Diagnosis:	Same as above
Procedure:	Lingual frenoplasty
Anesthesia:	General

Technique: The 4-year-old was brought to the operating room and was placed in the supine position. The patient was prepped and draped in the normal fashion and induced under general anesthesia. The patient was intubated with a pediatric tube with no problem. The ventral surface of the tongue with injected with 2% lidocaine with epinenphrine and retracted superiorly using a retraction suture placed through the tip of the tongue. A Bovie cautery was used to incise the lingual fenulum from the ventral surface of the tongue approximately 1 cm posteriorly. Using 3-0 chromic sutures, the ventral surface of the tongue was sutured in an interrupted fashion to obtain hemostasis and to prevent reattachment of the frenulum. The wound was covered with moist dressings and the patient was sent to recovery in good condition.

Assign the correct codes for this outpatient surgery.

ICD-9-CM and CPT Code(s): _____

ICD-10-CM Code(s): _____

6.26. **Pre-Procedure Diagnosis:**

Post-Procedure Diagnosis: Diverticulosis; diminutive sigmoid polyp at 20 cm (removed); internal hemorrhoids

Procedure: Colonoscopy

Anesthesia: Conscious Sedation

Procedure: After informed consent was obtained and history and physical examination performed, the patient was placed in the left lateral decubitus position. While being continuously monitored for heart rate, blood pressure, cardiac rhythm, and oxygen saturation, conscious intravenous sedation was established using intravenous Fentanyl and Versed. A digital rectal examination was unremarkable.

The Olympus video colonoscope was inserted into the rectum which revealed internal hemorrhoids. The colonoscope was then advanced through a sigmoid and left colons which revealed scattered diverticulosis. A diminutive 6- to 8-mm polyp was noted 20 cm from the anal verge and was removed using standard hot biopsy technique. The colonoscope was then advanced to the cecum, identified by the ileocecal valve and appendiceal opening. The colonoscope was advanced through the appendiceal opening and into the small bowel which was unremarkable.

The colonoscope was then withdrawn carefully inspecting the walls for mucosal abnormalities. Once back in the rectum retroflexion revealed internal hemorrhoids. The colonoscope was straightened and withdrawn. The patient tolerated the procedure well. There were no complications. She was sent to the Recovery Room in stable condition.

Plan: 1. The patient will remain on a high fiber diet.

               2. Will await histology of the benign appearing sigmoid polyp.

               3. Schedule the patient for surveillance colonoscopy in 36 months.

Assign the correct codes for this outpatient encounter.

ICD-9-CM and CPT Code(s): _____

ICD-10-CM Code(s): _____

6.27.   This 47-year-old man experienced acute odynophagia after eating fist. The patient felt a foreign body-like sensation in his proximal esophagus. He was evaluated with lateral, C-spine films, and soft tissue films without any evidence of perforation.

Procedure: EGD with foreign body removal

Findings: After obtaining informed consent, the patient was endoscoped. He was premedicated without any complication. Under direct visualization, an Olympus Q20 was introduced orally and the esophagus was intubated without difficulty. The hypopharynx was reviewed carefully, and no abnormalities were noted. There were not foreign bodies and no lacerations to the hypopharynx. The proximal esophagus was normal. No active bleeding was noted. The endoscope was advanced farther into the esophagus, where careful review of the mucosa revealed no foreign bodies and no obstructions. However, the gastroesophageal junction did show a very small fish bone, which was removed without complications. The endoscope was advanced into the stomach, where partially digested food was noted. The duodenum was normal. The endoscope was then removed. The patient tolerated the procedure well, and his postprocedural vital signs are stable.

ICD-9-CM and CPT code(s): _____

ICD-10-CM Code(s): _____

Evaluation and Management (E/M) Services

6.28.   A 45-year-old patient was found unconscious in a park and was brought to the emergency department by ambulance. A comprehensive physical examination was performed, and the medical decision making was of high complexity. The ED physician documents that he was unable to obtain a history due to the condition of the patient.

What is the correct E/M code assignment for the physician's services for this encounter?

a. 99284
b. 99285
c. 99285-52
d. 99291

6.29.   Dr. Jones saw Mr. Stone at the VA domiciliary after the patient had an episode of severe choking at the noon meal. He did not aspirate any food, but had a slight sore throat after the episode. The patient stubbornly refused to go to the clinic but agreed to be seen if the doctor came over. Mr. Stone has had several episodes of choking in the past few days, which he attributed completely to his sinus medication causing a very dry mouth. Dr. Jones documented a problem-focused interval history and an expanded problem-focused examination on this established patient. Medical decision making was of low complexity. Another medication was substituted. He was advised to drink liquids with his meals and take smaller bites. Give the correct codes for this visit.

ICD-9-CM and CPT Code(s):

a. 784.99, 783.3, 99335
b. 933.1, 99334
c. 933.1, 99335
d. 783.3, 99334

ICD-10-CM Code(s): _____

6.30.   A 59-year-old male established patient is scheduled for his routine physical examination; however, the physician finds a mass in the abdomen, schedules an abdominal CT scan, and orders laboratory for blood work and a UA. The physician performs a detailed history and an expanded problem-focused examination with medical decision making of moderate complexity. The patient has been a patient of this physician for several years. What E/M code(s) are assigned?

Code(s): _____

6.31. An elderly patient is brought to the emergency department by an ambulance due to a cardiac arrest suffered at home. The ED physician provides and documents critical care services to the patient for a total duration of 2 hours before the attending physician admits the patient to the cardiac care unit.

What codes are assigned for the ED physician? (Include E/M code(s).)

ICD-9-CM and CPT Code(s): _____

ICD-10-CM Code(s): _____

6.32. Summary of the clinic record of a family practice physician:

The patient is a 3-year-old male with Down's Syndrome who was seen in the office yesterday for bilateral otitis media. He was given a prescription for Septra liquid suspension. On repeat visit today, the mother reports that the patient complained of a "tummy ache" after the first dose and has vomited six times since being seen yesterday. PO intake is decreased but still sufficiently hydrated. Has not been able to keep down any antibiotics. A detailed history is documented.

Documentation states that the ears have increased redness with the right TM bulging more than yesterday. Considerable wheezing is noted on lung exam. No other significant findings are documented on the detailed exam.

The patient is treated with 500 mg of Ceftriaxone sodium, IM, and given a prescription for an albuterol metered dose inhaler with spacer. The patient and mother are taught the proper use of the inhaler.

The physician documents the diagnoses as:

1. Acute otitis media
2. First-time wheezer
3. Vomiting
4. Down's Syndrome

What codes would be reported for this visit (include E/M code)?

ICD-9-CM and CPT Code(s):

a. 381.4, 493.90, 787.03, 758.0, 99214, 96372, J0696
b. 382.9, 758.0, 99214, 94640, 96372, J0696 × 2 units
c. 382.9, 786.07, 787.03, 758.0, 99214-25, 94664, 96372, J0696 × 2 units
d. 382.9, 786.07, 787.03, 758.0, 99214-25, 96372, J0696

ICD-10-CM Code(s): _____

6.33. Dr. Smith sees his patient, Bob Jones, in the nursing home where he has resided for 11 months. Bob is pretty stable and happy, and Dr. Smith performs an annual physical examination and completes the minimum data set instrument. He performs and documents a detailed interval history, comprehensive examination, and performs medical decision making of and low complexity. Assign the appropriate CPT code.

> a. 99304
> b. 99308
> c. 99318
> d. 99306

6.34. An established patient sees his doctor in the office with complaints of chest pain. The physician admits the patient on December 1 under observation status at the local community hospital. The physician completes a comprehensive history that includes a complete review of all body systems and a complete past, family, and social history. The physician performs a comprehensive examination but finds no significant issues. The patient does admit to a great deal of stress at work. Medical decision making is of moderate complexity. On the second day of care, the physician continues to observe the patient when he conducts a detailed examination and medical decision making of moderate complexity. The patient is subsequently discharged home the next day with a diagnosis of mild depression. The patient was in observation status for three days.

What E&M codes would the physician report for the second day of care?

Code(s): _____

6.35. The patient was brought by ambulance to the ER after being shot in the head in a random drive-by shooting. Critical care services are provided by the physician for 125 minutes. During this time the physician performed CPR, reviewed ECG and blood gas results on the EHR, and intubated the young man. However, the patient died from his extensive injuries. What E/M codes are used to report the services supplied by the physician?

> a. 99292, 92950
> b. 99291, 99292, 92950
> c. 99291, 99292, 99090, 92950, 43752
> d. 99291, 99292, 92950

6.36. This established patient is seen for menstrual irregularities, as well as new symptoms of vaginal itching and skin rash. The visit included an expanded-problem focused history and physical examination as well as moderate complexity decision making. The physician diagnoses vaginal candidiasis and tinea corporis on this visit and provides treatment. The patient also provides continuing treatment for the patient's polycystic ovarian syndrome.

Assign the correct diagnosis and procedure codes:

ICD-9-CM and CPT: _____

ICD-10-CM: _____

Endocrine, Nutritional, and Metabolic Diseases and Immunity Disorders

6.37. A completion right thyroidectomy is performed after a previous right partial thyroidectomy was completed several years ago. All thyroid tissue is removed from the right side, and a total left thyroidectomy is performed. The parathyroid glands are separated from the thyroid tissue and replanted. What is the correct CPT code assignment for the services of the surgeon?

a. 60220-50
b. 60240
c. 60260-50, 60512
d. 60260-RT, 60220-LT, 60512

6.38. A 6-year-old child, an established patient, is seen in the pediatrician's office for routine immunization. The physician speaks with the child's father about national immunization recommendations, and the risks and benefits of vaccine provided, and gives follow-up instructions for possible side-effect treatment. The patient receives a DtaP immunization IM. Assign the appropriate CPT procedure code(s).

a. 90461, 90700
b. 99213, 90460, 90700
c. 90460, 90461, 90700
d. 90460

6.39. A 35-year-old man was referred to the endocrinology clinic for symptoms that involved headaches, deepening voice, and enlargement and coarsening of facial features, hands, and feet. This has been gradual over the past 3 years. The patient was referred by his dentist, who noticed increased spacing between his teeth over the same time period. Growth hormone levels tested by the endocrinology clinic were elevated for an adult male. Follow-up IGF-1 tests confirmed the diagnosis. The patient was scheduled for a CT scan of the brain to rule out pituitary tumor. Diagnosis after the second clinic visit was acromegaly and ruled out pituitary adenoma. Give the correct code(s) for the second clinic visit.

ICD-9-CM Code(s):

a. 253.0, 225.0
b. 253.0
c. 227.3
d. 253.0, 227.3

ICD-10-CM Code(s): _____

6.40. The following documentation is from the health record of a 54-year-old female patient:

CC: Refill of estrogen patch and follow-up.

HPI: Severe hot flashes have been controlled. Energy level is back to a reasonable level.

ROS: All other systems are reviewed and are negative.

She is able to meet her work commitments as a community college instructor.

Exam: Unremarkable.

Assessment: Menopausal symptoms controlled by estrogen patch. Refill for 6 months given. Return PRN.

Which of the following lists the correct codes for this clinic visit?

ICD-9-CM and CPT Code(s):

a. 627.2, V07.4, 99213
b. V07.4, V49.81, 99212
c. 627.2, 99213
d. V07.4, 99212

ICD-10-CM Code(s): _____

6.41.   This 45-year-old female diabetic patient comes in for her quarterly evaluation of her condition. She has type I diabetes, which has been in good control now. She has diabetic nephropathy and retinopathy. What diagnosis codes are assigned?

ICD-9-CM Code(s): _____

ICD-10-CM Code(s): _____

6.42.   From the hospital record of a patient requiring diabetic management:

Hospital Course: This 49-year-old female patient has a history of type I diabetes mellitus and is on 15 units of NPH and 10 of Regular in the morning, and 10 units of NPH and 5 of Regular in the evening. The patient started having symptoms of nausea and vomiting. The patient at the same time had increased frequency of urination and polydipsia. The patient was severely dehydrated on admission. There was no evidence of thrombophlebitis, varicosities, or edema on examination of the extremities. The patient was hydrated and, as a result, her blood sugar decreased from more than 600 to normal levels. The patient was discharged with the diagnosis of diabetic ketoacidosis, dehydration, polydipsia, and increased frequency of urination.

What diagnosis codes would be assigned for this admission for the physician's services?

ICD-9-CM Code(s): _____

ICD-10-CM Code(s): _____

6.43.   Assign the code(s) for a patient with type II diabetic gastroparesis who is presently on insulin.

ICD-9-CM Code(s):

a. 250.60, 536.3, V58.67
b. 250.60, 586.3, 337.1, V58.67
c. 250.61, 536.3
d. 250.62, 536.3, V58.67

ICD-10-CM Code(s): _____

6.44.   A 65-year-old female patient has a long history of type II diabetes mellitus with diabetic retinopathy. She is being seen today for her retinal ischemia and diabetic macular edema. What codes are assigned for this proliferative retinopathy?

ICD-9-CM Code(s):

a. 250.50, 362.07
b. 250.50, 362.06, 362.07
c. 250.50, 362.02, 362.07
d. 362.02, 363.07

ICD-10-CM Code(s): _____

Disorders of the Genitourinary System

6.45. **Procedure:** Transrectal prostatic biopsy under ultrasound guidance

Preoperative Diagnosis: Nocturia and hesitancy

Postoperative Diagnosis: Prostatic calcifications, BPH

History: Elevated PSA of 11.8. Digital rectal examination revealed a nodular prostate gland. Patient complains of frequent need to urinate during the night and hesitancy when urinating.

Procedure: The patient was placed in the left lateral position and endorectal scanning of the prostate gland was carried out utilizing the Toshiba Just Vision 400 ultrasound. Both axial and sagittal scanning probes were utilized.

The prostate gland was enlarged in size and shape with a gland volume of 112.5 cc. The seminal vesicles appeared symmetrical. The capsule was smooth and intact. There were no hypoechoic areas noted but nodules were seen throughout the entire left peripheral zone.

The Bard biopsy guide was then attached to the sagittal scanning probe. Biopsies were obtained utilizing a prostatic block through the left and right sides of the prostate gland including the apical, mid, and basilar portion of the peripheral as well as the lateral base and lateral apex for a total of 10 biopsies.

What codes are used to report this ambulatory surgery?

ICD-9-CM and CPT Code(s): _____

ICD-10-CM Code(s): _____

6.46. A patient in end-stage renal failure requires outpatient hemodialysis 3 times a week while awaiting kidney transplant. He has an A-V fistula in his left arm for vascular access. Which of the following code combinations is appropriate for reporting physician services for this 55-year-old male for the month of August?

ICD-9-CM and CPT Code(s):

a. 585.6, 90970
b. V56.0, 90960
c. 585.6, V56.8, 90999
d. 585.6, 90960

ICD-10-CM Code(s): _____

6.47. From the health record of a patient receiving endoscopy services:

The patient presents to the hospital outpatient department for follow-up cystoscopy for a history of high-grade bladder cancer. This was resected 7 years ago and was found to be grade III with superficial muscle invasion. A cycle of chemotherapy was provided, but no radiation. No recurrence has been noted since then. CT scan of the pelvis 6 months ago was negative for masses. Sometimes the patient experiences painful ejaculation, but no hematospermia has been found. Cytology to date has been negative, so a biopsy will not be performed because there has been 7 years without recurrence.

Cystoscopy examination today shows a normal anterior urethra and prostatic urethra. There is some lateral lobe prostatic hypertrophy, just barely touching in the midline. The bladder is nontrabeculated. There are no tumors, stones, or carcinoma in situ evident on examination. There is clear efflux from each orifice. The area of resection was around the right ureteral orifice, which appears a little atrophic, but patent.

Impression: Stable transitional cell of the bladder without recurrence with mild benign prostatic hypertrophy.

Which of the following code sets is appropriate for this case?

ICD-9-CM and CPT Code(s):

a. V67.6, V10.51, 600.00, 52000
b. 188.9, 600.0, 52000
c. 600.00, V10.51, 52010
d. V67.00, 188.9, 52000

ICD-10-CM Code(s): _____

6.48. The following documentation is from the health record of a 42-year-old female patient:

Preoperative Diagnosis:	Menometrorrhagia and endometrial polyp
Postoperative Diagnosis:	Same
Operation:	Diagnostic hysteroscopy Endometrial ablation Fractional dilatation and curettage
Specimens:	Endometrial curettings

Operative Findings: The uterus sounded to a depth of 8.5 cm. The cervical length was 4 cm and the cavity depth was 4.5 cm. Cavity width was 4 cm and the treatment cycle was 80 seconds. The power setting was 99.

Description of Procedure: The patient was brought to the operating room suite and general anesthesia was administered. The patient is placed in the dorsal-lithotomy position and her vagina and perineum were sterilely prepped and draped in the usual fashion.

The bladder was decompressed with an in-and-out catheter. The weighted speculum was placed into the vagina after bimanual pelvic examination had been performed revealing a midline positioned uterus. The anterior lip of the cervix was grasped with a single-tooth tenaculum. The uterus was sounded to a depth of 8.5 cm; however the internal cervical os could not be palpated with the uterine sound. Sure sound was therefore used to find a cervical length of 4 cm and a cavity length of 4.5 cm. This being accomplished, the diagnostic hysteroscopy was performed. Both tubal ostia were visualized. There was no evidence of intracavitary defect. Endometrial tissue was visible including polyps. Glycine was used as the distending media. The hysteroscope was withdrawn. The cervix was dilated to allow the admission of a #4 sharp curette. Uterine curettage was performed until a good uterine cry was noted. The polyp forceps was used to extract remaining fragments of tissue. The tissue was sent to Pathology for evaluation. Now the NovaSure instrument was placed and the settings accomplished giving a power setting of 99. After cavity assessment was passed, the ablation procedure was initiated. The ablation procedure treatment cycle lasted 80 seconds.

The array was closed, the instrument withdrawn, and then general anesthesia was reversed. The patient was taken to the recovery room in stable and satisfactory condition having tolerated the procedure well. All sponge, instrument, and needle counts were correct. The estimated blood loss was 3 cc.

What CPT code(s) would be assigned in this case?

Code(s): _____

6.49. This 35-year-old female has had 4 cesarean births in the past 6 years and has decided to proceed with sterilization.

Operative Report

Procedure: Laparoscopic tubal ligation with application of -Falope-Rings

Diagnosis: Multiparity; desired sterilization

Anesthesia: General

Under general anesthesia and in the supine lithotomy position, the patient was prepped and draped in the usual sterile fashion. A two-puncture laparoscopy was performed in the usual manner with insufflation through a Verres needle inserted infraumbilically. Through the first puncture, a trocar was inserted infraumbilically, followed by the laparoscope. A second trocar was inserted suprapubically in the midline, followed initially by a probe and then a Falope-Ring applicator. Both tubes were ligated in their midsegment. On the left side, two rings were applied because of the round position of the Falope-Ring director. The right tube was singly ligated. The operation was completed, and the trocar sites were closed with subcuticular sutures of 2-0 VICRYL. The patient was transferred to the recovery room in good condition.

What are the correct codes to assign for this service?

ICD-9-CM and CPT Code(s): _____

ICD-10-CM Code(s): _____

6.50. This 35-year-old man has had an eruption of molluscum contagiosum on the penis for several months. He finally sought medical attention. He was advised to have these lesions removed. He is here now for the procedure. The patient had destruction of a penile molluscum contagiosum performed by cryosurgery and laser surgery. What are the correct code(s)?

ICD-9-CM and CPT Code(s): _____

ICD-10-CM Code(s): _____

6.51.   This 60-year-old patient is admitted and taken to surgery for a laparoscopic radical nephrectomy with adrenalectomy. Surrounding lymph nodes are also removed. What is the correct CPT procedure coding for these procedures?

    a. 50545
    b. 50545, 60650
    c. 50548, 38570
    d. 50548, 60650, 38589

Infectious Diseases

6.52.   The patient is a 10-year-old girl who presents with a sore throat, fever of 101.4, swollen glands in the neck, and a red blotchy rash over the neck, face, chest, and back. She has significant nausea and has vomited 3 times since this morning and is complaining of severe pain when swallowing. A detailed history and examination are documented, with medical decision making of moderate complexity. The physician ordered a rapid strep test, which was performed in the office and was positive. Because of the significant nausea and questionable antibiotic compliance in the past, the physician administers 1.2 million units of Bicillin L-A (long-acting Penicillin G) via a deep intramuscular injection. The patient will be seen again in 5 days. Diagnoses were documented as strep throat with scarlatina.

Assign the codes, including E/M codes and laboratory codes, for this case.

ICD-9-CM, CPT, and HCPCS Code(s): _____

ICD-10-CM Code(s): _____

6.53.   The employees of this clinic who work in the patient care areas are receiving the vaccination for hepatitis B in the employee health clinic. What codes would be reported for this service given as an IM injection?

ICD-9-CM and CPT Code(s): _____

ICD-10-CM Code(s): _____

6.54.   This 5-year-old patient of ours is here in the office for her routine annual child exam. She has been healthy, but reports that she is challenged in K-4 to concentrate and pay attention. Mother would like to schedule an evaluation for possible attention deficit disorder. Active immunization with live measles, mumps, and rubella virus vaccine was given during her annual preventive medicine visit for this established patient. The physician requests a consultation with a psychologist for concentration deficit; they rule out attention deficit disorder.

What are the correct codes?

ICD-9-CM and CPT Code(s): _____

ICD-10-CM Code(s): _____

Disorders of the Skin and Subcutaneous Tissue

6.55. An elderly patient has an abscess formation around a pacemaker pocket on his chest wall that requires that the device be removed and the pocket reformed in another location. Which of the following code sets is appropriate for this outpatient surgical service? Do not assign E codes in this case.

ICD-9-CM and CPT Code(s):

a. 996.61, 682.2, 33222
b. 682.2, 33222
c. 996.61, 33233
d. 996.72, 682.2, 33999

ICD-10-CM Code(s): _____

6.56. This 18-year-old male patient has pustular acne that requires periodic opening and/or removal of milia and comedones from his face in the dermatology clinic on a recurring basis. These visits do not include medical history or examination by the physician—only the procedure.

Assign the correct codes for this encounter.

ICD-9-CM and CPT Code(s): _____

ICD-10-CM Code(s): _____

6.57. This 54-year-old female has noticed areas of raised skin on her face, mostly on her forehead. She states that they have grown quickly with the size almost doubling in 3 weeks. She has concerns that this may be skin cancer and wants an evaluation. She is scheduled for surgery, and the physician abraded 6 areas on the patient's face. They were determined to be keratoses. What codes would be assigned for the surgery episode of care?

ICD-9-CM and CPT Code(s): _____

ICD-10-CM Code(s): _____

6.58. A patient with significant second- and third-degree burns over his back and buttocks underwent debridement of approximately 175 sq cm of necrotic eschar tissue and application of 325 sq cm of Mediskin as a temporary wound closure. Assign the appropriate CPT code(s).

Code(s): _____

6.59. This patient received 45 sq cm of TranCyte to an ulcer of the lateral left foot. Assign the appropriate CPT procedure code(s).

Code(s): _____

6.60. From the record of a hospital inpatient:

This 49-year-old female is complaining of painful mouth ulcers for the last month. She has previously been treated with acyclovir and penicillin on two occasions. Although she indicates that she feels better, the patient continues to have ulcers with pain. She does deny fever, chills, dysphagia or lymphadenopathy.

Physical Exam: Reveals whitish patches measuring 1 mm × 1 mm on the buccal musoca and the hard palate. They are erythematous and inflamed.

Assessment: Aphthous ulcers and herpangina

Plan: Will start patient on oral clindamycin for buccal cellulitis and Amlexanox 5% as oral paste along with the Xylocaine mouth wash. Patient should follow up with me in 2 weeks.

Assign the correct code(s):

ICD-9-CM: _____

ICD-10-CM: _____

6.61. This is the record from an outpatient encounter.

Chief Complaint: Warts on the sole of the left foot

The 12-year-old patient is seen with complaints of painful warts on the sole of the left foot. He states that the warts first appeared about 3 weeks ago but have become progressively painful. The patient was seen in the office 2 months ago with chronic otitis media and he had no problems at that time with warts.

The physical examination of the bottom of the left foot reveals four separate lesions of the following sizes and locations: 4-mm verruca on the heel of the foot, two 3-mm verruca on the ball of the foot, and a 6-mm verrucous papule near the base of the big toe.

Initial impression: Plantar warts.

After consent from the mother, cryocautery was used to destroy each of the lesions. The patient experienced minor discomfort which abated soon after. The wounds were dressed and the patient was advised to make an appointment for 1 week.

Which codes are used to report this office visit?

ICD-9-CM and CPT Code(s): _____

ICD-10-CM Code(s): _____

Mental and Behavioral Disorders

6.62. A patient in a clinic received individual insight-oriented psychotherapy for more than 25 minutes. The physician also provided E/M services that included a problem-focused history, problem-focused examination, and straightforward level of medical decision making. What CPT code(s) would this physician report?

a. 90805
b. 90804, 99212
c. 90811
d. 90810, 99212

6.63. A young adult, who is self-referred, presents as a new patient in the clinic with complaints of an increasing inability to concentrate and complete tasks. He states that he has always been easily distracted and often leaves tasks uncompleted, but in recent years his restlessness has increased. He is perceived as unreliable at work and is concerned about future job advancements. The physician takes a comprehensive history and exam and performs medical decision making of moderate complexity. The physician's diagnosis is attention deficit disorder, DSM-IV 314.9, and the plan of treatment is to begin Ritalin and to follow up to assess dosage and efficacy. The physician documents that he spent 45 minutes in counseling with the patient.

What are the correct codes to report this encounter?

ICD-9-CM and CPT Code(s):

a. 314.00, 99214
b. 314.00, 99204
c. 314.01, 99204
d. 314.9, 99214

ICD-10-CM Code(s): _____

6.64. This 25-year-old man is seen by the psychiatrist for repeated attempts to stop smoking. An hour-long hypnotherapy session is completed to help eliminate the need for smoking. What CPT code(s) are assigned in this case?

Code(s): _____

6.65. Physician progress note states: This patient is a 75-year-old female who has severe Alzheimer's disease. The patient shows no acute change in mental status from her last visit. She requires continuous care because of her dementia, but the family is insistent on keeping her at home. She has made repeated attempts to leave and has wandered off in the past, hence the need for continuous care. She at times recognizes her daughter, the primary caregiver, but most of the time she is unaware of her identity. What diagnosis codes are reported for this visit?

ICD-9-CM Code(s): _____

ICD-10-CM Code(s): _____

Disorders of the Musculoskeletal System and Connective Tissue

6.66.   A patient had an osteopathic physician as a primary care provider. The patient suffered from sternoclavicular somatic dysfunction. An evaluation was done using a detailed history and an expanded problem-focused examination with low medical decision making. The physician performed osteopathic manipulation to the affected body region. What codes should be assigned to this office visit?

ICD-9-CM and CPT Code(s):

a. 739.7, 99213-25, 98925
b. 739.2, 98925
c. 786.59, 99212-25, 98925
d. 739.8, 99213

ICD-10-CM Code(s): _____

6.67.   From the health record of a young athlete:

Preoperative Diagnosis: Fracture of fibula, left

Postoperative Diagnosis: Left distal fibula fracture

Procedure: Reduction of fibular fracture

Indications and Description: This 14-year-old female gymnast felt pain in her leg after hitting the vault at the gym. She is unable to bear any weight on her left leg.

Physical examination revealed foot and ankle to be normal. The neurovascular status of the foot is normal. The ankle is nontender and not swollen. Findings are confined to the distal fibula, 2 inches proximal to the lateral malleolus. There is point tenderness in this area. An x-ray of the tibia and fibula shows a displaced comminuted fracture of the distal fibula.

The fracture was reduced, and the patient was put in a short leg splint molded for her from fiberglass, with extensive padding placed over the fracture site. Crutches were provided, and she is instructed not to place any weight on the foot. She was given a supply of Tylenol 3 for pain and will follow up at the clinic in 10 days.

Which of the following is the correct code combination assignment?

ICD-9-CM and CPT Code(s):

a. 824.8, E917.0, E849.4, E005.2, E000.9, 27788, Q4046
b. 824.2, E917.0, E849.4, E005.2, E000.9, 27788, 29515–51
c. 823.81, E917.0, E849.4, E005.2, E000.9, 27786, L4350
d. 824.4, E917.0, E849.4, E005.2, E000.9, 27810, 29515–51, L4396

ICD-10-CM Code(s): _____

6.68.   This 16-year-old was tackled during a football game 3 weeks ago and received fracture care with a cast for a displaced, comminuted fracture of the right fibula. He is coming in today for a walking cast, which was applied after a 2-view x-ray in the clinic. This converted an existing cast to one that did not require crutches. What are the codes that will appear on the CMS-1500 form that is sent to the insurance company?

ICD-9-CM and CPT Code(s): _____

ICD-10-CM Code(s): _____

6.69. The physician treats a patient who has osteomyelitis of the scapula following an injury. A piece of dead bone is removed from the body of the scapula.

What CPT code is assigned by the surgeon?

a. 23140
b. 23172
c. 23182
d. 23190

6.70. From the health record of a patient having hand surgery:

Operative Report

Preoperative Diagnosis: Foreign body on the left little finger at the metacarpophalangeal joint is a broken piece of glass.

Postoperative Diagnosis: Same.

Operation: Exploration of the MP joint of the left little finger with excision and removal of foreign body.

Indication of Surgery: The patient was a passenger in a vehicle that was struck by a large rock. The rock from a hillside hit the windshield, breaking the glass. She tried to brace herself with her left hand and sustained a laceration on the dorsum of the metacarpal phalangeal joint of the left little finger. The injury didn't seem significant at the time and she did not even see a physician. The wound subsequently healed, but she started noticing some pain in that region. Over three months later, she accidentally hit the metacarpal phalangeal joint of the left little finger against something and since then she has been complaining of severe pain and numbness. She had an x-ray of her left hand which revealed a foreign body in the metacarpal phalangeal joint of the left little finger. The patient was referred to me. I explained to the patient I need to open up the wound, explore the area, and remove the foreign body. The possible risks, benefits, and possible complications of the procedure were explained.

Technique: The patient was placed on the OR bed assuming the supine position. Blood pressure monitoring and pulse oximetry monitoring were in progress. The left hand and forearm were then prepped and draped. Initially, I tried to palpate the metacarpophalangeal joint until I found the area that had the most tenderness. This area is located at the dorsum of the MP joint of the left little finger proximal to the previously healed scar. This area was then marked out and infiltrated with 1% Carbocaine solution. An oblique incision was then made over the area parallel to the old scar. Incision was deepened and bleeders were fulgurated with high temperature. By careful sharp and blunt dissection, the foreign body was searched for. For a while, I could not find the foreign body. Therefore, the incision was extended distally towards the previous area of the laceration. After searching for some time, it was found that the dorsal digital nerve in this area was intact. It was retracted out of harm's way and the area near the extensor tendon towards the foot of the extensor tendon. The foreign body was wedged in the soft tissue of the joint capsule. It was a piece of broken glass and measures about 2 × 3 × 1 mm. It was completely extracted and removed. The wound was irrigated with a large amount of saline solution. Wound closure was accomplished with 5-0 nylon interrupted mattress sutures. Compression dressing was applied. The patient withstood the procedure well. She was advised to keep the hand elevated and keep it dry and clean. She was advised to use an ice compress and change dressing in 48 hours. The patient was placed on Vicodin 1 tablet q.4h p.r.n. for pain. She was cautioned not to take pain medicine if she was driving. She was instructed to return to my office in six days.

Assign the correct codes for this encounter.

ICD-9-CM and CPT Code(s): _____

ICD-10-CM Code(s): _____

6.71.   When back pain is due to a psychological condition, how is this diagnosis coded?

ICD-9-CM Code(s):

a. 724.5
b. 724.5, 307.89
c. 307.89
d. 307.89, 724.5

ICD-10-CM Code(s): _____

Neoplasms

6.72.   A non-Medicare patient with carcinoma of the oral cavity and lower lip is receiving daily intramuscular injections of interferon alfa-2a (3 million units) in the outpatient cancer center. Which of the following will be reported for this service? The payer does accept HCPCS Level II codes for drugs.

ICD-9-CM Code(s):

a. V58.12, 149.8, 96401, J9213
b. 149.8, 96372, J9213
c. 145.9, 140.9, 96372
d. V58.12, 96549

ICD-10-CM Code(s): _____

6.73.   This 32-year-old female with asthma and known cervical dysplasia is admitted for an endoscopic cervical biopsy with endocervical curettage. The procedure was performed without incident. The pathology report shows carcinoma in situ of the cervix. What diagnosis and CPT procedure codes are assigned?

ICD-9-CM and CPT Code(s): _____

ICD-10-CM Code(s): _____

6.74.   This patient had a history of carcinoma of the colon 5 years ago without reoccurrence or metastasis. After several tests he is admitted now for probable renal cell carcinoma, thought to be a new primary. Laparoscopic partial nephrectomy of the kidney was performed without incident. Frozen-section pathology report reveals a lipoma. What diagnosis and CPT procedure codes are assigned for the procedure performed in the hospital?

ICD-9-CM and CPT Code(s): _____

ICD-10-CM Code(s): _____

6.75. The patient had a 2.0-cm lesion removed from the neck, including 0.2-cm margins. The frozen section returned with a diagnosis of Merkel Cell tumor and clear margins.

What are the appropriate diagnosis and CPT procedure codes for this service?

ICD-9-CM and CPT Code(s):

a. 173.49, 11622
b. 209.32, 11623
c. 209.36, 11422
d. 216.4, 11423

ICD-10-CM Code(s): _____

6.76. This 42-year-old female patient has known ovarian carcinoma, and she is being admitted for right oophorectomy. Patient has type I diabetes mellitus, and during her stay we had a hard time controlling her blood sugar level. Right oophorectomy with lymph node sampling and peritoneal biopsies was completed to stage the cancer. Diagnosis: Ovarian carcinoma, without metastasis, and diabetes out of control. What are the correct diagnosis and CPT procedure codes for this admission?

ICD-9-CM and CPT Code(s): _____

ICD-10-CM Code(s): _____

Disorders of the Nervous System and Sense Organs

6.77. A patient has right trigeminal neuralgia, and gamma knife stereotactic radiosurgery is be performed. A Leksell stereotactic head frame was placed prior to the procedure, which consisted of a single shot to a total dose of 7,500 cGy delivered to the 50 percent isodose line.

What is the correct CPT code assignment for this service?

a. 61796, 20660
b. 61796, 61800
c. 64600
d. 61796

6.78. The following documentation is from the health record of a surgical patient.

A Medicare beneficiary has a procedure to promote nerve regeneration at a pain management center. The patient is placed in a prone position, and a midline incision overlying the affected vertebrae is made. The fascia is divided and the paravertebral muscles are retracted. The physician places the inductive electrode pads in the epidural space proximal to the damaged spinal segment. The pulse generator is sutured over the muscles, just below the skin, and closed with a layer closure.

What CPT procedure code is reported by the physician?

a. 63655
b. 63685
c. 63650
d. 63688

6.79.   From the health record of a patient having eye surgery:

Operative Report

Preoperative Diagnosis: Mild stage open-angle glaucoma, right eye; diabetes mellitus, type I

Postoperative Diagnosis: Same

Operation: Initial trabeculectomy, right eye

Anesthesia: Local

Procedure: Full-thickness lid speculums were placed. A fornix-based, conjunctival flap was performed in the superior temporal quadrant. An angulated blade breaker was used to make grooves at the site of the future scleral flap at approximately the 10 o'clock position. Next, a three-sided, partial-thickness, scleral flap was created using a #64 Beaver blade. A trabeculectomy was performed using a sharp blade. A peripheral iridectomy was performed. The scleral flap was irrigated and found to be free flowing. The conjunctiva was closed using two 8-0 collagen sutures at the 12 o'clock position and one 8-0 collagen at the nine o'clock position. Decadron 10 mg was injected subconjunctivally in the inferior fornix. Maxitrol ointment, patch, and shield were applied.

What are the correct codes for this procedure performed in the hospital surgery center?

ICD-9-CM and CPT Code(s):

a. 365.9, 365.71, 250.00, 66172–RT
b. 365.11, 365.71, 250.01, 65850
c. 250.51, 365.44, 365.71, 66170–52
d. 365.10, 365.71, 250.01, 66170–RT

ICD-10-CM Code(s): _____

6.80.   From the health record of a patient having office-based surgery:

Operative Report

Preoperative Diagnosis: Bilateral entropion

Postoperative Diagnosis: Bilateral entropion

Operation: Repair of entropion of right eye

Anesthesia: Local

Procedure: The patient was sterilely prepped and draped for ocular solution of 2 percent lidocaine, mixed in equal proportions with 0.75 percent Marcaine with the addition of Wydase, and a modified Van Lint technique was performed on the right eye. Incision was made in the inferior lid margin extended inferiorly. This consisted of a diamond shape, with 6-mm lengthwise incisions interconducted. Hemostasis was obtained using wet-field cautery. The incision was then sutured using a tapered needle. The first suture was placed through the approximate lash line, in addition to one suture through the area of the meibomian gland. Using the tapered needle, the tarsal plate was approximated and reapproximated. The incision was then reapproximated with subcuticular sutures. This was followed by implantation of approximately four interrupted skin sutures using 6-0 nylon.

What are the correct codes for this procedure performed in the hospital surgery center?

ICD-9-CM and CPT Code(s):

a. 374.00, 67921–RT
b. 374.00, 67921–50
c. 374.10, 67921–RT
d. 374.00, 67923

ICD-10-CM Code(s): _____

6.81. This 71-year-old male had a stroke 6 months ago. He is being followed during his therapy for the residuals of his stroke with evaluation of progress. He has right-sided hemiplegia and aphasia (right side is dominant). He also has hypertension and diabetes mellitus, type II. What diagnosis codes are assigned?

ICD-9-CM Code(s): _____

ICD-10-CM Code(s): _____

6.82. The patient presents to the ophthalmologist with a foreign body in the anterior segment of the right eye. The patient is a metalworker in a factory and had just taken off his protective eyewear when his co-worker's grinder malfunctioned. The metal fragment penetrated his eye. The eye was anesthetized and the metal shaving was removed with a magnet. How would this injury be coded (diagnosis codes?) What are the correct external cause and procedure codes?

ICD-9-CM and CPT Code(s): _____

ICD-10-CM Code(s): _____

6.83. **Preoperative Diagnosis:** Chronic otitis media

Postoperative Diagnosis: Same as above

Anesthesia: General

Procedure: Myringotomy, bilateral with insertion of tubes

Technique: The 10-month-old was brought to the operating room where general anesthesia was induced. An operating microscope was used to incise the anterior tympanic membrane of the right ear and suction any purulent effusion. None was noted. A ventilating tube was inserted into the eardrum. The procedure was repeated on the left ear in a mirror fashion. Ear drops were inserted into the auditory canal and the patient was sent to recovery.

Which codes were reported by the physician for this outpatient encounter?

ICD-9-CM and CPT Code(s):

a. 382.9, 69436-50
b. 381.00, 69421-50
c. 382.9, 69433-50
d. 382.9, 69436

ICD-10-CM Code(s): _____

Newborn/Congenital Disorders

6.84.   A neonatologist is treating a spontaneously delivered newborn with respiratory failure and erythroblastosis fetalis due to Rh antibodies. An exchange transfusion is required to stabilize this critically ill baby receiving services in the neonatal intensive care unit. The baby remains on CPAP to assist breathing and prevent further respiratory failure.

Which of the following code sets is reported by the neonatologist for this second day of care following birth?

ICD-9-CM and CPT Code(s):

a. 773.0, 770.84, 99469
b. V30.00, 99468, 36450, 94660
c. V30.00, 773.0, 770.84, 99469, 36450
d. 773.0, 770.84, 99469

ICD-10-CM Code(s): _____

6.85.   A 22-year-old patient presents for a closure of a patent ductus arteriosus. The patient's thorax is opened posteriorly and the vagus nerve is isolated away. The PDA is divided and sutured individually in the aorta and pulmonary artery.

What is the CPT code for this procedure?

a. 33813
b. 33820
c. 33822
d. 33824

6.86.   A newborn is born with a large gastroschisis and is transferred to a specialty hospital. The surgeon repairs the defect on the newborn's first day of life, without the use of a prosthesis.

Which of the following code set combinations is used to report the surgical service?

ICD-9-CM and CPT Code(s):

a. 569.89, 49580
b. 756.73, 49605
c. 569.89, 49600
d. 756.73, 49600

ICD-10-CM Code(s): _____

6.87. A hospital-based pediatric clinic is treating a newborn with talipes equinovarus by manipulation and short leg casting. Which of the following code sets is reported for a visit where the condition is evaluated with a problem-focused history and examination and parents' questions are answered, followed by foot and ankle manipulation and replacement of the plaster cast?

ICD-9-CM and CPT Code(s):

a. 754.69, 29450
b. 736.71, 29405
c. 754.51, 29405
d. 754.51, 99212–25, 29450

ICD-10-CM Code(s): _____

6.88. From the health record of a newborn delivered in a birthing room setting:

This infant was born in the New Beginnings Birthing Center adjacent to Children's Hospital at 10:58 a.m. on September 1. He weighed 8 lb, 5 oz and was 21 inches long with Apgar scores of 9 and 9. Dr. Smith performed a history and examination immediately following the vaginal delivery with no abnormal findings. Parents declined circumcision or administration of hepatitis B. The patient was discharged at 6:30 p.m. with his mother.

Which of the following code sets is appropriate for Dr. Smith's services on September 1?

ICD-9-CM and CPT Code(s):

a. V30.2, 99460, 99238
b. V30.00, 99463
c. V30.2, 99460
d. V30.2, 99463

ICD-10-CM Code(s): _____

Pediatric Conditions

6.89. A 6-month-old infant, born prematurely, presents for his monthly injection for RSV. The nurse documents Synagis 40 mg, IM.

Which of the following CPT/HCPCS code sets is correct for reporting this office visit?

a. 99212, 90378, 96372
b. 90378, 90471

c. 99212, J1459
d. 90378, 96372

6.90. This 5-year-old female patient presents to the office for bilateral ear drainage, fever, and ear pain. The patient is in foster care and brought in by the new foster mother. There is a large perforation in the left eardrum visible. She was given Augmentin twice a day for 7 days and will be seen in follow-up.

Diagnosis: Acute suppurative otitis media. An expanded problem-focused history and examination were performed, with medical decision making of moderate complexity.

What are the correct diagnosis and CPT procedure codes (including E/M) for this case?

ICD-9-CM and CPT Code(s): _____

ICD-10-CM Code(s): _____

6.91. The same patient in item 6.85 is scheduled for tubes now after the acute otitis media has resolved.

Surgery Center Report

Preoperative Diagnosis: Chronic recurrent suppurative otitis media

Postoperative Diagnosis: Same

Operation: Bilateral myringotomy, placement of permanent ventilating tube

Anesthesia: General

Procedure: A standard myringotomy incision was made and a copious amount of serous fluid suctioned from the middle ear cleft. A Goode T-tube was placed without problems. The procedure was then repeated on the left side in the same manner.

What are the diagnosis and procedure codes (including E/M) reported by the surgeon for this procedure? The procedure was performed in the hospital same-day surgery center.

ICD-9-CM and CPT Code(s): _____

ICD-10-CM Code(s): _____

6.92. This 7-year-old child with an acute attack of his childhood asthma is taken to ER. Spirometry, both pre- and post-bronchodilator, reveal continued bronchospasm with intractable wheezing. An expanded problem-focused history and examination were performed with moderate medical decision making. He is subsequently admitted to the hospital. What diagnosis and procedure codes (including E/M) are assigned by the ER physician?

ICD-9-CM Code(s): _____

ICD-10-CM Code(s): _____

CPT Code(s): _____

Conditions of Pregnancy, Childbirth, and the Puerperium

6.93. This 29-year-old female has had 2 spontaneous abortions because of incompetent cervix. Because of this, she had a cervical cerclage placed in the third month of this pregnancy. She is coming in now to have the cerclage removed under general anesthesia. She was taken to surgery, and the cerclage was removed without complication. She was discharged that evening. There are no signs of labor, and the membranes are intact. She was instructed on the signs of labor and will see me in the office in 2 days. Estimated due date is in 2 weeks, but labor could begin at any time.

What are the correct code assignments for this case?

ICD-9-CM and CPT Code(s):

a. 654.53, 59871
b. 654.53 (The cerclage removal is part of the global package.)
c. 622.5, with appropriate E/M procedure
d. 622.5, 59871

ICD-10-CM Code(s): _____

6.94. The following documentation is from the health record of a 24-year-old female patient.

Preoperative Diagnoses:	1. Term intrauterine pregnancy at 39 3/7 weeks
	2. Polyhydramnios
	3. Failure to progress
Postoperative Diagnoses:	1. Term intrauterine pregnancy at 39 3/7 weeks
	2. Viable male infant. Apgars: 8/9 at one and five minutes respectively. Birth weight 7 lbs, 10 oz.
Operation:	Primary cesarean section with low-transverse uterine incision
Anesthesia:	Spinal
Estimated Blood Loss:	500 cc.
Complications:	None

Description of Procedure: The patient was brought to the surgical delivery room suite and anesthesia was administered. The patient was placed in a supine position with left lateral uterine displacement. The abdomen was sterilely prepped and draped in the normal fashion for cesarean section.

After ascertaining the adequacy of the anesthetic level with an Allis test, a Pfannenstiel incision was made approximately three finger breaths above the pubic symphysis and carried down to the level of the fascia. The fascia was dissected off in the midline, and the peritoneum was carefully entered. The bladder was retracted inferiorly with a DeLee retractor and then a bladder flap was created. The DeLee retractor was repositioned to further retract the bladder inferiorly.

A transverse curvilinear incision was made in the lower uterine segment and extended upward and laterally using blunt dissection. Fetal membranes were ruptured and a viable male infant was delivered from a vertex presentation in an atraumatic fashion. The oropharynx and nares were suctioned on the operative field. The umbilical cord was doubly clamped and cut. The infant was handed off to the awaiting pediatric personnel.

Cord blood was obtained after a segment of cord was clamped and saved for cord blood gases pending Apgars. The placenta was delivered by manual extraction. The uterus was explored to remove any remaining fragments of membranes. The uterus was exteriorized. The uterine incision was reapproximated using No. 1 chromic suture in a running and locking fashion. A second layer of No.1 chromic suture was placed in a Lembert fashion to imbricate the first layer, creating a double layer closure. The uterine incision was inspected and hemostasis confirmed.

The uterus was returned to the abdominal cavity. The uterine incision was inspected once again for hemostasis. All blood and clots were cleared from the lateral gutters and then a final inspection confirmed hemostasis of the uterine incision. The rectus muscles were brought together with three simple interrupted 2-0 Vicryl sutures. Hemostasis was confirmed at the level of the rectus muscles and then the fasciad was reapproximated using two separate 0-Vicryl sutures in a running fashion. The subcutaneous tissues were irrigated and the skin was reapproximated with surgical steel staples. A sterile dressing was applied. The patient was taken to the recovery room in stable and satisfactory condition having tolerated the procedure well.

What is the correct CPT code assignment for this service?

Code(s): _____

6.95.   This 26-year-old G1P1 female at 12 weeks gestation, has been spotting and on bed rest. She awoke this morning with severe cramping and bleeding and her husband brought her to the hospital. After examination, it was determined that she has had an incomplete early spontaneous abortion. She was taken to surgery, and a dilation and curettage was performed. There were no complications from the procedure. She is to follow up with me in the office. She has had 4 antepartum visits during her pregnancy.

What is the correct code assignment?

ICD-9-CM and CPT Code(s):

a. 637.91, 59812
b. 634.91, 59812, 59425
c. 634.91, 58120
d. 634.92, 58120, 59425

ICD-10-CM Code(s): _____

6.96.   This 30-year-old female comes to the clinic because of excessive vomiting for the last 3 days. She is estimated to be in her 24th week and has had no problems with vomiting in her early pregnancy. What is the correct diagnostic code assignment for this case?

ICD-9-CM Code(s): _____

ICD-10-CM Code(s): _____

6.97. This 29-year-old female is admitted to the hospital with pneumonia due to *Pneumocystis carinii*. She is in her 30th week of pregnancy and has AIDS. What diagnosis codes are assigned?

ICD-9-CM Code(s): _____

ICD-10-CM Code(s): _____

6.98. **Procedure:** McDonald's cerclage placement

Postoperative Diagnosis: Intrauterine pregnancy at 14 weeks; patient has a history of cervical incompetence

Anesthesia: Epidural

History: The patient is a 31-year-old gravida 4, para 2. A positive HCG was noted approximately six weeks ago. Ultrasound reveals an intrauterine pregnancy in the second semester. Her previous pregnancies were brought to term using cerclage.

Findings: Preoperatively the internal os was approximately 1.2 cm dilated. The posterior cervix was approximately 2 cm long and the interior cervix was approximately 1.1 cm long.

The patient was placed in the dorsal lithotomy position and prepped and draped for cerclage. A Mersilene band was used with one needle placed in at the 6 o'clock position and brought out at the 3 o'clock position and replaced at the same position and brought out at the 12 o'clock position. A second needle was taken in at 3 o'clock and brought out at 9 o'clock and then replaced and brought out in the 12 o'clock position.

The Mersilene band was then tied at the 12 o'clock position and the internal os was closed. At the end of the procedure the knot could be felt at the appropriate position and the internal os was closed to digital examination.

The procedure was without complications, and the patient was taken to the PACU in good condition.

What codes are used to report this outpatient encounter?

ICD-9-CM and CPT Code(s): _____

ICD-10-CM Code(s): _____

6.99. **History of Present Illness:** This is a 31-year-old, G4P0 who presents today for follow-up of a suspected spontaneous abortion. She had a history of having had elective abortions at ages 17 and 19. At age 27 she experienced a spontaneous abortion and became pregnant again approximately 9 weeks ago. She presents today after experiencing blood loss, cramping, and pain during the early hours of the morning.

Physical Examination: Abdomen is soft and non-tender but vaginal vault does show remnants of bloody discharge. Ultrasound showed no fetal heart tones or movement. A dilation and curettage is performed to treat this incomplete spontaneous abortion. The diagnosis and procedure codes for this encounter would include:

ICD-9-CM and CPT Code(s):

a. 634.91, 59820
b. 634.92, 59820
c. 634.81, 59812
d. 634.91, 59812

ICD-10-CM Code(s): _____

Disorders of the Respiratory System

6.100. A patient is respirator-dependent and has a tracheostomy in need of revision due to redundant scar tissue formation surrounding the site. Under general anesthesia and after establishing the airway to maintain ventilation, the scar tissue is resected and then repair is accomplished using skin flap rotation from the adjacent tissue of the neck. What codes will be used to report this procedure performed in the hospital short-stay surgery area?

ICD-9-CM and CPT Code(s):

a. 519.00, V46.11, 31614
b. V55.0, V46.11, 31614
c. V55.0, 31610
d. 519.00, 31613

ICD-10-CM Code(s): _____

6.101. This 60-year-old patient was admitted with emphysematous nodules. A thoracoscopic wedge resection was performed in the left lung to remove the lung nodules. A resection was done in the upper and lower lobes. Which of the following answers is correct?

ICD-9-CM and CPT Code(s):

a. 518.89, 32666, 32667
b. 492.8, 32666
c. 518.89, 32505
d. 492.8, 32666, 32667

ICD-10-CM Code(s): _____

6.102. From the health record of a patient newly diagnosed with a malignancy:

Preoperative Diagnosis: Suspicious lesions, main bronchus

Postoperative Diagnosis: Carcinoma, in situ, main bronchus

Indications: Previous bronchoscopy showed two suspicious lesions in the main bronchus. Laser photoresection is planned for destruction of these lesions because bronchial washings obtained previously showed carcinoma in situ.

Procedure: Following general anesthesia in the hospital same-day surgery area, with a high-frequency jet ventilator, a rigid bronchoscope is inserted and advanced through the larynx to the main bronchus. The areas were treated with laser photoresection.

Which codes are reported for this service?

ICD-9-CM and CPT Code(s):

a. 231.2, 31641
b. 162.2, 31641, 31623–59
c. 231.2, 31641, 31623–59
d. 162.2, 31641

ICD-10-CM Code(s): _____

6.103. This 80-year-old male presented to the ER with acute pulmonary edema after experiencing a 3-day history of increasing shortness of breath and cough. He was admitted to the critical care unit with a diagnosis of congestive heart failure and treated with Procardia, Nitro Paste, and Lasix with resolution of his respiratory distress.

The patient responded to treatment with increasing nitroglycerin and Lasix. The patient was also given intravenous fluids and low-dose dopamine to maintain an adequate wedge pressure and cardiac output.

Final Diagnosis: Acute pulmonary edema with congestive heart failure.

What diagnosis code(s) are reported?

ICD-9-CM Code(s): _____

ICD-10-CM Code(s): _____

6.104. This 82-year-old nursing home patient presents with aspiration pneumonia. The patient aspirated food particles. Treatment included clindamycin 600 mg IV q 6 hours. He also has superimposed staphylococcal pneumonia. The condition resolved with treatment, and patient transferred back to the nursing home. What is the correct diagnosis code assignment?

ICD-9-CM Code(s): _____

ICD-10-CM Code(s): _____

6.105. Under conscious sedation, administered by the surgeon, the patient underwent a bronchoscopy with biopsy of the walls of the left upper lobe bronchus and left mainstem bronchus, dilation of the left mainstem bronchus, and placement of a bronchial stent in the left mainstem bronchus. Assign the appropriate CPT codes.

a. 31622, 31625, 31636, 99144
b. 31628, 31632, 31636
c. 31625, 31636
d. 31625, 31636, 99144

6.106. **Procedure:** Direct microlaryngoscopy using general anesthesia

Diagnosis: Dysphonia

Technique: This 22-year-old patient was taken to the outpatient surgical suite where general anesthesia was administered. A Jako laryngoscope was inserted with an operating microscope to perform a laryngoscopy. The vocal cords were examined and no evidence of abnormality was discovered. They were within normal limits. The entire endolarynx was also well visualized and showed no evidence of subglottic stenosis. No other abnormalities were noted. The procedure was terminated and the patient sent to PACU in good condition.

What codes are used to report this outpatient encounter?

ICD-9-CM and CPT Code(s): _____

ICD-10-CM Code(s): _____

6.107. After an injury to the chest, this patient requires a thoracentesis using a water seal for accumulated air in the pleural cavity. What is the correct procedure code assignment for this case?

    a. 32420
    b. 32421
    c. 32422
    d. 32960

Trauma and Poisoning

6.108. Assign the correct diagnosis codes for a 29-year-old patient with deep third-degree burns of the chest and right leg. He was the victim of a house fire in a single family home. He has third-degree burns over 25 percent of his body.

ICD-9-CM Code(s): _____

ICD-10-CM Code(s): _____

6.109. The patient in question 6.102 was treated with skin grafting over a period of time until his burns healed. Six months later, he is being seen with severe scarring due to third-degree burns of his right leg and chest received in a house fire, in a single family home. What diagnosis codes are assigned for this case?

ICD-9-CM Code(s): _____

ICD-10-CM Code(s): _____

6.110. This 79-year-old patient had a gastrostomy performed because of dysphagia due to a stroke. He has been doing fairly well but is now admitted with extensive cellulitis of the abdominal wall. Examination reveals that the existing gastrostomy site is infected. The physician confirms that the responsible organism is *Staphylococcus aureus*. What diagnosis codes are assigned?

ICD-9-CM Code(s): _____

ICD-10-CM Code(s): _____

6.111. What is the correct CPT code assignment for a 36-square-centimeter adjacent tissue transfer performed on the hip to cover a large open wound?

CPT Code(s): _____

6.112. What diagnosis codes are reported for an encounter where the patient is seen for a crushing injury of the left toes, foot, and ankle? He was crushed in a metal rolling mill machine at work.

ICD-9-CM Code(s): _____

ICD-10-CM Code(s): _____

Part III
Advanced Coding Exercises

Chapter 7

Case Studies from Inpatient Health Records

Note: Even though the specific cases are divided by setting, most of the information pertaining to the diagnosis is applicable to most settings. If you practice or apply codes in a particular type of setting, you may find additional information in other sections of this publication that may be pertinent to you.

Every effort has been made to follow current recognized coding guidelines and principles, as well as nationally recognized reporting guidelines. The material presented may differ from some health plan requirements for reporting. The ICD-9-CM codes used are effective October 1, 2012, through September 30, 2013. The current standard transactions and code sets named in HIPAA have been utilized, which require ICD-9-CM Volume III procedure codes for inpatients. The 2013 draft editions of ICD-10-CM and ICD-10-PCS are utilized in this chapter.

Instructions: Cases are presented as either multiple choice or fill in the blank.

- For multiple-choice cases:
  - Select the letter of the appropriate code set.
- For the fill-in-the-blank cases:
  - Assign the MS-DRG, where indicated.
  - Assign present on admission (POA) indicator for each ICD-9-CM diagnosis code.
    - Y: Yes (POA)
    - N: No (Not POA)
    - U: Unknown (Documentation is insufficient to determine if condition is POA.)
    - W: Clinically undetermined (Provider is unable to clinically determine whether or not the condition was POA.)
    - Leave blank for the exercises in this book all codes that are exempt from POA reporting. See the Exempt List as published in the *ICD-9-CM Official Guidelines for Coding and Reporting*. These codes are exempt because they represent circumstances regarding healthcare encounters or factors influencing health status that do not represent a current disease or injury, or are always present on admission.

ICD-9-CM Coding Instructions:

- Sequence the ICD-9-CM principal diagnosis in the first diagnosis position.
- Assign all reportable secondary diagnosis codes including V codes and E codes (both cause of injury and place of occurrence).
- Sequence the ICD-9-CM principal procedure code in the first procedure position.
- Assign all reportable secondary ICD-9-CM procedure codes.

ICD-10-CM and ICD-10-PCS Coding Instructions:

- Sequence the ICD-10-CM principal diagnosis code in the first diagnosis position.
- Assign all reportable secondary ICD-10-CM codes.
- Sequence the principal ICD-10-PCS code in the first procedure position.
- Assign all reportable secondary ICD-10-PCS codes.

The scenarios are based on selected excerpts from health records. In practice, the coding professional should have access to and refer to the entire health record. Health records are analyzed and codes assigned based on physician documentation. Documentation for coding purposes must be assigned based on medical record documentation. A physician may be queried when documentation is ambiguous, incomplete, or conflicting. The queried documentation must be a permanent part of the medical record.

The objective of the cases and scenarios reproduced in this publication is to provide practice in assigning correct codes, not necessarily to emulate complete coding, which can be achieved only with the complete medical record. For example, the reader may be asked to assign codes based on only an operative report when in real practice, a coder has access to the entire medical record.

The *ICD-9-CM Official Guidelines for Coding and Reporting*, published by the National Center for Health Statistics (NCHS), includes Present on Admission (POA) Reporting Guidelines in Appendix I. These guidelines supplement the official conventions and instructions provided within ICD-9-CM. Adherence to these guidelines when assigning ICD-9-CM diagnosis codes is required under the Health Insurance Portability and Accountability Act (HIPAA) of 1996. Additional official coding guidance can be found in the American Hospital Association (AHA)'s *Coding Clinic for ICD-9-CM* publication.

Disorders of the Blood and Blood-Forming Organs

7.1.   The following documentation is from the health record of an 87-year-old female patient.

Discharge Summary

History of Present Illness: The patient is an 87-year-old female who was admitted from a nursing home with dehydration and pleural effusion, as well as urinary tract infection and thrombocytopenia with petechial hemorrhage. On admission, she was found to have a platelet count of 77,000 and a hematology consultation was done. The patient denied any bleeding diathesis in the past. She stated that she had recent bruising of the hands related to needle sticks but otherwise has not had any past history of any bleeding disorder. She stated she was taking aspirin on a regular basis. No specific history of hematuria, hematemesis, gross rectal bleeding, or black stools.

Past Medical History: Significant for congestive heart failure, diabetes

Medications: Coreg, isosorbide, aspirin, Actos, digoxin, glyburide, hydralazine, furosemide, Ditropan, and potassium

Family History: No family history of any bleeding disorder

Physical Examination: She is an elderly-appearing white female, somewhat short of breath, using supplemental oxygen. Examination of the head and neck revealed no scleral icterus. Throat was clear. Tongue was papillated. There was no thyromegaly or JVD. There was no cervical supraclavicular, axillary, or inguinal adenopathy. Chest examination revealed rales, bilaterally. There were decreased breath sounds at the right base. There were coarse rales heard in the right midlung field. Heart examination showed rhythm was irregularly irregular. Abdomen examination was difficult to perform. I was unable to palpate the liver or spleen. Bowel sounds were active. Extremities revealed no clubbing, cyanosis, or edema. There were diffuse ecchymoses, especially in the dorsum of the right hand.

Laboratory Studies: Hematocrit was 43, white blood cell count 9,000 with 82 percent neutrophils, and the platelet count 77,000. The MCCV was 102. Creatinine was 1.7. Bilirubin was 1.7. The alkaline phosphatase was 122. AST 498, ALT 493, and albumin 3.6. The prothrombin time was 18 seconds and the PTT was 25 seconds. The chest x-ray showed a right pleural effusion.

Course in Hospital: The patient was admitted and started on IV fluids. Her diuretics were increased, and she showed a good response with a resolution of her pleural effusion and better control of her congestive heart failure. Hematology consult recommended holding platelet transfusion unless there was evidence of active bleeding. No platelets were given during this admission.

The patient was discharged back to the nursing home on day 6 in improved condition to continue with the same medication regimen as previous to hospitalization.

Final Diagnoses:
1. Pleural effusion from congestive heart failure
2. Dehydration
3. Primary thrombocytopenia with petechial hemorrhage and hematoma of the eyelids and arms and hands
4. Urinary tract infection
5. Type II diabetes mellitus

Which of the following code sets would be correct for this hospitalization?

a. 428.0, 276.51, 287.30, 599.0, 250.00
b. 428.0, 276.51, 287.5, 599.0, 250.00
c. 428.0, 511.9, 276.51, 287.30, 599.0, 250.00
d. 276.51, 511.9, 428.0, 287.30, 782.7, 599.0, 250.00

ICD-10-CM Code(s): _____

Optional MS-DRG Exercise (for users with access to MS-DRG software or tables)

What is the correct MS-DRG for this case? _____

Which of the following is an incorrect statement regarding the MS-DRG assignment on this case?

a. MS-DRG assignment in this case is based on the principal diagnosis; the secondary codes do not impact the DRG.
b. A principal diagnosis of CHF results in a higher-paying DRG than a principal diagnosis of dehydration.
c. This patient's LOS exceeded the average length of stay for the assigned DRG.
d. All of the above are true.

7.2.   The following documentation is from the health record of a 34-year-old male patient.

Admission Diagnosis: Sickle cell pain crisis.

Discharge Diagnosis: Sickle cell pain crisis/Staph (Staphylococcus) aureus bacteremia.

Secondary Diagnosis: Sickle cell disease, priapism, chronic lower back pain secondary to sickle cell diagnosis, asthma, gastroesophageal reflux disease (GERD), and hemorrhoids.

Consults: None.

Procedures: PICC line placement, bone scan, and transesophageal echocardiogram (heart and aorta).

Hospital Course: The patient is a 34-year-old African-American male with a history of sickle cell disease who presented with back pain and whole body pain, a remote history of some diarrhea and nausea, and some fevers and chills. Blood cultures taken on admission and during his first night as an inpatient grew four out of four bottles of Staph. aureus. The patient received 1 gm of ceftriaxone in the Emergency Department and received approximately six days of vancomycin IV as an inpatient. Thereafter he was switched to Ancef 1 gm IV g.8 hours.

In order to find a source for the patient's Staph. bacteremia, a transesophageal echocardiogram was done which did not show evidence of any cardiac vegetations. A bone scan was also done which did not show any deep-seated abscesses or any evidence of osteomyelitis. In light of the fact that the patient had Staph. bacteremia of unknown source, Infectious Disease was consulted. As per their recommendation, the patient is to be on five weeks of IV Ancef.

At the time of admission, the patient was placed on a PCA pump. He was rapidly weaned off of this and he was also placed on some oxygen and was bolused with fluids and kept on maintenance fluids. The patient's clinical status improved rapidly. He was soon weaned off the oxygen, fluids, and pain medications.

At the time of discharge, the patient is afebrile and stable. A PICC line was placed in order to ensure access for the next five weeks, during which he will receive his IV antibiotics. Home care and home IV teaching was arranged for the patient and his family.

Follow-Up: Hematology was contacted and follow-up will be arranged within the next two weeks. Follow-up will also be arranged with Infectious Disease in five weeks. Home medications include folate 1 mg p.o. q.d.; Flexeril 10 mg p.o. b.i.d.; Ancef 2 gm q.12 IV times five weeks; Phenergan 12.5 mg p.o. q.4 p.r.n. nausea; and Zantac 150 mg p.o. b.i.d. The patient was told to return for fevers, chills, sweats, nausea, vomiting, or bone or muscle pain.

Disposition is to home with home care.

Code Assignment Including POA Indicator

ICD-9-CM Principal Diagnosis: _____

ICD-9-CM Additional Diagnoses: _____

ICD-9-CM Procedure Code(s): _____

Issues To Clarify: _____

ICD-10-CM Code(s): _____

ICD-10-PCS Code(s): _____

7.3. The following documentation is from the inpatient record of a patient with anemia.

Discharge Summary

Date of Admission:	11/19/XX
Date of Discharge:	11/21/XX

Discharge Diagnoses:
1. Anemia in chronic kidney disease.
2. Chronic kidney disease, stage 3.
3. Diabetes mellitus, type 2.
4. Hypertension.
5. Coronary artery disease.
6. Congestive heart failure.
7. Hypokalemia.

Attending Physician for Service:	Family Practice Service.
Consultations:	None.
Procedures:	None.

Hospital Course: The patient is a 66-year-old gentleman with multiple medical problems including coronary artery disease, diabetes mellitus, and chronic kidney disease, who presented to the Emergency Department at Anytown Hospital on 11/19/XX complaining of shortness of breath. He had been seen in the office earlier that week and seemed to be doing reasonably well at that point in time.

On admission he said that over the last two to three days his shortness of breath had been increasing, and he had orthopnea and a nonproductive cough. He denied chest pain at that point in time. He denied other symptomatology.

In the Emergency Department he was noted to have significant anemia with hemoglobin of 7.0 and a hematocrit of 21.2 with an MCV of 78.3. He was given two units of packed red blood cells via peripheral vein and admitted to the Transitional Care Unit to rule out myocardial infarction and to receive blood.

Problems

1. **Anemia.** Initial H&H of 7.0 and 21.2. He received two units of packed red blood cells and at discharge his H&H was 9.1 and 27.0, respectively. His reticulocyte count was pending at discharge. Iron level was 51, total iron binding capacity was 371, and ferritin level was 14. He had been on iron as an outpatient. This was stopped secondary to diarrhea, which he felt was probably from the iron. We will restart this at this time consisting of Niferex one p.o. q day. Follow his H&H as an outpatient. I would consider him for erythropoietin therapy at some point in time.

2. **Cardiac.** History of coronary artery disease and congestive heart failure. No past history of CABG. He had one elevated troponin on day 1 of hospitalization. He had had two normal troponins previous to this and two post this. I am uncertain of the significance of this one elevation of his troponin to 1.6. He had no chest pain throughout. Electrocardiogram showed no changes. He was briefly started

on heparin. This was subsequently discontinued the following day. We will send him home on his regular cardiac regimen consisting of Digoxin, an ACE inhibitor, diuretics consisting of Lasix and Carbatolol. He will also be given p.r.n. nitrates. From a congestive heart failure perspective on admission he was felt to have mild congestive heart failure. He diuresed well, and once he was transfused, his shortness of breath, and orthopnea improved significantly.

3. **Hypokalemia**. The day after admission revealed this and his potassium was replaced. Being we were restarting his Lasix therapy, we will send him home on potassium supplementation as well.

4. **Diabetes mellitus**. Well-controlled. Continue Glucotrol at 5 mg p.o. b.i.d.

5. **Hypertension**. Controlled. Continue Lotensin, Coreg, and will add Lasix as above.

6. **Gastrointestinal**. He had weakly heme-positive stools on admission. He has had this recently and has actually undergone upper and lower endoscopy twice this year already. He has had no complaints of melena or bright red blood. I am wondering if this was not secondary to trauma during the rectal examination. We will continue to follow for now.

Code Assignment Including POA Indicator

ICD-9-CM Principal Diagnosis: _____

ICD-9-CM Additional Diagnoses: _____

ICD-9-CM Principal Procedure: _____

ICD-9-CM Additional Procedures: _____

ICD-10-CM Code(s): _____

ICD-10-PCS Code(s): _____

Disorders of the Cardiovascular System

7.4.   The following documentation is from the health record of a 66-year-old male patient.

Discharge Summary

Admission Date: 6/19/XX

Discharge Date: 6/28/XX

History of Present Illness: This patient is a 66-year-old man admitted on 6/19 because of unstable postinfarct angina. He underwent cardiac bypass surgery here 15 years ago. He did well until 1989, when he developed angina and underwent angioplasty here. On 6/9, he was awakened with severe chest pain and was taken to a nearby community hospital where he was found to have a small anterior wall ST elevation myocardial infarction, with the CPK only slightly elevated.

Because of this small infarction, he was referred here for consideration for further coronary arteriography. He was discharged from the hospital on 6/16. On 6/19, as the patient was walking from the car to the office, he developed quite significant chest pain and was therefore admitted to rule out further infarction.

Hospital Course: He was taken to the cardiac catheterization laboratory the day after admission. At that time, complete left heart catheterization, left ventricular cineangiography, coronary arteriography, and bypass visualization were performed. We found that his left ventricle showed severe anterior hypokinesis, although it did still move. The left main coronary artery was narrowed by about 70 percent.

The bypass to the circumflex looked good, but the bypass to the left anterior descending had a very severe stenosis in the body of the graft. There was a very large, marginal circumflex artery that had an orificial 80 percent stenosis. I felt that he was not a candidate for angioplasty but should have bypass surgery. He was seen in consultation by Dr. Reed, who agreed with this, so he was taken to the operating room on 6/21 for that procedure.

Using extracorporeal circulation, the left internal mammary artery was anastomosed to the left anterior descending coronary artery and a venous graft was placed from the aorta to the marginal circumflex. It was found that the old venous graft to the main circumflex was in excellent condition with very soft, pliable walls, so that vessel was left intact. There were no complications of this surgery.

His postoperative course was singularly uncomplicated. He never had any arrhythmia problems; his wounds healed nicely. He had a tiny left pleural effusion that never needed to be tapped. He was walking about the ward participating in the cardiac rehab program at the time of discharge.

Discharge Instructions: Discharge medications will simply be aspirin grains 5 q. d., Tylenol with Codeine 1 or 2 p.r.n. for pain, Lopressor 50 mg a day, and Colace, as necessary. He was instructed to contact his private physician upon return home for resumption of his medical care. He is to call me here at the medical center if there are any questions or problems that he wishes to discuss.

Discharge Diagnoses:
1. Unstable angina (intermediate coronary syndrome)
2. Recent incomplete anterior wall myocardial infarction
3. Coronary atherosclerosis, three vessel
4. Successful double-bypass surgery

What are the correct codes for this admission?

a. 414.01, 414.05, 410.12, 411.1, V45.82, 36.11, 36.15, 39.61, 37.22, 88.53, 88.57
b. 414.01, 414.05, 410.12, 411.1, V45.81, 36.12, 39.61, 37.22, 88.53, 88.57
c. 414.00, 414.05, 410.11, 411.1, 36.11, 36.15, 39.61, 37.22, 88.53, 88.57
d. 414.01, 414.05, 410.12, 411.1, 412, V45.81, 36.11, 36.15, 39.61, 37.22, 88.53, 88.57

ICD-10-CM Code(s): _____

ICD-10-PCS Code(s): _____

Optional MS-DRG Exercise (for users with access to MS-DRG software or tables)

Indicate the principal diagnosis. _____

Which of the codes affects the MS-DRG assignment on this case?

_____

True or False: For this MS-DRG, the presence of a complication/comorbid condition affects the MS-DRG assignment?

7.5   Discharge Summary

Date of Admission: 4/19

Date of Discharge: 4/24

Discharge Diagnosis: Acute myocardial infarction
Hyperlipidemia
Complete heart block
Upper gastrointestinal hemorrhage
Arteriosclerotic heart disease

Admission History: This is a 45-year-old white male with a history of hyperlipidemia and tobacco use. He presented to the hospital with an acute myocardial infarction. He was treated with intravenous TPA and had a reperfusion. The patient continued to have chest pain with an inferior ST elevation on EKG.

Course in Hospital: The patient sustained an acute myocardial infarction. The patient presented with an acute myocardial infarction and underwent catheterization. The patient was found to have stenosis of the mid right coronary artery and right distal coronary artery. The left coronary branches have minimal noncritical disease. The left ventricular ejection fraction was approximately 45% with inferior wall hypokinesis.

The patient had a successful stent PTCA to the mid-RCA with a stent. I initially attempted to dilate with a balloon, but the results were inadequate and we proceeded to place a 4.0-mm J&J stent. The patient continued to have anginal symptomatology and for this reason was taken to the OR for CABG × 2. He did well after the CABG × 2 without any anginal symptoms.

The patient also had gastrointestinal bleeding following the PTCA. The patient developed retching and hematemesis and anemia for which he required blood transfusion. The probable cause of the nausea and vomiting was a reaction to anesthesia. Upper endoscopy revealed no evidence of peptic ulcer disease.

At the present time the patient has been treated with aspirin and Ticlid and has been doing very well. The plan is to discharge him home with follow-up in my office next week.

Instructions on Discharge: Follow up in 1 week in my office. Medications include: aspirin 1 tablet per day, Ticlid 250 mg twice per day, Tagamet 400 mg twice per day, and sublingual nitroglycerin as needed for chest pain. Condition upon discharge is stable. Activity is restricted until cardiac rehabilitation.

History and Physical

Admitted: 4/19

Acute myocardial infarction

Complete heart block

Ventricular ectopy

Possible ASHD

Reason for Admission: Pain in chest

History of Present Illness: This is a pleasant 45-year-old male with a history of hyperlipidemia and previous tobacco use. He also has a family history of coronary artery disease. He denies any prior history of coronary artery disease, myocardial infarction, or CVAs. The patient has been essentially very healthy, except for occasional skipped heartbeat in the past for which he has never taken any medications. The patient is presently on no medications.

Two days ago, he started complaining of a dull chest ache that appeared to radiate to his left arm and lasted for a few minutes. He was brought to the emergency department and was noted to have an acute inferior myocardial infarction with complete heart block. I was consulted to evaluate the patient and proceeded with administration of TPA therapy and IV Atropine for complete heart block. At the present time the patient is in sinus rhythm and is presently receiving IV TPA. He denies any melena, hematochezia. Denies any shortness of breath, PND, orthopnea.

Past Medical History: He denies any history of hypertension or diabetes. He has a history of high cholesterol. He states that he had his cholesterol checked approximately 3 months ago and it was around 310. He used to smoke tobacco, one pack a day for 20 years. He quit smoking 6 months ago. He denies any history of coronary artery disease, myocardial infarction, or cerebrovascular accident.

He has a history of heart palpitations that he describes as skipped heartbeat in the past for which he is not taking any medications. He has never had an evaluation.

He has a history of kidney stones two years ago. He denies any history of peptic ulcer disease. He has a history of hemorrhoidal bleeding in the past. The last episode of bleeding was 6 or 7 months ago.

The patient denies any trauma or recent surgery.

Allergies: Patient has no known drug allergies

Chronic Medications: None

Social History: He quit tobacco 6 months ago and denies alcohol abuse. He is a construction worker.

Review of Systems: Denies melena, hematochezia, hematemesis, and he denies change in weight

Physical Examination: This is a pleasant gentleman who appears slightly diaphoretic and is expressing having mild chest pain which is better from admission. He is presently receiving IV TPA. Vital signs are as follows: Blood pressure is 100/70; heart rate in the 80s. The neck shows no JVD, no carotid bruits. The lungs are clear and heart is regular rate with S4 gallop rhythm and no murmurs. The abdomen is soft and nontender. Extremities show no edema. The pulses of his femoral and dorsalis pedis are 2+ bilaterally. Neurological examination reveals an alert and oriented male × 3.

Laboratory Data: SMA-7, sodium 138, potassium 3.7, BUN 7, creatinine 0.9. CBC showed a white blood cell count of 12. Hematocrit 37, hemoglobin 13. Platelet count is 312. His EKG showed complete heart block with significant ST elevation in the inferior leads with reciprocal changes in the anteroseptal leads, consistent with an acute inferior wall myocardial infarction. His chest x-ray is pending.

Impression and Plan: Acute myocardial infarction that appears to have started around 10:30 in the morning. He presented very early to the emergency department and was treated aggressively with intravenous TPA, intravenous aspirin, intravenous nitroglycerin.

We will continue the TPA and begin lidocaine. We will obtain cardiac enzymes and admit to CCU. The patient will need cardiac catheterization evaluated within 48 hours. If symptoms recur or patient does not have evidence of reperfusion, will need urgent cardiac catheterization. If heart block occurs, will treat with intravenous Atropine on a p.r.n. basis. We will check a cholesterol and lipid profile in the hospital.

Consultation

Date: 4/20

Chief Complaint: Vomiting blood

Review of Systems: This 45-year-old white male was seen in consultation because of GI bleeding. The patient was admitted 1 day ago with acute myocardial infarction. He was treated with TPA and later went to cardiac catheterization where he was found to have a lesion of the mid RCA and distal RCA. Today the patient exhibited hematemesis with retching. He has no past history of ulcer disease or GI bleeding.

Physical Examination: Physical examination reveals an adult male lying in bed. Blood pressure is 120/80, pulse 60. HEENT: Pale. Lungs: Clear. Heart: Regular rate and rhythm. Abdomen: Benign.

Laboratory: WBC is 12, hemoglobin 12, and hematocrit 37

Impression: Upper GI bleeding; rule out ulcer disease

Recommendation: We will perform an upper endoscopy to be performed today after informed consent is obtained. Further recommendations are to follow.

Progress Notes

4/19   This is a 45-year-old white male with a history of increased cholesterol, no prior coronary artery disease, MI, or CVA. He presented with acute ischemia and heart block. He was given IV TPA; 1–1 1/2 hours after TPA he had severe chest pain with elevated ST inferior leads. He was treated emergently for urgent catheter and PTCA.

Post Catheter/Stent

Procedure: Left heart catheter, coronary angio, left ventricular angiography

Results: Normal LCA, 99% mid-RCA and 70 stenosis distal RCA, successful stent PTCA to mid RCA with excellent results

4/20   **Cardiac:** Patient continues to have pain. Will prepare for CABG when patient stable from GI perspective.

GI: The patient experienced vomiting with flecks of blood after the cardiac catheterization. In light of apparent acute blood loss anemia, will check for peptic ulcer. Probable reaction to anesthetics.

Endoscopy Note:

Preop: Gastrointestinal bleeding

Postop: Gastrointestinal bleeding, etiology unknown

Procedure: EGD

Complications: None

4/21   Patient is scheduled for the OR today. Bleeding stable.

OP Note:

Preop: Critical stenosis of the mid-RCA and distal RCA

Postop: Same

Operation: CABG × 2

Complications: None

4/22   Patient recovering well. No chest pain or shortness of breath. The wound looks good. Will monitor blood loss anemia. The patient declines blood transfusion.

4/23   Chest clear, no chest pain, abdomen is soft with bowel sounds. Will transfer to the floor.

4/24   Wound healing well, patient OOB ambulating, no chest pain, lungs clear.

4/25   Will discharge today. Patient to follow up in 1 week.

Operative Report

Date: 4/21

Preoperative Diagnosis: Critical stenosis of mid right coronary artery and distal right coronary artery

Postoperative Diagnosis: Same

Operation: Coronary bypass × 2 using saphenous vein from aorta to right mid coronary artery and distal right coronary artery

Anesthesia: General

Under general anesthesia with arterial and pulmonary artery monitoring with sterile prep and drape, a sterile midline sternotomy was performed. The pericardium was opened. Purse-string sutures were placed in the ascending aorta and the right atrium. Extracorporeal circulation was undertaken at this point. The greater saphenous vein was harvested from the right leg endoscopically. The patient was then placed on cardiopulmonary bypass. Cardioplegia was affected. The right coronary artery was dissected. Using a 6-0 Prolene suture an end-to-side anastomosis was created between the right mid coronary artery and the aorta. A second opening for end-to-side anastomosis was performed from the aorta to the distal right coronary artery. Following spontaneous contraction of the heart, the patient was removed from cardiopulmonary bypass. Approximating the pericardium then began closure. Hemostasis was obtained. The sternum was approximated with a parasternal wire and fascia and skin with vicryl. The patient tolerated the procedure well and was transferred to the recovery room in stable condition.

Endoscopy Report

Date: 4/20

Pre-gastrointestinal bleeding; rule out ulcers

Post-upper gastrointestinal bleeding; stomach and duodenum appear unremarkable

Meds: Demerol 50 mg IV
Versed 3 mg IV

Procedure: Esophagogastroduodenoscopy

The patient was sedated and the scope inserted into the hypopharynx. There was fresh blood oozing from an area in the hiatal hernia pouch just below the gastroesophageal junction. The scope was passed further down to visualize the remainder of the stomach and the duodenum. All areas appeared unremarkable with no other ulcers or lesions identified. The patient tolerated the procedure well. He did have some retching and vomiting after the scope was removed.

Cardiac Catheterization Report

Date: 4/19

Procedure: Left heart catheterization

Left ventricular angiography using low osmolar contrast

Coronary angiography using low osmolar contrast

PTCA with stent to mid right coronary artery

After obtaining informed consent the patient was taken to the cardiac catheterization laboratory. He was prepped and draped in the usual fashion and 2% Xylocaine was used to anesthetize the right groin. 6-French sheaths were introduced into the right femoral artery and vein, and a 6-French multipurpose catheter was used for left heart catheterization, coronary angiography, and left ventricular angiography. I then proceeded to perform a stent/PTCA to the mid RCA. An HTF wire was used to cross the RCA stenosis and a 4.0-mm J&J stent was placed in the mid right coronary artery with excellent results. The final angiogram was obtained and the guiding catheterization was removed. The sheaths were securely sutured and the patient tolerated the procedure well without complications.

Findings

1. Left heart catheterization revealed an elevated resting left ventricular end-diastolic pressure of 18 mm Hg.

2. Left ventricular angiography revealed mild to moderate inferior wall hypokinesis with overall mildly depressed left ventricular systolic function and an estimated global ejection fraction of 45%.

3. Coronary angiography (using single catheter): The left coronary artery arises normally from the left sinus of Valsalva. The left main artery, left anterior descending coronary artery and its branches, and the circumflex artery and its branches have minimal irregularities.

   The right coronary artery arises normally from the right sinus of Valsalva. There is a 99% very eccentric stenosis in the large mid right coronary artery and a 70% stenosis of the distal right coronary artery.

Impression: Arteriosclerotic coronary artery disease was found. There was a successful implantation of 4.0-mm J&J stent in the mid right coronary artery. This site was predilated with a 4.0-mm balloon, and then followed by the insertion of a stent.

The mid right coronary artery shows excellent results. Pending the patient's progress we may have to proceed with CABG. The patient will remain on aspirin, Coumadin, and nitrates in the hospital. He will remain on intravenous heparin while his PT levels are adjusted.

Radiology Reports

Date: 4/19

Chest, Supine: There is no gross evidence of acute inflammatory disease or congestive heart failure.

Impression: No acute disease

Date: 4/21

Diagnosis: The patient appears to have undergone sternotomy. The heart appears normal. The endotracheal tube is in place as is the Swan-Ganz catheter.

Impression: Stable postoperative chest

EKG Reports

Date: 4/19

Impression: Elevated ST changes. Cannot eliminate the possibility of ischemia. Complete heart block is also noted.

Date: 4/20

Impression: Acute inferior myocardial infarction. Complete heart block has resolved.

Code Assignment Including POA Indicator

ICD-9-CM Principal Diagnosis: _____

ICD-9-CM Additional Diagnoses: _____

ICD-9-CM Procedure Code(s): _____

ICD-10-CM Code(s): _____

ICD-10-PCS Code(s): _____

7.6. A patient is admitted with severe atherosclerosis of the left common carotid artery. He undergoes a percutaneous angioplasty of the artery, along with percutaneous infusion of streptokinase into the left common carotid artery to assist with clot resolution. A carotid artery stent was also inserted to ensure that the artery would remain open. Assign the appropriate procedure code(s) to report this procedure.

ICD-9-CM Code(s):

a. 00.61, 99.10, 00.63, 00.40, 00.45
b. 00.61, 99.10, 00.64, 00.40, 00.45
c. 00.61, 00.63, 99.10
d. 00.61, 00.63

ICD-10-PCS Code(s): _____

7.7. Joe Jones was admitted to the hospital with severe angina. At cardiac catheterization he was found to have major atheromatous involvement of the left anterior descending coronary artery, with near-total occlusion, but well-preserved flow in the remainder of the coronary arteries. Because only one vessel was involved, the attending physician decided on a percutaneous treatment and stent placement. Mr. Jones underwent percutaneous angioplasty of the LAD with placement of two sirolimus-eluting stents. Intracoronary Urokinase administered to assist with clot dissolution. Assign the appropriate procedure codes for the hospital to report this inpatient procedure. Do not assign codes for the cardiac catheterization for this exercise.

ICD-9-CM Code(s):

a. 00.66, 00.40, 36.07, 36.07, 99.10
b. 00.66, 36.07
c. 00.66, 00.40, 00.46, 36.07, 99.10
d. 36.09, 00.40, 00.46, 36.06, 99.10

ICD-10-PCS Code(s): _____

7.8. A patient with severe arterial disease involving the lower abdominal aorta and the iliac bifurcation is admitted to the hospital as an inpatient for endovascular repair. Incisions are made over each femoral artery, and a catheter with modular attachments is inserted via the right femoral artery. The catheter carries a self-deploying endovascular prosthesis, which consists of an aortic component with a modular bifurcated prosthesis to extend into each of the iliac arteries. Via the femoral incisions, the components are aligned and are noted to be secure. The small incisions are closed, and the patient is taken to the recovery area for further observation. Assign the appropriate procedure code(s) to describe this procedure.

ICD-9-CM Code(s):

a. 38.44
b. 39.79
c. 39.71
d. 39.7

ICD-10-PCS Code(s): _____

7.9 **History and Physical:** The patient is a 67-year-old male who was transferred from Down-the-Street Hospital, where he was admitted six days ago with chest pain, shortness of breath, elevated cardiac enzymes, and EKG changes indicating an anterolateral ST elevation myocardial infarction. He subsequently underwent a cardiac catheterization, which revealed significant four-vessel disease. He was transferred here for a coronary artery bypass procedure.

Past History: Type 2 diabetes (diet controlled), hypercholesterolemia, and status post appendectomy

Medications: See transfer list

Allergies: None known

Physical Exam

General: Normal appearing male in no acute distress

Cardio: Rate and rhythm regular

Lungs: Normal

Tests: Chest x-ray normal; EKG nonspecific T-wave changes

Impression and Plan: Anterolateral myocardial infarction, coronary artery disease, diabetes mellitus, and hypercholesterolemia; patient will undergo CABG tomorrow

Operative Report

Preoperative Diagnosis: CAD

Postoperative Diagnosis: Same

Procedure: CABG × 4; saphenous vein graft of obtuse marginal, diagonal artery and posterior descending artery; left internal mammary artery to the left anterior descending artery. Cardiopulmonary bypass.

Description of Procedure: After obtaining adequate anesthesia, the patient was prepped and draped in the usual fashion. A primary median sternotomy incision was made, and the pericardium was opened. The left internal mammary artery was dissected as a pedicle using electrocautery and small hemoclips at the same time that the greater saphenous vein was harvested endoscopically from the left lower extremity. Cardiopulmonary bypass was instituted, and the patient was taken to a mild degree of hypothermia.

The aorta was cross-clamped, and electrical arrest effect was administered via cold blood cardioplegia. The saphenous vein graft was placed end-to-side with the posterior descending artery, and then a separate graft was placed to the obtuse marginal artery and finally a separate graft was placed to the diagonal artery. Each anastomosis was done with running 7-0 Prolene suture and verified no bleeders were present. The left internal mammary artery was subsequently brought through a subthalamic tunnel and placed end-to-side with the left anterior descending coronary artery.

Following completion of the grafts, warm blood cardioplegia was administered. During this time, two atrial and ventricular pacing wires were attached to the heart's surface; in addition, mediastinal tubes also were placed. The cross clamps were released following this, and sinus rhythm returned spontaneously. The patient was weaned from cardiobypass without incident.

After all grafts were checked for diastolic flow, which revealed no problems, the incisions were closed. The patient was taken to the recovery room in good condition and will be monitored in the intensive care unit for complications.

Progress Notes

Day 1: Patient progressing well; all vital signs are stable. Will transfer to step-down unit today.

Day 2: Heart rate stable and incision healing nicely. If patient continues to progress will be ready for discharge in a few days.

Day 3: Stable; patient ambulating in hallway without difficulty.

Day 4: Continues to progress in ambulation; ready for discharge tomorrow.

Day 5: Discharge patient today to follow up with myself next week.

What is the correct code assignment for this admission?

ICD-9-CM Code(s):

a. 410.01, 414.01, 250.00, 272.0, 36.13, 36.15, 39.61
b. 414.01, 410.01, 250.00, 272.0, 36.13, 36.15, 39.61
c. 414.00, 410.02, 995.89, 250.00, 36.13, 36.15, 39.61
d. 414.01, 410.01, 272.0, 250.00, 36.14, 39.61

ICD-10-CM Code(s): _____

ICD-10-PCS Code(s): _____

7.10.   The following documentation is from the health record of a patient admitted with significant aortic and mitral valve stenosis.

Surgery Date: 03/13/XX

Preoperative Diagnosis: Severe aortic and mitral valve stenosis

Postoperative Diagnosis: Severe aortic and mitral valve stenosis

Operative Procedure: Aortic valve replacement using a 19-mm bovine pericardial valve prosthesis; mitral valve replacement using a 26-mm bovine pericardial valve prosthesis; transesophageal echocardiogram; cardiopulmonary bypass.

Anesthesia: General endotracheal

Description of Procedure: Patient brought to the OR and placed on the OR table in the supine position. Arterial line and Swan-Ganz catheter were placed, general endotracheal anesthesia induced, and the patient prepped and draped in usual fashion. Transesophageal echocardiogram was then performed.

Next the chest was opened through a midline median sternotomy incision. The patient was heparinized and aortic and single right atrial cannules were inserted in the usual fashion. Retrograde cardioplegia line was placed through the right atrium in the coronary sinus. The patient was next placed on cardiopulmonary bypass and cooled to 27 degrees centigrade. During the cooling process, the aorta was cross-clamped and 1000 ml of cold cardioplegic solution was given. Inspection of the mitral valve revealed a severely diseased mitral valvular apparatus with calcification in the annulus. A few of the secondary and primary chordae were able to be preserved but the entire anterior leaflet was removed along with decalcifying the annulus. 2-0 Ti-Cron pledgeted sutures were then placed circumferentially in the annulus. Next a26-mm bovine pericardial valve prosthesis was seated and sutures were placed through the sewing ring of the valve. The atriotomy was closed using double row of 4-0 Prolene sutures.

Transverse aortotomy was then performed and inspection of the aortic valve revealed a trileaflet aortic valve. Excision of the three leaflets was then carried out. The annulus was sized and found to accommodate a 19-mm bovine pericardial valve prosthesis. Next 2-0 Ti-Cron simple sutures were placed circumferentially in the annulus and then through the sewing ring of the valve. The valve was seated, sutures were tied and there was good seating of the valve. The aortotomy was then closed using double row of 4-0 Prolene sutures. A de-airing cannula was placed in the ascending aorta and the heart was filled with blood to remove the air. While the lungs were ventilated with the patient in head-down position, light pressure was applied to the carotids. The aorta cross-clamp was removed. The patient was then rewarmed to 37 degrees centigrade. Once the patient was rewarmed with adequate cardiac output and pulse, was weaned from cardiopulmonary bypass The aortic and right atrial cannulas were removed and protamine was administered. Following adequate hemostasis, the entire mediastinum was irrigated with copious amounts of warm antibiotic solution. Two mediastinal chest tubes were placed for postoperative drainage. Aingle ventricular pacing wire was placed. Sternotomy was then closed in standard fashion after all instrument and sponges were accounted for. The patient was then taken to the cardiac postprocedural intensive care unit in stable condition.

Which of the following is the correct code set for this inpatient procedure?

ICD-9-CM Code(s):

a. 396.0, 35.11, 35.12, 39.61, 88.72
b. 396.0, 35.22, 35.24, 39.61, 88.72
c. 424.0, 424.1, 35.22, 35.24, 88.72
d. 394.0, 424.1, 35.22, 25.24, 88.72

Disorders of the Digestive System

7.11. The following documentation is from the health record of an 81-year-old female patient.

Operative Report

Diagnoses: Acute cholecystitis with gallstone, bile duct obstruction, acute pancreatitis.

251

Operation: Cholecystectomy; exploration of common bile duct; insertion of feeding tube; intraoperative cholangiogram performed under fluoroscopy

History: The patient is an 81-year-old female admitted 48 hours ago with evidence of acute gallstone pancreatitis. The patient had some thickening of her gallbladder wall and pericholecystic fluid. The patient had marked elevation of amylase and was given 48 hours of medical therapy with chemical clearance of her pancreatitis. The patient was thought to be a candidate for open exploration of her biliary tract, with concomitant cholecystectomy and possible common duct exploration.

Description of Procedure: After discussion with the patient and her family and obtaining informed consent, she was taken to the operating room where, after induction of general anesthesia, the abdomen was prepped and draped in a standard fashion. Following this, a right upper quadrant incision was used to gain access to the abdominal cavity. Manual exploration revealed no abnormalities of the uterus, ovaries, colon, or stomach. The pancreas was enlarged and edematous in the area of the head. Attention was then turned to the right upper quadrant, where the gallbladder was noted to be somewhat distended. This decompressed with a 2-0 VICRYL purse string stitch using the trocar. The cystic artery was dissected free and double clipped proximally, singly distally, and divided. The duct was then dissected free and subsequently clipped proximally.

Low osmolar cholangiogram with fluoroscopy was then obtained by opening the cystic duct and placing a cholangiogram catheter. The common bile duct measured roughly 1.5 cm in size. The duct tapered out in the area of the intraduodenal portion of the common duct to near-occlusion. The gallbladder was removed by transecting the cystic duct and removing it in a retrograde fashion. The gallbladder contained several stones.

Following removal of the gallbladder, attention was turned to the common bile duct, which was opened. No stones were retrieved initially from the bile duct. A biliary Fogarty was passed distally and, with some difficulty, was negotiated into the duodenum. On return, no calculus material was obtained. Palpation of the distal duct revealed thickening because of the pancreatic inflammation, which was noted to improve somewhat over the inside portion of the C-loop to the duodenum. The patient was felt to have bile duct obstruction from some other primary duct process other than a stone or inflammation.

Following this, cholangiography revealed some mild emptying of the distal common duct into the duodenum. With the overall picture, it was thought that the patient might benefit from a feeding jejunostomy, because she might well sustain postoperative or perioperative complications of respiratory insufficiency or perhaps other imponderables. As such, jejunum was identified roughly one foot beyond the ligament of Treitz, and 2-0 VICRYL purse-string stitches × 2 were placed. The jejunotomy was performed, and a 16 French T-tube was then placed and brought out through a stab wound in the left upper quadrant. The tube was anchored anteriorly with interrupted 2-0 silk stitches and externally with 2-0 stitches. Jackson-Pratt drain was placed through a lateral stab wound in the right upper quadrant and used to drain the duodenotomy and choledochotomy. This was anchored with several 3-0 silk stitches.

Following this, the wound was irrigated with Kantrex irrigation, 1 g/L, and the wound was closed by closing the posterior rectus sheath with running #1 VICRYL suture. The sub-q was irrigated and the skin was closed with staples. The wound was then dressed, and the patient was taken to the recovery room postop in stable condition. Estimated blood loss was 400 cc. Sponge and needle counts were correct × 2.

Code Assignment

ICD-9-CM Principal Diagnosis: _____

ICD-9-CM Additional Diagnoses: _____

ICD-9-CM Principal Procedure: _____

ICD-9-CM Additional Procedures: _____

ICD-10-CM Code(s): _____

ICD-10-PCS Code(s): _____

7.12.   The patient is a 56-year-old male who was admitted with a history of hematemesis for the past 36 hours. He also had some tarry black stools and was noted to have a giant gastric ulcer which was actively bleeding. Patient was subsequently referred for surgical intervention.

Final Diagnosis:
1. Acute gastric ulcer
2. Chronic pancreatitis
3. Liver cirrhosis due to alcoholism
4. Cirrhosis due to chronic hepatitis C

Procedure Performed: Subtotal gastrectomy with Billroth II anastomosis

Operative Procedure: The patient was brought to the operating room and placed on the table in a supine position, at which time general anesthesia was administered without difficulty. His abdomen was then prepped and draped in the usual sterile fashion. An upper midline incision was made. The peritoneum was then entered using the Metzenbaum scissors and hemostats. A retractor was placed, and he was noted to have a cirrhotic liver with micronodular cirrhosis. The left lobe of the liver was mobilized at that point, and the retractors were placed. On palpation of the stomach along the lesser curvature at approximately the mid portion, there was a large gastric ulcer located in the body of the stomach. At this point, the gastrocolic omentum was taken off the greater curvature of the stomach to the level just above the pylorus. Additionally, the lesser omentum was taken down off the lesser curvature of the stomach to the level of the pylorus. The body of the stomach was then transected approximately 3 cm above the ulcer. At that point, the stomach was reconstructed in a Billroth II fashion by bringing the jejunum through the transverse colon mesentery. Two stay sutures were placed to align the jejunum along the posterior wall of the stomach, and a GIA stapler was used to create the anastomosis without difficulty. The stomach and jejunum were then pulled below the transverse colon mesentery, and this was tacked in several places using 3-0 silk sutures. A feeding jejunostomy tube was then placed distal to this using the feeding jejunostomy kit without difficulty. The abdomen was then irrigated thoroughly using normal saline solution. Hemostasis was achieved using Bovie electrocautery. The midline incision was then closed using #1 PDS in a running fashion. The skin was closed using skin staples. A sterile dressing was applied. The patient was extubated in the operating room and returned to the Intensive Care Unit in guarded condition.

Code Assignment Including POA Indicator

ICD-9-CM Principal Diagnosis Code(s): _____

ICD-9-CM Additional Diagnoses Code(s): _____

ICD-9-CM Principal Procedure Code(s): _____

ICD-9-CM Additional Procedures Code(s): _____

ICD-10-CM Code(s): _____

ICD-10-PCS Code(s): _____

Optional MS-DRG Exercise (for users with access to MS-DRG software or tables)

Which MS-DRG is appropriate for this case? _____

Excluding the principal diagnosis, what other code affects the MS-DRG assignment for this admission? _____

7.13.   Discharge Summary

Principal Diagnosis: Morbid obesity

Principal Procedure: Open Roux-en-Y gastric bypass, removal of gastroplasty ring, gastric (G) tube prior placement

History of Present Illness: The patient is a 55-year-old white female with a history of gastroplasty ring placement in 1979 who comes to Dr. Smart for revision by doing a Roux-en-Y gastric bypass because of recurrence of her morbid obesity. Her morbid obesity is complicated by gastroesophageal reflux disease (GERD) and obstructive sleep apnea (OSA).

Past Medical History: (1) Morbid obesity. (2) OSA. (3) GERD.

Past Surgical History: (1) Gastroplasty in 1979. (2) Laminectomy.

Allergies: Keflex

Medications: Pepcid q. d.

Physical Examination: Vital signs: Afebrile, vital signs stable. General: No acute distress. CV RRR. PULMONARY CTAB. Abdomen: Soft, nontender, nondistended.

Impression: A 55-year-old white female with a history of gastroplasty, needing a revision into a Roux-en-Y gastric bypass after morbid obesity not secured.

Hospital Admission: The patient was admitted through same-day surgery and taken to the operating room for open Roux-en-Y gastric bypass with removal of a gastroplasty ring, liver biopsy, and G tube placement. Afterward, she was taken to the ICU because of her obstructive sleep apnea. She was monitored closely, did very well, and afterward, she was transferred to the floor. She was full advanced to activities of daily living through our gastric bypass protocol. She advanced to gastric bypass soft diet by postoperative day four. She did well with this. On postoperative day five, she was deemed ready to go home. She understands her discharge instructions and will be given pain medications as well as continue prescription for Zantac for her GERD and for marginal ulcer prophylaxis.

Condition on Discharge: Stable on postoperative day five from open Roux-en-Y gastric bypass

Disposition: The patient was discharged home with family.

Medications: Resume previous home medications. The patient can resume her Pepcid, or she can continue taking Zantac 150 b.i.d.

Follow-up: The patient will follow up with Dr. Smart.

Diet on Discharge: Gastric bypass soft diet. She has been instructed by a dietician two times already.

Operative Report

Preoperative Diagnosis: Morbid obesity with gastroplasty dysfunction

Postoperative Diagnosis: The same

Operation: Revision gastroplasty to Roux-en-Y gastric bypass and liver biopsy.

Indications: This 55-year-old lady had undergone a Silastic ring gastroplasty by another surgeon in 1979 at a weight of more than 250 lb. She had done well for a long time and then had started regaining her weight and also developed significant gastroesophageal reflux disease. A gastric endoscopy done preoperatively showed that the Silastic ring of her gastroplasty had eroded into the gastric lumen with a wide outlet from the pouch and also with a separate dehiscence of the staple line. In the interim, she had developed sleep apnea but did not have hypertension or diabetes. Following the endoscopy and because of being on disability related to a laminectomy and to spinal problems, the excess weight seemed to aggravate her disability and seemed a justifiable reason for a surgical intervention.

Description of Procedure: With the patient supine on the operating table and under satisfactory general anesthesia, we attempted a right and then left subclavian line but had difficulties with the wire guide. Subsequently, a neck central line was placed and the abdomen was prepped and draped in a sterile manner. An upper midline incision was made and carried through the fat by tearing and through the fascia with the cautery. There were adhesions immediately of omentum to the anterior abdominal wall and also to the lower abdominal wall where a paramedian incision had been. These were all lysed, which was not difficult. A Tru-Cut needle was used to obtain a biopsy from the left lobe, which was moderately fatty by examination. The gallbladder was emptied sufficiently to know that there were no stones. The uterus and ovaries were surgically absent. We began by lysing adhesions on the undersurface of the left lobe of the liver to the stomach until we were able to uncover the old gastric pouch and appreciate the location of the staple line. I could also appreciate where the Silastic ring was, separate from the nasogastric tube, which was brought inside. We dissected around the distal esophagus and brought a long Penrose drain around it for retraction purposes. I held up the portion of the stomach near the lesser curve where the Silastic ring was palpable, and we used the cautery to enter into the lumen to find the ring. Its suture was cut and the ring was removed and sent to pathology. The opening made for the gastrotomy was closed with interrupted 2-0 silk sutures. We then dissected a little more proximal to this location along the lesser curve to go around the serosa of the stomach to its backside. A 12 French Robinson catheter was put along this tract and turned around to come to hold the lesser omentum on traction. We also divided some of the gastrocolic omentum to gain access from the lateral side to the posterior lesser sac. We then used a 45-mm blue load endoscopic autosuture stapler to staple and transect the stomach at the lesser curve transversely to create the posterior part of our pouch. When this was done, there was still a small hole into the distal stomach and perhaps into the proximal pouch where the staples had found the tissue too thick to seal completely. On the gastric pouch side, this was managed by an over-and-over suture of 2-0 Prolene from one edge to the other. On the gastric side, this was managed with interrupted 2-0 silk sutures. We then dissected behind the stomach up to the angle of His and eventually were able to pass the 12 French Robinson catheter through the angle of His and around the stomach to represent the pathway for the stapler to go at a later time. We lifted the omentum upward and identified the ligament of Treitz. The jejunum was divided a measured 7.5 inches beyond that ligament, and the mesentery at that level was divided using the endoscopic stapler. The small bowel was then measured from that point to the cecum, which proved to be 204 inches, and we selected a 72-inch Roux limb length. The side-to-side jejunojejunostomy was created with the biliopancreatic limb and the Roux limb using an outer running 3-0 Prolene seromuscular layer and an inside GIA stapled anastomosis. The Prolene was continued over the holes made for the stapler and also used to invert the stapled edge of the biliopancreatic limb. The aperture between the two mesenteric leaves was closed with a couple of 3-0 silk sutures. We then made a channel through the omentum up to the transverse colon and then across the gastrocolic omentum to allow the Roux limb to lie easily antecolic up near the pouch. When this placement was assured, the Roux limb was fixed to the end of our pouch with three interrupted 3-0 silk seromuscular sutures. The cautery was used to make an opening in the jejunum in the gastric wall and the posterior part of the anastomosis was done with interrupted 3-0 VICRYL suture. An opening was made in the Roux limb through which a 10-mm Hegar dilator was passed through the jejunal and gastric sides of the anastomosis. That anastomosis was then sutured with the VICRYL over the dilator and then further reinforced with interrupted 3-0 silk seromuscular sutures. When this was done, we removed the dilator and passed the nasogastric tube through the anastomosis to lie in the Roux limb. The end of the Roux limb was then oversewn with a running 3-0 Prolene suture. After this, we used the 60-mm blue load endoscopic stapler to begin to transect the gastric pouch from the remainder of the stomach, going vertically towards the angle of His. It ultimately took three 45-mm cartridges after the first 60-mm cartridge in order to complete this, but it was done satisfactorily. We used 2-0 Prolene to oversew that vertical staple line throughout its length. We also used the 2-0 Prolene to oversew the gastric staple line throughout its length. The anastomosis in the pouch looked fine, and we made sure that the nasogastric tube was movable within the pouch. We then created a gastrostomy to the distal stomach, with a 2-0 silk purse-string suture near the greater curve. A 22 French Foley catheter was brought through a left upper quadrant stab wound and on into the stomach, and the balloon was filled. A purse-string suture was tied, and a couple of

2-0 silk sutures between stomach and abdominal wall were placed. After this, we irrigated the abdomen with an antibiotic solution containing Kantrex and bacitracin. All of the bowel and omentum was laid back in its normal position, and there was no tension on the Roux limb. The fascia was then closed with a running #1 loop PDS suture. The subcutaneous fat was cleaned with antibiotic solution and the skin was closed with 3-0 VICRYL dermal sutures and 3-0 VICRYL subcuticular sutures. The patient tolerated the procedure well and was taken to the SICU. Estimated blood loss was 350 mL, and the sponge count was correct.

Code Assignment

ICD-9-CM Principal Diagnosis: _____

ICD-9-CM Additional Diagnoses: _____

ICD-9-CM Principal Procedure: _____

ICD-9-CM Additional Procedures: _____

ICD-10-CM Code(s): _____

ICD-10-PCS Code(s): _____

Optional MS-DRG Exercise (for users with access to MS-DRG software or tables)

What is the MS-DRG assignment for this admission? _____

Which of the following would change the MS-DRG assignment of this admission?

a. Secondary diagnosis of a complication/comorbid condition or a major complication/comorbid condition
b. Additional procedure codes
c. If one of the current diagnoses was not present on admission
d. All of the above

Endocrine, Nutritional, and Metabolic Diseases and Immunity Disorders

7.14.   This 56-year-old female was admitted for resection of an adrenal mass. The patient has had hypertension and palpitations of several years' duration treated with Toprol under good control. Ultrasound was done in consideration of the possibility of a mass, and catecholamine studies have been normal. A 4- to 5-cm right adrenal mass was identified. Dr. White had obtained a 24-hour urinary free cortisol, ACTH, and short suppression tests, all of which confirmed the presence of Cushing's syndrome. The patient was not diabetic. She did report weight gain, some shift in body configuration, and easy bruising of several years' duration. The easy bruising was identified on examination in the hospital.

Surgery: A 5-cm, well-circumscribed round cortical tumor was resected from the adrenal gland via an open approach. Pathology report confirmed that the tumor was benign.

Allergies: No known drug allergies

Medications on Discharge: Hydrocortisone, rapidly tapering dose, currently on 40 mg daily; Toprol 50 mg q. a.m.; Prevacid 30 mg q. d.; Lipitor 10 mg q. a.m.; Prempro 0.625/2.5

Physical Exam: Vital signs stable. HEENT: Sclerae and conjunctivae clear. Neck: Supple. No palpable thyroid. Lungs: Somewhat decreased breath sounds currently. There is mild splinting with deep breathing. Abdomen: Tenderness in the incision area. She has active bowel sounds at this time. Extremities: No definite bruises currently. No edema noted.

Discharge Diagnosis: Right adrenal tumor with Cushing's syndrome secondary to tumor

Plan: The patient appears to have tolerated the surgery well. She will require steroid replacement. Excess cortisol output is presumed entirely due to her tumor, and her ACTH was suppressed previously. As with exogenous steroid therapy, there will be contralateral adrenal suppression. The patient will be tapered rapidly to replacement hydrocortisone levels. We will try the remaining hydrocortisone withdrawal over the next 6 months or so, depending on her ACTH and cortisol responses. She is discharged to home with follow-up in my office in 1 week.

Which of the following is the correct code set for this hospitalization?

ICD-9-CM Code(s):

a. 239.7, 255.0, 401.9, 785.1, 07.21
b. 194.0, 401.9, 785.1, 07.22
c. 227.0, 255.0, 401.9, 785.1, 07.21
d. 227.0, 255.0, 07.29

ICD-10-CM Code(s): _____

ICD-10-PCS Code(s): _____

Optional MS-DRG Exercise (for users with access to MS-DRG software or tables)

Which of the following MS-DRGs is correct for this admission?

a. 644, Endocrine Disorders with CC
b. 615, Adrenal and Pituitary Procedures without CC/MCC
c. 614, Adrenal and Pituitary Procedures with CC/MCC
d. 628, Other Endocrine, Nutritional and Metabolic OR Procedures with MCC

7.15. The following documentation is from the health record of a 57-year-old male patient.

Discharge Diagnoses: 1. Lung cancer currently undergoing chemotherapy with Taxol and carboplatin with dexamethasone
2. Type II diabetes, with neuropathy and nephropathy, not controlled
3. Hyperlipidemia
4. Hepatomegaly

History: This patient is a 57-year-old man who presented for outpatient chemotherapy. He had surgery for lung cancer in September and is now undergoing chemotherapy with Taxol and carboplatin, including dexamethasone as part of his chemo and prophylaxis for nausea. He has done very well with the chemotherapy. When he presented for outpatient treatment on the day of admission, he was found to be hypoglycemic. He is a known type II diabetic. His diabetes is complicated by neuropathy and nephropathy. Due to his blood glucose levels, it was decided to postpone this chemo session, and he was admitted for control of his diabetes. Dr. Johnson consulted with the patient to manage his diabetes regimen. He has been on 70/30 insulin, 25 units in the morning and 15 units in the evening. He had problems in the hospital with hypoglycemia several times the first day, with blood sugar levels ranging from 30 to greater than 450. An IV insulin drip was started, and he also had q. 1 hour Accu-Cheks. His hepatomegaly has enlarged from the last time that I saw him. Question whether this is fatty infiltration due to poor diabetes control, or whether there is now some involvement with metastatic carcinoma. The patient also continued his oral medications for hyperlipidemia during the hospital stay.

Laboratory Data: Sodium 128, potassium 5.5, chloride 89, CO_2 34, BUN 13, creatinine 0.8, glucose range 30–460, with final glucose of 210. Calcium 9.4, WBC 9.8, hemoglobin 11.6, hematocrit 34.3, platelets 277,000

Plan: One difficulty here is the cyclic nature of his chemo treatment regimen, likely to produce major shifts in his glucose, which is already difficult to control. The patient will need to monitor his glucose levels closely. He is discharged on 70/30 insulin, 35 units in the morning and 20 units in the evening. Dr. Johnson will be managing his diabetes, and the patient has instructions to call his nurse on a daily basis for the next week. He is to follow up with me for further chemotherapy in the oncology clinic next week.

Code Assignment Including POA Indicator

ICD-9-CM Principal Diagnosis: _____

ICD-9-CM Additional Diagnoses: _____

ICD-9-CM Procedure Code(s): _____

Issues To Clarify: _____

ICD-10-CM Code(s): _____

ICD-10-PCS Code(s): _____

7.16. The following documentation is from the health record of a 52-year-old patient.

Discharge Summary

Admission Date: 11/14/XX

Discharge Date: 11/17/XX

Discharge Diagnosis:
1. Diabetic ketoacidosis
2. Dehydration
3. Congestive heart failure
4. Aortic valve stenosis
5. Urinary tract infection due to *E. coli*
6. Hyperkalemia

7. Peripheral vascular disease
8. Hypertension
9. Hyperlipidemia
10. Chronic renal insufficiency
11. Old myocardial infarction
12. Tobacco use
13. Coronary atherosclerosis with native coronaries

Admitting Diagnosis:
1. Diabetic ketoacidosis
2. Diabetes mellitus Type I
3. Dehydration
4. Congestive heart failure
5. Hyperkalemia
6. Hyperlipidemia
7. Hypertension
8. Tobacco abuse
9. Severe peripheral vascular disease
10. Atherosclerotic coronary artery disease
11. Urinary tract infection
12. Renal insufficiency
13. History of CVA

Present Illness: A 52-year-old white female with known diabetes mellitus Type I, CVAs, cellulitis, hypertension, chronic renal insufficiency, hyperlipidemia, poorly compliant diabetic. Most recently in hospital from September 3 to September 8 with cellulitis, congestive heart failure, poorly controlled diabetes with diabetic ketoacidosis. Discharged home. She was supposed to be following up with her primary care physician doing b.i.d. Accu-Cheks. She was nauseated for the previous two weeks. As soon as she got nauseated, she quit checking her blood sugar level. She cancelled her doctor's appointment because she was "too sick to go." She had decreased appetite and was feeling poorly overall. She came to the emergency room with a blood sugar of 737. She had ketones 200 to 250. Her blood urea nitrogen was 75, creatinine 1.8. Her potassium is 6.1, chloride 5, bicarb at 13. Patient is a poor historian, although she is awake and alert at the time of evaluation, on an insulin drip. Overnight her nausea had resolved. The nausea probably occurred because she was in the beginning stages of diabetic ketoacidosis.

Hospital Course: The patient was put on insulin drip. Blood sugars got down. She was put on q.i.d. Accu-Cheks. Once her blood sugar level came down to the 100s, potassium was lowered. I had a very lengthy discussion with patient about the need for keeping doctor's visits and checking blood sugars. The patient was placed on Cipro. Her electrocardiogram showed a prolonged Q T. The patient went to ultrasound and had sludge and possible small stones in her gallbladder, and it was felt that she was able to be discharged home improved.

Discharged Medications/Instructions: Insulin 70/30, 20 units in the a.m., 20 in the p.m., Rezulin 400 mg q. a.m., Tenormin 50 q.d., Plavix 75 q.d., Monoket 10 mg b.i.d., Lasix 20 mg b.i.d., aspirin 325 q. a.m., Zocor 20 once a day, Oxycotin 20 b.i.d., Prozac 20 q. a.m., Vasotec 5 mg q. a.m., Propulsid 10 mg at Ac and HS, Bactrim DS one tablet every 12 hours. She is to see her primary care physician in one week. She is to call if she has any difficulties.

Disposition: Discharged home

History and Physical

Past Medical History: The patient has history of renal insufficiency with a blood urea nitrogen of 30 to 40 with a creatinine of 1.2 to 1.4. She has had a CVA, severe peripheral arterial disease. Echocardiogram done shows aortic stenosis, mitral leaflet thickening, normal left ventricular size, normal diabetes. Smokes three to four packs of cigarettes a day. She has hypertension. She has hyperlipidemia. She is dehydrated. She has a history of atherosclerotic coronary artery disease.

Medications: At the time of admission included Rezulin 40 mg q.d., Prozac 20 q.d., Propulsid 10 a.c. and h.s., Vasotec 2.5 two every morning, Atenolol 50 q. a.m., Plavix 75 q. a.m., Lasix 20 milligrams b.i.d., Novolin 70/30 20 units every a.m., aspirin 325 q. a day, vitamin E, iron, Oxycotin 20 a.m. and h.s., Zocor 20 mg at dinner. The patient has no known drug allergies.

Social History: She is married but her husband lives out of state and works there. She has one daughter. She does not drink and has smoked about 3 to 4 packs a day since a teenager.

Physical Exam: At the present time, the patient is afebrile, vital signs are stable. She is awake and alert, oriented times 3.

HEENT: Pupils equal, round, reactive to light and accommodation, extraocular muscles intact, oropharynx benign

Neck: Supple without adenopathy or jugular venous distention

Lungs: Clear to auscultation

Heart: Reveals a regular rate and rhythm without murmurs, gallops, or rubs

Abdomen: Soft, nontender, positive bowel sounds, no masses noted

GU: Deferred

Extremities: No edema. She has a baseline edema currently. Pulses are absent, pedal pulses.

Laboratory: At the time of admission, her glucose was 737, blood urea nitrogen 75, creatinine 1.8, acetone greater than 200, less than 250, sodium 136, potassium 6.1, chloride 95, bicarb of 13. Her hemoglobin was 13.9 and hematocrit of 44.1, white blood cell count of 9.2 with a left shift showing 80.2 percent neutrophils, 16.2 percent lymphocytes. Platelets were 241,000. Urinalysis shows positive nitrites, greater than 1,000 glucose, 30 protein, 15 ketones, trace hemoglobin. She had 13 white blood count per high power field. Rare red per high power field, 2+ bacteria. Gram stain on her u/a showed no organisms seen.

Impression(s):
1. Diabetic ketoacidosis
2. Diabetes mellitus type I
3. Dehydration
4. Congestive heart failure
5. Hyperkalemia
6. Hyperlipidemia
7. Hypertension
8. Tobacco abuse
9. Severe peripheral vascular disease, arterial in nature
10. Atherosclerotic coronary artery disease

11. Urinary tract infection
12. Renal insufficiency

Plan: Admit, hydrate. She has been on insulin drip, we will d/c this now and change to q. 4 Accu-cheks and continue sliding scale. Hopefully on 16th be able to reinstitute her routine meds. Her potassium has now come down to the mid 4's secondary to her hydration and her sugar being driven intracellular with the insulin drip. I have impressed upon the patient the need for checking blood sugars and keeping M.D. appointment versus death in the future. The patient is on Cipro for her urinary tract infection. Further workup as indicated during hospital stay.

Exam: 9005 EK EKG REG
Compared with 9/25/07 no change

Impression: Normal EKG

Code Assignment Including POA Indicators

ICD-9-CM Principal Diagnosis: _____

ICD-9-CM Additional Diagnoses: _____

Issues To Clarify:_____

ICD-9-CM Diagnosis Code(s): _____

ICD-10-CM Code(s): _____

Disorders of the Genitourinary System

7.17. The following documentation is from the health record of a 48-year-old female patient.

Discharge Summary

Discharge Diagnoses

1. Dysfunctional uterine bleeding
2. Anemia

Therapies

1. Transfusion of four units of packed red blood cells
2. Fractional D&C
3. ThermaChoice balloon endometrial ablation

Discharge Medications: Tylenol III and iron supplementation

Hospital Course: The patient presented to the emergency department with complaints of heavy vaginal bleeding which had progressively gotten worse over the previous three months. Prior to the patient's admission, she was using seven maxi pads in an hour. Assessment at that time showed that she was hemodynamically stable. However, she did have a hemoglobin of 8.5 and was continuing to bleed. She was admitted for IV premarin therapy and transfusion.

The patient has a mechanical heart valve and for this reason, she was on Coumadin. A PT with INR was obtained to make sure that the patient was not supra therapeutic.

However, she was in the normal range. Despite the Premarin, the patient did continue to bleed. After the first two units of blood were transfused, her hemoglobin was only 8.8. She was given two additional units via peripheral vein and scheduled for a D&C and a balloon ablation of her endometrium. This was performed. The procedure was uncomplicated. She was discharged home to follow up in the office.

History & Physical Exam

Admission: For surgery

Present Illness: This is a 48-year-old gravida 10, para 7 who had been seen in the office with complaints of some bleeding after being menopausal for approximately one year. On examination, her uterus was found to be slightly enlarged, six to eight weeks' sized, the adnexa were non palpable. An ultrasound was performed which showed the endometrial thickness was 25 rom and had a complex echogenicity to it. Uterus measured $10.5 \times 8.2 \times 6.1$ cm, right ovary $3.7 \times 3.8 \times 3.5$ cm, left ovary $3.1 \times 2.1 \times 3.2$ cm. There is no evidence of fluid in the cul-de-sac. An endometrial biopsy was performed which showed a small amount of proliferative-type endometrium with breakdown consistent with dysfunctional uterine bleeding. She was scheduled to have a D&C later this month. However, the patient presented to the Emergency Department with complaints of very heavy vaginal bleeding requiring the use of seven maxi pads in an hour. The patient was found to be hemodynamically stable, blood pressure and pulse were in the normal range. However, hemoglobin was found to be 8.5. She was bleeding rather heavily; there was a large amount of clot in her vagina. She was admitted for a blood transfusion. She received two units of packed red cells via peripheral vein and was also started on IV Premarin 25 mg every six hours. The patient has a history of having a mechanical heart valve for which she takes Coumadin; the fear was that perhaps she was overly anticoagulated. However, a PT with INR was found to be in the therapeutic range. Due to the patient's heavy bleeding, I felt that a D&C with some kind of therapeutic intervention was warranted. In this particular circumstance, an endometrial ablation would serve the patient very well. Plan is to perform a D&C with a balloon thermo-ablation.

Past Medical History: Significant for mechanical valve placement

Surgery: Valve replacement

Current Medications: Lasix, Lanoxin, Coumadin. Allergies: No drug allergies

Obstetrical History: Gravida 10, para 7

Social History: No tobacco, alcohol, or drugs

Family History: Significant for diabetes in her mother

Physical Exam: Blood pressure 120/80, weight 224

HEENT: Moist mucous membranes without thyromegaly or lymphadenopathy

Breasts: Symmetrical without additional mass, nipple discharge

Lungs: Clear to auscultation

Heart: Regular rate and rhythm

Abdomen: Soft, no mass. No lesions are seen on the vulva, vagina or the cervix. Uterus is approximately six to eight weeks' sized. The adnexa were not palpable.

Assessment and Plan: 48-year-old gravida 10, para 7 with dysfunctional uterine bleeding. Plan is to perform a D&C (dilation and curettage) with a ThermaChoice balloon ablation. The patient is currently in-house and this is scheduled for Thursday morning at 8 a.m.

Operative Report

Pre-Operative Diagnoses

1. Dysfunctional uterine bleeding
2. Anemia

Post-Operative Diagnoses: Same

Operations: Fractional D&C and Therma-Choice balloon endometrial ablation

Anesthesia: General with endotracheal tube intubation

Complications: None

Estimated Blood Loss: Less than 50 cc. Drains: None

Specimen(s) to Lab

1. Endocervical curettings
2. Endometrial curettings

Operative Procedure: The patient was taken to the Operating Room and under adequate general anesthesia. She was prepped and draped in the dorsolithotomy position for a vaginal procedure. The uterus was sounded to approximately 9–10 cm. Using Pratt cervical dilators, the cervix was dilated to the point that a Sims sharp curette could be inserted. A Kevorkian curette was first used to obtain endocervical curettings and the Sims sharp curette was passed to obtain endometrial curettings. After the curettings were obtained, the Therma-Choice system was assembled and primed. The catheter with the balloon was placed inside the endometrial cavity and slowly filled with fluid until it stabilized at a pressure of approximately 175 to 180 mmHg. The system was then preheated, and after preheating to 87 degrees C, eight minutes of therapeutic heat was applied to the lining of the endometrium. The fluid was allowed to drain from the balloon and the system was removed. The procedure was then discontinued.

All sponge, instrument, and needle counts were correct. The patient tolerated the procedure well and was taken to the Recovery Room. She will be discharged home when stable.

Pathology Report

Endocervical mucosa with squamous metaplasia, negative for dysplasia

Inactive endometrium with features of non-cycling endometrium

No evidence of hyperplasia or malignancy

Code Assignment Including POA Indicator

ICD-9-CM Principal Diagnosis: _____

ICD-9-CM Additional Diagnoses: _____

ICD-9-CM Procedure Code(s): _____

Issues To Clarify: _____

ICD-10-CM Code(s): _____

ICD-10-PCS Code(s): _____

Optional MS-DRG Exercise (for users with access to MS-DRG software or tables)

What are the results when you group this case with the code for acute blood loss anemia versus anemia due to blood loss?

MS-DRG assignment with the acute blood loss anemia code:

_____

MS-DRG assignment with the anemia due to blood loss code:

_____

Which MS-DRG is appropriate for this case? _____

7.18.   The following documentation is from the health record of a 92-year-old female patient.

Admission Diagnoses

1. Fever
2. Delirium

Discharge Diagnoses

1. Left lower extremity cellulitis
2. Probable urosepsis with streptococcal bacteremia
3. Status post acute renal failure likely secondary to acute tubular necrosis
4. Insulin-requiring diabetes mellitus
5. Probable chronic obstructive pulmonary disease
6. Hypothyroidism
7. Hypertension

Consultations: Infectious Disease

Procedures Performed

1. Doppler ultrasound of the left lower extremity which showed no evidence of DVT
2. Transthoracic echocardiogram which showed normal left ventricular function

Hospital Course: The patient is a 92-year-old white female with past medical history significant for hypertension, hypothyroidism, and insulin requiring diabetes mellitus who was brought to the Emergency Room for evaluation of fever and dyspnea. The patient at that time was a poor historian; however, family corroborated abrupt onset of symptoms with no clear source. Generally the patient has been healthy although she is minimally active and most of her activities of daily living consist of ambulating around her bedroom with the assistance of family.

In the Emergency Room the patient was febrile to 40:C. Urinalysis was significant for pyuria with evident bacteria. No focal infiltrate was seen on chest x-ray. The patient had marked leukocytosis with a white count of 25,000, 80 polys and 15 band forms. She was admitted for intravenous antibiotics. She was treated with Ceftriaxone and by the following morning was noticeably brighter and more alert. She remained afebrile for the duration of her hospital course. Also on the morning of first hospital day, blood cultures were reported as positive for gram positive cocci in chains. This was subsequently confirmed as group C streptococcus which was Penicillin sensitive. Urinalysis grew out mixed flora. It was somewhat unclear as to the specific source of the patient's bacteremia. It is somewhat unusual for a UTI to yield this organism. The patient had some mild erythema on her left lower extremity and had marked discomfort to touch over both of her ankles, which she attributed to her "diabetes." She remained on Rocephin and was actually tolerating near normal diet.

On the evening of the second hospital day, the patient complained of increased pain and was noted to be increasingly incoherent. She had been placed on nasal cannula overnight for have markedly increased erythema in her left lower extremity concerning for desaturation. On evaluation by cross covering physician, she was noted to have markedly increased erythema in her left lower extremity concerning for possible DVT. Doppler ultrasound showed no evidence of clot. She was started on Vancomycin for improved gram positive coverage. Respiratory status remained stable. However, the patient was minimally arousable later that morning. She had been administered a 1-mg dose of morphine for leg pain. Chest x-ray showed increased interstitial edema possibly consistent with heart failure. The patient received Narcan with some improvement in her mental status. Arterial blood gas showed evidence of significant CO_2 retention with pH of 7.19, pCO_2 70, p02 50, serum bicarbonate of 26. She was diuresed and administered nebulizer treatments. She was moved to the Medical Intensive Care Unit for possible ventilation with BiPAP. Echocardiogram showed no wall motion abnormalities and no left ventricular dysfunction. Chemstix remained greater than 100 mg/dL. The patient had prompt improvement in her respiratory status with diuresis and prevision of Narcan. No further invasive ventilation was necessary.

Of note during these events the patient's family was in close attendance including her three daughters and grandson. There was extensive consultation with them regarding any advanced directives that the patient might have specified previously. It was the consensus of the family that reasonable attempts at aggressive intervention were indicated as long as there was a possibility of a reversible etiology for her problems. Fortunately the patient's condition stabilized.

For the remainder of her hospital course, intervention focused on improving her pulmonary status as well as renal function. Her creatinine had increased from prior baseline of 1.2 up to 1.7 with noticeable drop-off in her urine output. The patient had received intravenous antibiotics during her hospital course but had not had any noticeable hypotensive episodes. She was receiving diuretics, which complicated calculation of her urine sodium; however, overall picture appeared consistent with acute tubular necrosis. Renal ultrasound was obtained and showed no evidence of hydronephrosis or obstruction. She was restarted on her oral Indapamide and continued to have steady improvement in her pulmonary status. She did not require any supplemental oxygen following resolution of her pulmonary edema.

Infectious Disease was consulted with regards to her cellulitis and was concerned that it was not resolving as would be expected with a streptococcal organism. Therefore she was continued on Vancomycin for an additional five days and by the time of this dictation erythema had completely resolved and the patient was consistently alert, sitting up in bed and actually ambulating around her room. Leukocytosis resolved and, as noted above, renal function normalized. The plan was to continue her on oral Dicloxacillin for an additional 10 days of oral antibiotic therapy. Only additional intervention was provision of a combined albuterol Atrovent inhaler given the patient's signs of chronic interstitial lung disease. This appeared to improve her ventilatory status as she had no further episodes of nocturnal desaturation. The patient at this time is stable for discharge.

I briefly discussed her hospital course with her primary physician, who will continue to follow her. Family is requesting the assistance of home health nurse for overall assessment over the next two weeks while the patient continues to recuperate at home. Other peripheral issues addressed during this hospitalization included the patient's probable iron deficiency anemia. Recent colonoscopy and endoscopy showed evidence of diverticular disease but no other pathology. The patient has had upper GI bleeding. She was guaiaced during this admission, had stable hematocrit. B-12 and folate were checked and were within normal limits. Other issue was the patient's diet and she was evaluated by a speech therapist who noted that she did fine without any aspiration as long as she was provided with somewhat *thickened* feeds and had her usual foods provided. It was particularly requested that she be given pills, tablets, and capsules with a spoonful of pudding, applesauce, or yogurt instead of fluid. It was also recommended that she continue to have thickener available. The family was aware of these recommendations and is extraordinarily attentive to the patient's needs.

Medications on Discharge: Insulin NPH 10 units qam; Synthroid .05 mg po qd; Aspirin 325 mg po qd; Lorazepam 0.5 mg po qhs; Iron 324 mg po tid; Colace 100 mg po qd; Dulcolax 10 mg prn constipation; Combivent MDI 2 puffs bid; Indapamide 2.5 mg po qd; Dicloxacillin 125 mg po qid × 10 days

Follow-up: The patient's family has been instructed to call for appointment.

Diet: Soft mechanical 1,800 calorie ADA

Activities: The patient may ambulate to a chair with assistance.

Special Instructions: The patient should seek prompt medical attention for any recurrent fever, increased erythema in her lower extremity, or mental status changes as reported by the family.

Code Assignment Including POA Indicator

ICD-9-CM Principal Diagnosis: _____

ICD-9-CM Additional Diagnoses: _____

ICD-9-CM Procedure Code(s): _____

Issues To Clarify:_____

ICD-10-CM Code(s): _____

ICD-10-PCS Code(s): _____

7.19.   The following documentation is from the health record of a 14-year-old male patient.

Discharge Summary

The patient is a 14-year-old male with a history of renal failure and failed left kidney transplant. The patient was admitted for his second kidney transplant.

Prior to surgery, the patient underwent hemodialysis, through the existing AV fistula. The transplant was accomplished within 48 hours of the harvesting of the donor organ. Tissue samples confirmed adequate donor match. The previously transplanted, now failing, kidney was first removed; then the new kidney was placed.

One postoperative dialysis session was required before the transplanted kidney was functioning adequately. Postoperatively, the patient was watched carefully for signs of rejection. Patient's postoperative course was relatively uneventful.

The patient was discharged, to be followed weekly in the office.

Which of the following code sets will be reported for the above admission?

ICD-9-CM Code(s):

a. 996.81, 586, 55.53, 55.69, 39.95 × 2
b. 586, 996.81, 55.69, 39.95 × 2
c. 586, V42.0, 55.53, 55.69, 39.95
d. 584.9, V42.0, 55.69, 39.95

ICD-10-CM Code(s): _____

ICD-10-PCS Code(s): _____

7.20.   The following is from the health record of a 77-year-old female.

Discharge Summary

Admission Date:	04/12/XX
Discharge Date:	04/15/XX
Discharge Diagnosis:	1. Acute renal failure
	2. Congestive heart failure
	3. Chronic obstructive pulmonary disease (COPD)
	4. Leg cellulitis, resolved
	5. Seizure disorder
	6. Venous insufficiency
	7. Osteoarthritis
	8. Morbid obesity
	9. Acute ankle arthritis, likely pseudogout
Discharge Medications:	Resume home medications
Procedures:	None
Consults:	None

Present Illness: This is a 77-year-old female transferred to the acute care ward from a subacute unit for treatment of renal insufficiency. She was originally admitted with a BUN of 32, creatinine 1.4. While on the subacute unit she was diuresed for congestive heart failure and developed acute renal failure. Her BUN rose to 78, creatinine to 2.3. She was transferred to the trauma care unit (TCU) for IV fluids and monitoring for her redevelopment of congestive heart failure. She was developing some rales with IV fluids on the subacute unit. She was monitored closely over the next 3 days. As her BUN and creatinine fell she seemed to tolerate it fairly well symptomatically, having some rales. She had a BUN of 60 and a creatinine of 1.3 on the day of discharge. She was released by the cardiologist that day when he felt she was in no significant congestive heart failure and her BUN and creatinine were improving. She should follow up with the cardiologist in the near future for follow-up electrolytes and reevaluation of her congestive heart failure.

While the patient was on the TCU, she also developed some ankle pain. It was somewhat swollen and was given a dose of steroids. She had quick resolution to the pain and swelling and likely this was an episode of pseudogout.

History and Physical Exam

Admission Date: 04/12/XX

Chief Complaint: Acute renal failure.

Present Illness: This is a 77-year-old white female who was transferred down from the subacute unit to the acute care unit for increasing renal insufficiency. The patient was originally admitted on 03/28 with a BUN, creatinine of 32 and 1.4. The patient has been treated with I.V. Ancef and I.V. Lasix for cellulitis and pulmonary edema. Yesterday, her BUN and creatinine were found to be 78 and 2.3. She was transferred to the acute care unit for I.V. fluids and to monitor her renal function. This a.m., she complains of right ankle pain. She denies any trauma to the right ankle, but she does give a history of generalized osteoarthritis. She reports that there is excruciating pain with weight bearing and with any movement. In addition, she reports that the right ankle is very tender to touch.

Past Medical History:		
	1.	Obesity
	2.	Renal failure
	3.	Bilateral lower extremity cellulitis
	4.	Hypertension
	5.	Anemia
	6.	COPD
	7.	Seizure disorder
	8.	Intertrigo

Current Medications:		
	1.	Lotrisone, b.i.d. topical to breast and groin
	2.	Prinivil, 40 mg po q.day
	3.	Dilantin—mg po b.i.d.
	4.	Benadryl, 25 mg q. 4 hours prn
	5.	Catapres, 0.1 mg prn
	6.	Hydrocortisone cream, 1% topical b.i.d. prn
	7.	Tylox, 1–2 tabs po q.i.d. prn
	8.	Norvasc, 5 mg po q.day

Allergies: No known drug allergies

Review of Systems: The patient reports that she does have arthritis in her back and multiple joints. She denies a history of gout. She denies sporadic fevers, chills, cough, abdominal pain, GI or GU complaints.

Social History: The patient is a smoker; she has smoked two packs per day for the previous 20 years.

Physical Exam: BP 140/70, pulse 100, respirations 24, temperature 97.5. In general, this is an obese white female in no acute distress. HEENT: Atraumatic, normocephalic. Pupils equal, round, and reactive. Oropharynx is clear. Neck: Supple; no lymphadenopathy; trachea midline. Lungs: Lungs reveal few crackles, right base. Heart: Regular rate and rhythm; Sl, S2, no murmur, click, gallop, or rub. Abdomen: Protuberant, positive bowel sounds, and nontender. Extremities: Chronic venous changes bilaterally with trace edema. Right lateral malleolus is very tender to palpation, range of motion is limited by pain. There is no calf or thigh tenderness.

Laboratory Data/Clinical Tests: Glucose 98, BUN 76, creatinine 2.1, calcium 8.2, sodium 134, potassium 4.4, chloride 94, total CO_2 30

Assessment/Plan

1. Renal failure. This is most likely prerenal secondary to overdiuresis. We will hold her diuretics and continue with general I.V. fluids. Her BUN, creatinine is slightly improved today since yesterday with this therapy. Urine electrolytes and eosinophils are currently pending.

2. Right ankle pain. Etiology not completely certain. There is no history of trauma. I question if this could possibly be an inflammatory arthritis monoarticular such as gout or pseudogout. We will check a sed rate and a rheumatoid factor. We will hold off on giving the patient any nonsteroidal anti-inflammatories, in light of her renal failure. We'll continue with the Tylox and give her a trial of SoluMedrol. We'll also check a foot x-ray.

3. Cellulitis. This is stable, off of her antibiotics.

4. Hypertension. We will continue her current treatment.

Which of the following is the correct code assignment?

ICD-9-CM Code(s):

a. 584.9, 428.0, 496, 345.90, 459.81, 721.90, 715.89, 278.01, 275.49, 712.37, 401.9
b. 403.90, 584.9, 428.0, 496, 345.90, 459.81, 721.90, 715.89, 278.01, 275.49, 712.37
c. 586, 428.0, 496, 345.90, 459.81, 721.90, 715.89, 278.01, 275.49, 712.37
d. 404.90, 584.9, 428.0, 496, 345.90, 459.81, 721.90, 715.89, 278.01, 275.49, 712.37

ICD-10-CM Code(s): _____

Optional MS-DRG Exercise (for users with access to MS-DRG software or tables)

True or False: The assigned MS-DRG for this admission contains a CC or MCC.

Infectious Diseases

7.21. The following documentation is from the health record of a 71-year-old male patient.

Discharge Summary

History and Physical Findings: This 71-year-old male is a nursing home resident as a result of a cerebrovascular accident 2 years ago. He has had numerous hospital admissions for pneumonia and other infectious complications. On the day of admission (4/21), the patient was noted to be clammy, with tachypnea, to have decreased level of responsiveness, and to show increased fever. He was seen in the ER, where evaluation revealed the presence of probable urosepsis. The patient was also found to have renal insufficiency with BUN and creatinine elevated. His WBC count was 23,000 with decreased hemoglobin and hematocrit. He was admitted for treatment of *Escherichia coli* septicemia. Physical examination revealed an elderly male who was aphasic and with a right hemiplegia from a previous CVA. The heart had a regular rhythm. The lungs were clear. The abdomen was soft.

Significant Lab, X-Ray, and Consult Findings: Follow-up chemistry showed progressive decline in the BUN and creatinine to near-normal levels. Initial white blood cell count was 23,700. Final blood count was 9,000. The urinalysis showed white cells too numerous to count. The urine culture had greater than 100,000 colonies of *E. coli* and group D strep, which revealed the cause of the UTI. Repeated blood cultures grew *E. coli* with the same sensitivities as that of the urine. There were no acute abnormalities noted. EKG showed sinus tachycardia and low lead voltage, otherwise was normal and unchanged.

Course in Hospital: The patient was initially started empirically on Primaxin. He underwent fluid rehydration and his electrolytes were followed closely. Electrolytes improved through his hospital stay. He was continued on IV Primaxin until the date of discharge, when he was changed to Cipro by tube. All of the bacteria grown in the urine and in the blood were sensitive to the Cipro. The chest x-ray showed no change from previous admissions, and he was followed closely with additional oxygen as needed. The patient does have a history of chronic obstructive lung disease and has required intermittent oxygen therapy at the nursing home. At this time, the patient had reached maximal hospital benefit. He was switched to oral antibiotics. He was to continue on tube feedings, which he was tolerating quite well. The patient was discharged back to the nursing home on 5/4.

Discharge Diagnoses: *E. coli* septicemia
UTI
Renal insufficiency
Chronic obstructive lung disease
CVA with right hemiplegia

Code Assignment Including POA Indicator

ICD-9-CM Principal Diagnosis: _____

ICD-9-CM Additional Diagnoses: _____

Issues To Clarify: _____

ICD-10-CM Code(s): _____

Optional MS-DRG Exercise (for users with access to MS-DRG software or tables)

What is the correct MS-DRG for this case?

_____

7.22. The following documentation is from the health record of a 34-year-old male.

Discharge Summary

History of Present Illness: The patient is a 34-year-old male who was transferred to the hospital with the diagnosis of rule out AIDS. The patient dates the onset of his current illness to two months prior to admission when he had a tooth extraction. The patient doesn't know whether he was treated with antibiotics at that time; however, he does note that the socket was packed. The patient states that after the above tooth extraction, he developed a fever with shaking chills, night sweats, and anorexia. He lost about 12 pounds. He also notes the onset of mild right flank pain associated with foam in urine and urinary frequency. There was no hematuria, dysuria, incontinence, urinary retention, hesitancy, or slow stream. The patient also complains of occasional diarrhea but no melena or bright red blood per rectum. Medications on transfer are Codeine, Lasix, Amphojel, Mylanta, Penicillin, Ranitidine, Halcion. Social history is remarkable for continuous IV drug abuse, both heroin and cocaine. There's no history of homosexual activity. He doesn't drink alcohol but smokes a half-pack of cigarettes a day.

Pertinent Lab, X-Ray, and Consult Findings: This patient is a 34-year-old, well-developed, well-nourished male in no acute distress. Mucous membranes are moist. There is a questionable white area at the outer aspect of the right lower gingiva near second tricuspid. There are small mobile submandibular and posterior cervical nodes. The patient also has bilateral inguinal adenopathy and two left epitrochlear nodes. Chest x-ray showed minimal blunting of both costophrenic angles, no definite effusions are noted. There are confluent patches of infiltration in the left midlung field spanning from the hilum to the periphery as well as in the right lower lung. These findings are nonspecific, but could very well fit in with the diagnosis of Pneumocystis carinii pneumonia. Urinalysis negative. CBC: Hemoglobin 9.0, hematocrit 27.2, MCV 87, WBC 5.1, 11 lymphs, S monos, platelets 206,000. Sodium 130, potassium 3.98, chloride 112, C02 10, BUN 50, creatinine 4.7, glucose 82, calcium 7.0, albumin 0.80. Sputum culture showed normal respiratory flora with normal Enterobacter aerogenes. Urine culture showed no growth.

Hospital Course by Problem List

Problem #1. Acquired immunodeficiency syndrome: The patient's history was significant for weight loss. Social history significant for IV drug abuse. Physical examination revealed diffuse lymphadenopathy. Laboratory data revealed neutropenia with lymphopenia. Serological test was positive for HIV.

Problem #2. Pneumocystic carinii pneumonia: The patient underwent bronchoscopy and brushings from the left and right lower lobes revealed changes consistent with pneumocystic carinii and reactive bronchial cells and pneumocytes. The patient was treated with two weeks of intravenous Septra therapy. However, there was no improvement in his clinical status. After two weeks of therapy, the patient was still afebrile. His chest x-ray did not improve and WBC count progressively declined to a low of 2.5. The infectious disease service recommended Pentamidine therapy at that point. The patient became afebrile.

Problem #3. Chronic renal failure: The patient's renal failure deteriorated during his hospitalization prior to transfer. Workup was negative and the etiology remains unclear. The patient's renal function remained stable throughout this hospitalization. At the time of transfer, his BUN and creatinine were 50 and 5.0, respectively. He was started on Bicitra therapy to correct the metabolic acidosis felt secondary to his renal failure.

Problem #4. Nephrotic syndrome secondary to renal failure: The patient was found to have edema, hypoalbuminemia, proteinuria, and high triglyceride levels, all consistent with the diagnosis of nephrotic syndrome. The patient did have a renal biopsy done prior to transfer to this hospital and the results per phone report are as follows: Interstitial nephritis, no deposits over capillary loops, no immunofluorescence of CMV. The patient was treated with bed rest, a low-sodium, high-protein fluid restriction diet. In spite of this therapy, the patient's albumin level had not improved at the time of transfer.

Problem #5. Chronic normocytic normochromic anemia secondary to external hemorrhoid bleeding. The patient required transfusion of two units of packed red blood cells via a peripheral vein. Otherwise, his hematocrit remained relatively stable throughout the admission. Physical examination revealed swollen hemorrhoids with stool heme negative.

The patient was transferred in stable condition to the local hospital. Medications at the time of transfer were Bicitra, Pentamidine, Restoril, Lorazepam.

Which of the following is the correct code assignment for this admission?

ICD-9-CM Code(s):

a. 042, 136.3, 276.2, 581.89, 585.9, 280.0, 305.61, 305.51, 455.5, 305.1, 33.24, 99.04
b. 042, 136.3, 276.2, 581.89, 585.9, 280.0, 455.5, 33.24, 99.04
c. 042, 136.3, 581.89, 585.9, 280.0, 305.61, 305.51, 305.1, 33.24, 99.04
d. 136.3, 042, 581.89, 585.9, 280.0, 305.61, 305.51, 305.1, 33.24, 99.04

ICD-10-CM Code(s): _____

ICD-10-PCS Code(s): _____

7.23.   The following documentation is from the health record of a two-year-old boy.

Discharge Summary

Admission Date: 7/18/20XX

Discharge Date: 7/20/20XX

Admitting Diagnosis: Fever of unknown origin

Discharge Diagnosis: 1. Primary herpetic gingivostomatitis
2. Kawasaki's disease
3. Strep pharyngitis

History: The patient is a 2-year-old male who presented to the ER this evening from his primary medical doctor's office with 4 days of fever, rash, cracked lips, and drooling. Mom states that he has had a decreased activity level, decreased p.o. intake, and increased irritability. He has received Tylenol and Motrin at home. Mom denies vomiting or diarrhea. He has had a sick contact at day care. He also has dysphagia and rhinorrhea.

Past Medical History: Significant for a VSD that has not been repaired. He is followed by a cardiologist and the abnormality is currently stable.

Physical Exam: This young male is quite irritable. He has bulbar conjunctival injection without discharge. His tympanic membranes are dull bilaterally. His tonsils are enlarged. He also has an exudate in his oropharynx. Heart shows regular rate and rhythm with a IV–VI systolic murmur at the left lower sternal border. He has a diffuse maculopapular rash on his lower extremities, trunk, back, and diaper area. He also has perineal desquamation.

Hospital Course: Patient presented to the ER with a 4- to 5-day history of fever, rash, cracked lips, drooling, and sore throat. Due to lymphadenopathy, perineal desquamation, bilateral bulbar conjunctivitis, and rash found on physical exam, he was treated for Kawasaki's disease with IVIG 2 g/kg and aspirin 80 mg per day. He was also tested for herpes due to the perioral, paranasal, and oral lesions. His test came back positive for herpes I virus and he was treated with Kefzol. Cardiologist performed an echocardiogram to evaluate his VSD. His lesions slowly improved and are largely healed at this time. He remained afebrile for the past 4 nights. His medications were changed to oral form. He is no longer taking antibiotics, and he will be continued on oral acyclovir. Follow-up with cardiologist is in 4 weeks.

Which of the following is the correct code set for this hospitalization?

ICD-9-CM Code(s):

a. 523.10, 054.9, 745.4, 446.1, 034.0
b. 054.2, 745.4, 034.0, 446.1, 785.6, 372.30, 782.1
c. 054.2, 745.4, 446.1, 034.0
d. 054.2, 446.1, 034.0

ICD-10-CM Code(s): _____

7.24.   History

The patient is a 78-year-old female who was initially admitted to the intensive care unit for sepsis and urinary tract infection and decreased level of consciousness. After admission to the intensive care unit, the patient was found to have a massive right-sided cerebrovascular accident, which was felt to be secondary to an embolic phenomenon. The patient also had severe mitral regurgitation, moderate tricuspid regurgitation, and aortic insufficiency. CT of the head revealed an acute left middle cerebral arterial infarction involving the temporal and parietal lobes with localized mass effect and mild midline shift. No hemorrhage was seen.

The patient's sepsis was treated with IV antibiotics as was her urinary tract infection. Discussion was undertaken with the patient's next of kin as to the patient's resuscitation status. The patient was made a Do Not Resuscitate. Decision was made to keep the patient comfortable, and she was transferred to a medical bed. The patient's antibiotics were adjusted by an infectious disease group. Her renal failure which was determined to be due to her sepsis was followed by nephrology. Neurology was consulted for the patient's cerebrovascular accident. They did an EEG, which showed marked slowing; however, there was no total absence of brain activity. Cardiology consultation was obtained because of new onset atrial fibrillation. Cardiology felt that no aggressive intervention was needed; however, she would be given medicine to control her ventricular rate. The patient remained unresponsive. She was started on tube feeding and her antibiotics were continued. The patient was noted to have some thrombocytopenia as well as her continued renal failure and anemia. Diuresis was attempted with IV diuretics by nephrology in an attempt to help the patient's congestive heart failure. The patient was retaining copious amounts of fluid despite the diuretics. Her prothrombin time eventually normalized. Her blood sugar was elevated, and she was placed on insulin once per day at bedtime to cover her tube feedings. The patient was found without audible or visible respirations and no heart tones. She was pronounced dead at 12:40, and her body was released to the funeral home.

Which of the following code sets would be assigned by the hospital for this admission?

ICD-9-CM Code(s):

a. 038.9, 995.91, 599.0, 434.11, 394.1, 397.0, 398.91, 427.31, 287.5, 285.9
b. 995.91, 599.0, 586, 434.11, 424.0, 397.0, 428.0, 427.31, 287.5, 285.9
c. 038.9, 995.92, 599.0, 586, 434.11, 396.3, 397.0, 398.91, 427.31, 287.5, 285.9
d. 434.11, 038.9, 995.92, 586, 428.0, 424.0, 397.0, 427.31, 287.5, 285.9

ICD-10-CM Code(s): _____

Optional MS-DRG Exercise (for users with access to MS-DRG software or tables)

What is the correct MS-DRG for this case?

a. 064, Intracranial Hemorrhage or Cerebral Infarction with MCC
b. 871, Septicemia without mechanical ventilation 96+ hours with MCC
c. 872, Septicemia without mechanical ventilation 96+ hours without MCC
d. 868, Other Infectious and Parasitic Disease Diagnoses with CC

7.25. Discharge Diagnosis

1. *Escherichia coli* and *Staphylococcus aureus* urinary tract infection with sepsis
2. Sepsis syndrome
3. Advanced dementia
4. Hypothyroidism
5. Hypertension
6. Protein calorie malnutrition
7. Dysphagia

Discharge Medications: Levoxyl 88mcg p.o. q. a.m., Paxil 20mg p.o. q. a.m., Namenda 10mg p.o. q. a.m., Ativan 0.5 q. 8 hours agitation, Augmentin 500 mg p.o. b.i.d. for 15 days, and Megace 400 mg p.o. b.i.d.

Discharge Disposition: Improved and home with home healthcare.

History of Present Illness: The patient is an 85-year-old female who was apparently brought into the emergency room by her family this evening for multiple problems. According to the family, she has not been eating recently and has been getting extremely weak. She has been unable to stand without assistance for quite some time now. The patient, although awake and alert, will not answer any questions. All history is obtained from the computer records, as well as the ER staff and ER physician. Initial workup reveals significant urinary tract infection. She is also most likely septic secondary to her presentation given her hypotension and acute encephalopathy.

Laboratory/Radiology: Admission labs significant for a white blood cell count of 9.8, hemoglobin 14.9, platelets of 328,000 with a BUN of 29 and creatinine of 1.4. Urinalysis was small bilirubin, 15 mg ketones, large blood, 100 mg protein, positive nitrates, large leukocytes, and too many WBCs to count, with many bacteria and many red cells. CT of the head was normal. Portable chest x-ray showed hyperexpanded lung fields but no mass.

Hospital Course: The patient was admitted to the general medical floor with the diagnosis of sepsis. After discussion with family, she was made DNR III and was hydrated and started on IV ciprofloxacin. She has a significant advanced dementia and does not speak but was somewhat more encephalopathic secondary to her sepsis, and this improved to her baseline. Her BUN and creatinine normalized, and she was continued on her usual medications for dementia. Her hydrochlorothiazide was held, but she was continued on her Toprol. Levoxyl was held and a TSH was within normal limits. She was continued on her Paxil. Subsequently, her urine culture grew out *E. coli*, pan sensitive, and *S. aureus*, pan sensitive, and she was changed from ciprofloxacin to Augmentin 500mg p.o. b.i.d., which she tolerated well. Speech therapy was consulted, and an MBS was performed. Diet with thin liquids was recommended. She does have protein calorie malnutrition.

Disposition: The daughter has been contacted because the patient is stable for discharge. She is discharged to her daughter's care with physical and occupational therapy.

Code Assignment Including POA Indicator

ICD-9-CM Principal Diagnosis: _____

ICD-9-CM Secondary Diagnosis: _____

ICD-10-CM Code(s): _____

Behavioral Health Conditions

7.26.   In the following case scenario, a 26-year-old white male was admitted after being transferred from the outpatient evaluation service with severe homicidal and suicidal ideation. Admitting diagnosis was severe major depressive disorder with psychotic features. Pharmacologic treatment was initiated and suicide precautions were instituted. After a thorough neuropsychological, personality, and behavioral psychologic evaluation, the risks and benefits of ECT were reviewed. Due to the severity of the psychotic episode and the patient's delusional state, it was determined that ECT was warranted. Extensive efforts were made to secure informed consent from the patient, and a course of single seizure unilateral ECT was begun.

ECT was administered three times per week, and the course of therapy was completed in a three-week period. On the fourth treatment of ECT, postictal observation was notable for cardiac arrhythmia, which subsided without sequelae. Otherwise, the patient tolerated the therapy well and responded quickly with resolution of the psychotic features and overall improvement in the acute phase of his depressive disorder. Suicide precautions could be lifted after the fifth treatment with ECT. After establishing adequate therapeutic levels of lithium, the patient was discharged to be managed as an outpatient.

Discharge Diagnosis: Severe major depressive disorder with suicidal ideation, stabilized after a course of ECT.

Which is the correct code set for reporting this case scenario?

ICD-9-CM Code(s):

a. 296.24, V62.84, V62.85, 94.27, 94.22, 94.08
b. 296.23, V62.84, V62.85, 94.27, 94.22, 94.08
c. 296.24, V62.84, V62.85, 427.9, 94.26, 94.22, 94.08
d. 296.23, V62.84, V62.85, 997.1, 427.9, 94.27, 94.22, 94.08

ICD-10-CM Code(s): _____

ICD-10-PCS Code(s): _____

7.27. The following documentation is from the health record of a 56-year-old male patient.

Final Diagnosis

Axis I: Chronic schizophrenia, paranoid type with acute exacerbation, improved
Axis II: None
Axis III: Cardiomyopathy secondary to hypertension
            COPD
            Type II diabetes mellitus
Axis IV: Psychosocial and environmental stressors are severe
Axis V: Admission GAF 25 to 30
            Discharge GAF 55

Physical Examination: For pertinent findings on medical examination, see the medical doctor's dictation.

Pertinent Laboratory Results: Electrolyte panel within normal limits. Digoxin level was 0.6, hemoglobin A1C 6.5, triglycerides 138, CBC unremarkable. TSH 1.3, urinalysis negative. EKG showed normal sinus rhythm.

Hospital Course: This is a 56-year-old male who was admitted due to decompensating at his apartment where he thought people were trying to get into his apartment, and he continued to decompensate with his paranoia and persecutory-type delusions, so that it was felt he needed longer hospitalization. During this time he also switched his medications from Zyprexa to Seroquel to Risperdal, and then he was admitted on Prolixin. We reviewed his records, and it appears he did quite well on Risperdal so he went back to taking that, and he was titrated up to 30 mg q. h.s. of Risperdal and 100 mg of trazodone. These two medications helped significantly to eliminate his delusions and paranoid ideation. He slept better. Patient started going on therapeutic passes that went well. His sister reports that he is doing the best that she has seen him in quite some time. During his stay here his mother passed away from a long medical illness, and he was able to go to the funeral and dealt with that loss in an appropriate way. He continued to show improvement and was placed on Level E. He continued to go to psychosocial programming. A discharge meeting was held, and it was agreed that he could get most of his services through the outpatient program. It was felt by everyone that the patient was stable enough to be discharged, and discharge was scheduled.

Pertinent Findings on Mental Status at Discharge: 45 minutes spent in the final examination with the patient. Appearance: Pleasant, white male who looks his stated age. Behavior is cooperative, fair eye contact. Speech is of normal rate and volume. Not rapid or pressured. Mood euthymic, affect appropriate. Thought process is goal directed, decreased paranoid ideation. Negative for racing thoughts and flight of ideas. Thought content: He denies signs of active psychosis, denies current suicidal or homicidal intent. Insight and judgment improved. Impulse control is fair.

Prognosis: Fair. The main problem is that the patient is on so many medications for his medical problems. He did do well with the pill organizer and self-medications, but his mental illness may be exacerbated if his medical conditions are not well controlled.

Discharge Medications: Digoxin 0.25 mg q. d, Glucotrol 2.5 mg a.m. and 7.5 mg q. 5:00 p.m., potassium 10 mEq q. a.m., Spironolactone 25 mg q. a.m., an aspirin 325 mg q. a.m., Lasix 10 mg q. d., lisopril 2.5 mg q. d., Atrovent inhaler two puffs q. i.d., isosorbide dinitrate 10 mg t.i.d., beclomethasone inhaler four puffs b.i.d., Risperdal 3 mg q. h.s., Colace 100 mg b.i.d., and trazodone 100 mg q. h.s.

Aftercare Recommendations: The patient will be discharged to his apartment. Social services will follow the patient. He will follow up with a psychiatrist and medical care through the outpatient program. Also, a home health nurse will come to see the patient.

Which of the following code sets is correct for reporting this inpatient hospitalization?

ICD-9-CM Code(s):

a. 295.34, 425.4, 401.9, 496, 250.01, 94.25
b. 295.32, 402.90, 496, 250.01, 94.25
c. 295.34, 402.90, 496, 250.00, 94.25
d. 295.84, 402.90, 496, 250.00, 94.25

ICD-10-CM Code(s): _____

ICD-10-PCS Code(s): _____

7.28. The following documentation is from the health record of a 17-year-old male patient.

History of Present Illness: The patient is a 17-year-old white male who was brought to the ED after being found passed out in the town park. The patient was in restraints and accompanied by two police officers. The patient was combative and aggressive, threatening physical harm to himself as well as the physician and hospital staff. The patient has a long history of alcohol and drug abuse, was in the local treatment center, and walked off campus two days ago.

Allergies: NKDA

PMH: Attention deficit hyperactivity disorder (ADHD), drug and alcohol dependence, aggressive behavior

Family History: Noncontributory

ROS: As above

Physical Examination: Vital signs: Temp. 100.1 degrees; BP 144/88 mm Hg; General: Alternating between lethargy and combativeness; HEENT: Pupils pinpoint, 1 mm bilaterally; Skin: Cool, clammy to touch, feet and hands cold, slightly diaphoretic; Heart: Rate tachy, no murmurs; Lungs: Clear, respiratory rate 28 and shallow; Abdomen: Benign; Neurological: Mental status as above; follows commands inconsistently, responds to voice; Cranial nerves: Pupils as noted, gag intact; Motor: Moving all four extremities with equal power; Sensory: Responds to touch in all four extremities; deep tendon reflexes +3 throughout, but plantar reflexes down going bilaterally.

Laboratory: U/A shows 2+ blood, done after Foley catheter was placed; drug screen positive for amphetamines; ETOH 0.30; ABG within normal limits; EKG sinus tachycardia

Hospital Course: Family was contacted, IV fluids were initiated, and the patient was admitted to ICU with suicide protocol, Ativan 1 to 2 mg IV q. 2 hours p.r.n. He was maintained on soft restraints with checks every 15 minutes and monitored with telemetry and neuro checks through the night. By the morning he was no longer tachycardic. By hospital day three he was medically stable, but still saying he wants to "kill himself." Psychiatric consult requested; see dictated report.

Disposition: Discharge to psych. Psychiatric liaison service agreed to accept him in transfer to the inpatient adolescent psychiatric unit at children's hospital.

Discharge Diagnoses: Drug overdose with amphetamines and alcohol
Apparent suicide attempt
Continued verbalization of suicidal ideation

Which of the following code sets would be correct for this case?

ICD-9-CM Code(s):

a. 969.72, 785.0, 304.40, E950.3, 980.0, 303.00, E950.9, 314.01, 312.00
b. 785.0, E939.7, 305.90, 314.01, 312.00
c. 969.72, 785.0, 304.00, E980.3, 303.00, 314.01, 312.00
d. 785.0, 303.00, 304.40, 969.7, E950.3, 980.0, E950.9, 314.01, 312.00

ICD-10-CM Code(s): _____

Disorders of the Musculoskeletal System and Connective Tissue

7.29.   **Preoperative Diagnosis:**   Bucket-handle tear left medial meniscus

   Postoperative Diagnosis: Bucket-handle tear left medial meniscus

   Procedure: Arthroscopic partial medial meniscectomy

Indications: The patient is a 16-year-old male who tore his left medial meniscus while playing football at the local high school football field. The patient is a wide receiver for the high school football team and was tackled resulting in the torn medial meniscus. I saw and treated the patient initially in the emergency room three weeks ago for this injury.

Technique: After induction with general anesthesia, a standard three-portal approach of the knee was evaluated. Mild synovitic changes were noted in the suprapatellar pouch. No chondromalacia changes were noted. The anterior portion of the medial meniscus had a flap tear, which was removed.

After all instruments were withdrawn, 4-0 nylon horizontal mattress stitches were used to close the wound, and pressure dressings were applied. The patient was awakened and taken to the recovery room in good condition.

Code Assignment Including POA Indicator

ICD-9-CM Principal Diagnosis: _____

ICD-9-CM Additional Diagnoses: _____

ICD-9-CM Procedure Code(s): _____

ICD-10-CM Code(s): _____

ICD-10-PCS Code(s): _____

7.30.   **Preoperative Diagnosis:**   Primary osteoarthritis of right knee

   Postoperative Diagnosis: Primary osteoarthritis of right knee

   Procedure: Right posterior stabilized total knee arthroplasty

Implants: DePuy Sigma System size 4 right posterior stabilized femoral component, size 3 modular tibial tray with 8 mm noncrosslinked polyethylene spacer and 35 mm × 8.5 mm thick patella. Antibiotic cement was used.

Procedure Description: After obtaining informed consent, the patient was brought to the operating room whereupon the smooth induction of right femoral block and general anesthesia was performed. The patient was positioned in supine fashion on the operating room table, and all bony prominences were well-padded. A bump was placed under the right hip, and a tourniquet was placed on the right proximal thigh. A gram of Kefzol was given intravenously. The right lower extremity was prepped and draped in standard sterile fashion for arthroplasty including an alcohol pre-prep.

After exsanguinations of the extremity with an Ace wrap, the tourniquet was inflated to 300 mg Hg. An approximately 6-inch longitudinal incision was made about the anterior aspect of the knee centered on the inferior pole of the patella. The skin and subcutaneous tissue were dissected sharply down to the level of the fascia, and a medial parapatellar incision was made in the fascia with the medial most split proximally. The patella was everted, and the knee was flexed. Care was taken to protect the patellar tendon insertion. The osteophytes about the femoral notch were removed and a partial resection of the posterior patellar fat pad was carried out. The femoral canal was entered with a drill, and the sword with distal femoral cutting guide were attached set for a resection of 10 mm. The lateral femoral condyle was noted to be eroded distally and posteriorly; however, a 10-mm cut was sufficient for the distal cut.

Using anterior-referenced system, the femur was sized to a size 4. Rotation was set at 3 degrees external rotation. This was checked using the epicondylar axis. The four-in-one cutting guide was then applied, and the distal femoral anterior and posterior cuts as well as the chamfer cuts were completed. Care was taken to protect the collateral ligaments during these cuts. The femoral notch was then completed using the notch-cutting guide supplied with the system. Once that was done, attention was turned to the tibia. Using an external referenced guide, a tibial cut was made with a zero degree posterior slope with 2 mm off the low (lateral) side. This resection resulted in a similar amount of resection medially and laterally. The tibia was exposed using a Homan placed posteriorly and laterally. The osteophytes were removed laterally and posteriorly.

At this point the osteophytes about the posterior femoral condyles were removed using a curved osteotome under direct visualization. The tibia was then sized to a size 3. A thin cut was then made for the modular tibial tray system. An 8-mm posterior stabilized trial spacer, size 3 tibia tray, and size 4 femur were then applied. The knee was taken through a range of motion. Following this, stability was symmetric medially and laterally. The patella was then prepared. The osteophytes were removed with a rongeur, and the thickness was measured to be 25 mm. An 8.5-mm resection was made down to 16.5 mm and a 16.5 × 35 mm patellar trial was applied after the cut was completed. Stability of this component was then trialed, and it was found to be excellent.

The trial components were removed, and the knee was copiously irrigated with normal saline. The final components were then cemented into place in the sizes mentioned above. Order of cement was patella, tibia, femur. The tibial tray was placed and the knee brought out into full extension to compress the tibial and femoral components. Again, antibiotic gentamicin-containing cement was used. The wound was then cleared of excess cement and bony debris and irrigated one final time. It was then closed in layers over a ConstaVac drain. Number 1 Vicryl was used for the extensor fascia and Scarpa fascia in a simple interrupted fashion, 3-0 Monocryl was used for the subcutaneous tissue in a simple buried fashion, and staples were placed at the level of the skin.

A sterile dressing was placed. The ConstaVac drain extension and reservoir were attached and activated, and a compressive wrap was placed from the toes to the thigh. The tourniquet was released for a total tourniquet time of 112 minutes. EBL was minimal. Postoperatively the patient was taken to the recovery room in stable condition.

Which of the following is the correct code assignment?

ICD-9-CM Code(s):

a. 715.16, 81.54
b. 715.36, 81.47
c. 715.16, 81.55
d. 715.36, 81.54

ICD-10-CM Code(s): _____

ICD-10-PCS Code(s): _____

7.31.   The following documentation is from the health record of an ORIF patient.

Operative Report

Preoperative Diagnosis: Displaced comminuted fracture of the lateral condyle, right elbow

Postoperative Diagnosis: Same

Procedure: Open reduction, internal fixation

Description: The patient, with malignant hypertension and type I diabetes mellitus, was anesthetized and prepped with Betadine, sterile drapes were applied, and the pneumatic tourniquet was inflated around the arm. An incision was made in the area of the lateral epicondyle through a Steri-Drape, and this was carried through subcutaneous tissue, and the fracture site was easily exposed. Inspection revealed the fragment to be rotated in two planes about 90 degrees. It was possible to manually reduce this quite easily, and the judicious manipulation resulted in an almost anatomic reduction. This was fixed with two pins driven across the humerus. These pins were cut off below skin level. The wound was closed with some plain catgut subcutaneously and 5-0 nylon in the skin. Dressings were applied to the patient and tourniquet released. A long arm cast was applied.

Which of the following is the correct code assignment?

ICD-9-CM Code(s):

a. 812.52, 401.9, 250.01, 79.32
b. 812.42, 401.0, 250.01, 79.31
c. 812.42, 401.0, 250.01, 78.52
d. 812.52, 401.9, 250.00, 79.32

ICD-10-CM Code(s): _____

ICD-10-PCS Code(s): _____

7.32.   ## Discharge Summary

Admission Date: November 15, 20XX

Discharge Date: November 20, 20XX

Description: The patient is a 49-year-old male who was admitted on November 15. He underwent revision laminectomy and stabilization of his lumbar spine with a Dynesys system. The patient tolerated the procedure well and had an uneventful hospital course, except experienced acute pain after the surgery requiring additional physical therapy and pain control.

By postoperative day 5, he was tolerating a regular diet, had obtained pain control, and cleared physical therapy. He was subsequently discharged home with written instructions. He is to follow up in 3 weeks after discharge. He was given Percocet and Flexeril for pain and spasms, as needed.

History and Physical

Admit Diagnosis: Recurrent herniated disc

Procedure: Lumbar laminectomy, disc stabilization with Dynesys

History of Present Illness: 49-year-old male with left leg and back pain. Diagnosed with recurrent disc herniation

Past Medical History: Status post laminectomy and diskectomy 2 years ago

Physical Examination

Neck: Supple

Heart: Regular rate and rhythm

Lungs: Clear to auscultation

Neuro: Left leg weakness, numbness, and pain

Skin: No lesions, masses, or rashes

Assessment and Plan: Recurrent HNP L5 to S1

Operative Report

Preoperative Diagnosis: Radiculopathy and degenerative disc disease at L5–S1 with recurrent disc herniation at L5–S1

Postoperative Diagnosis: Same

Procedure Performed: Revision L5 laminectomy, revision S1 laminectomy and diskectomy, stabilization of L5 to S1 with flexible rod Dynesys system

Anesthesia: General

Blood Loss: Minimal

Complications: Intraoperative dural tear, which was repaired with watertight seal with interrupted 4-0 Nurolon sutures

Description of the Procedure: Under sterile conditions, the patient was brought to the operating room and was placed under general endotracheal anesthesia and placed in a prone position. Lumbar spine was then prepped and draped in the usual sterile manner with a Betadine prep. A lateral x-ray was obtained with an 18-gauge spinal needle placed for level localization. Based upon the x-ray, a direct posterior approach to the lumbar spine was performed. This was carried down to the transverse process of L5 and the sacral ala bilaterally. After adequate exposure, complete laminectomy was performed in a subperiosteal fashion with a combination Leksell and Kerrison rongeurs at the L5 and S1 levels. Mobilization of the left S1 and L5 nerve roots was performed, although there was a significant amount of scar tissue. There was a large free L5-S1 recurrent disc fragment, which was removed with a pituitary rongeur. There was a small dural tear within the axilla of the L5 nerve root repaired with watertight seal with interrupted 4-0 Nurolon sutures. After adequate decompression, attention was brought to stabilization. Using the usual internal and external landmarks, pedicle screws were placed in the L5 and S1 pedicles bilaterally. These were drilled, probed, dilated, and then a combination of 7.2 mm × 40 mm screws and 7.2 mm × 45 mm screws were placed in the L5 and S1 pedicles bilaterally. AP and lateral x-rays were obtained, noting appropriate placement of the screws. Measuring of the cord device was performed bilaterally. The cord was placed in the usual fashion, tensioned, and then finally tightened. The wound was copiously irrigated with bacitracin solution. No drain was utilized. The fascia was closed with interrupted 0 VICRYL suture. The subcutaneous tissue and skin were closed in three sequential layers. The patient was awakened in the operating room, extubated, and brought to the recovery room in satisfactory condition.

Code Assignment Including POA Indicator

ICD-9-CM Principal Diagnosis: _____

ICD-9-CM Additional Diagnoses: _____

ICD-9-CM Procedure Code(s): _____

ICD-10-CM Code(s): _____

ICD-10-PCS Code(s): _____

Neoplasms

7.33.   Discharge Summary

Date of Admission: 2/3

Date of Discharge: 2/4

Discharge Diagnosis: Malignant ascites from metastatic adenocarcinoma of the colon

Course in Hospital: This 59-year-old white female patient was admitted for continuous infusion chemotherapy with 5-FU and Leucovoran. Patient had a central venous catheter placed in the superior vena cava which was used for the chemotherapy treatment. This was done under the care of Dr. ZXY. The patient tolerated her chemotherapy very well. She had no complications throughout her hospital course, and she was discharged to be followed further as an outpatient by her oncologist.

Instructions on Discharge: Follow up in the office

History and Physical

Admitted: 2/3/20XX

Reason for Admission: Chemotherapy

History of Present Illness: The patient is a 59-year-old white female with peritoneal carcinomatosis and malignant ascites from colon carcinoma. She is admitted for continuous chemotherapy. The patient has a sigmoid colostomy and has had multiple abdominal surgeries for carcinoma; the first one was an anterior and posterior repair in 1982. She had six weeks of radiation therapy completed two years ago and has been on weekly chemotherapy consisting of 5-FU and methotrexate recently. Because of increasing abdominal girth, she was admitted in June and diagnosed with malignant ascites and carcinomatosis. At that time, she had an extensive evaluation including an upper gastrointestinal series, barium enema, CT scan, and ultrasound of the abdomen. She was told she had adhesions causing a partial obstruction. No further surgery was pursued. For the past week, she has complained of frequent vomiting. Her weight has decreased another six pounds. She denies any abdominal pain. She has occasional diarrhea for which she takes Questran. She has had no blood in her colostomy drainage.

Past Medical History: No hypertension, myocardial infarction, diabetes, or peptic ulcer disease. Anterior and posterior repair in 1982, colectomy, cholecystectomy, appendectomy, hysterectomy with bilateral salpingo-oophorectomy for uterine fibroids in 1968.

Allergies: None

Chronic Medications: Pancrease three times a day; Questran as needed for diarrhea; Os-Cal 2 × a day, 250 mg

Family History: Mother died at age 80. Father died of colon cancer at age 60.

Social History: Prior to that time, she smoked a pack a day for 20 years. She denies any alcohol intake. She works in the shipping department.

Review of Systems: Unremarkable

Physical Examination: An alert, white female in no acute distress

General Appearance

    Skin, Head, Eyes, Ears, Nose, Throat: Pupils are equal, reactive to light and accommodation. Extraocular movements are intact. Fundi are benign. Tympanic membranes are normal.

    Mouth: No oral lesions are seen.

    HEENT: Within normal limits

    Neck: Carotids are plus 2 with no bruits. Thyroid is normal. There is no adenopathy at present.

    Lungs: Clear

    Heart: Regular sinus rhythm. No murmur, rub, or gallop.

    Breasts: A small, approximately 3-mm, cystic lesion the medial aspect of her left breast at around eight o'clock. It is freely movable and nontender. There are no axillary nodes.

    Abdomen: Distended. Sigmoid colostomy present. Right lower quadrant induration is present. There is no abdominal tenderness. There is no hepatosplenomegaly. Bowel sounds are normal.

    Pulses: Femorals are plus 2 with no bruits. There are good pedal pulses bilaterally.

    Genitalia: Normal

    Rectal: Deferred

    Extremities: No edema

    Neurologic: Deep tendon reflexes are plus 2 throughout

Laboratory Data: Pending

Impression

    Peritoneal carcinomatosis from colon cancer

    Small left breast cyst

Plan: The patient will be admitted for continuous chemotherapy.

Progress Notes

2/3 Patient tolerating chemo well. No complaints offered.

2/4 Patient well hydrated, nausea and vomiting under control. Will discharge.

Code Assignment Including POA Indicator

ICD-9-CM Principal Diagnosis: _____

ICD-9-CM Additional Diagnoses: _____

ICD-9-CM Procedure Code(s): _____

ICD-10-CM Code(s): _____

ICD-10-PCS Code(s): _____

7.34. Discharge Summary

Date of Admission: 1/3

Date of Discharge: 1/7

Discharge Diagnosis: Recurrent carcinoma, left lung

This is a 63-year-old female who is two years status post left upper lobe resection for adenocarcinoma. Pathology at that time revealed a positive bronchial margin of resection. She was treated with postop radiation and has done extremely well. She has remained asymptomatic with no postoperative difficulty. Follow-up serial CT scans have revealed a new lesion in the apical portion of the left lung, which on needle biopsy was positive for adenocarcinoma. She was admitted specifically for a left thoracotomy and possible pneumonectomy.

Past Medical History: Positive for tobacco abuse 2 PPD × 30 years in the past. Significant for a right parotidectomy and also significant for hypertension, degenerative joint disease of lumbar spine, and chronic pulmonary disease. The patient also suffered a stroke in the left brain with resulting hemiparesis three years ago. Medications on discharge: Tenormin 25 mg once a day, Calan SR 240 mg twice a day, Moduretic one tablet q. day, K-Dur 10 meq q. day, Proventil MDI 2 puffs PO q.i.d. p.r.n., Azacort MDI 2 puffs PO t.i.d., Vioxx 25 mg PO daily.

Physical Examination: Revealed a well-healed right parotid incision. No supraclavicular adenopathy. She has a healed left posterior lateral thoracotomy scar. Impression is that of local recurrence, status post left upper lobectomy. She is to undergo a left pneumonectomy.

Operative Findings and Hospital Course: There was a large mass in the remaining lung, extensive mediastinal fibrosis, bronchial margin free by frozen section. Following surgery she was placed in the intensive care unit postoperatively. The chest tube was removed on postoperative day number two.

She experienced some EKG changes consistent with acute nontransmural MI. Cardiology was consulted, and she was started on nitroglycerin and IV heparin. She was eventually weaned from her oxygen therapy.

She was started on regular diet and was discharged in good condition. Her wound was clean and dry.

Instructions on Discharge: Discharged home with instructions to follow up with cardiology next week. Also follow up with me in the office.

History and Physical

Admitted: 1/3

History of Present Illness: Patient is a 63-year-old right-handed female with history of recurrent adenocarcinoma of apical segment of left upper lobe of lung. She has received radiation therapy to her chest. She weighs 123 pounds. She also has chronic obstructive pulmonary disease.

Review of Systems: She can climb two flights of steps with minimal difficulties. She has a significant underbite. She has stiffness in lower spine, worse in the a.m. She has hypertension and took her Tenormin 25 mg, Calan SR 240 mg this a.m.

Past Surgical History: She had a right parotidectomy seven years ago and was told they needed to use a "very small" ETT. Two years ago she underwent a left upper lobe resection at this facility. Previous medical records are being requested.

Allergies: She is allergic to sulfa. Postoperatively last time she received Demerol. She also had hallucinations in the ICU for several days. She blames the hallucinations on the Demerol. The only allergy sign was hallucinations.

Physical Examination: Revealed a well-healed right parotid incision. No supraclavicular adenopathy. She has a healed left posterior lateral thoracotomy scar. Impression is that of local recurrence, status post left upper lobectomy. She is to undergo a left completion pneumonectomy, muscle flap coverage of bronchial stump. The patient has hemiparesis in the right extremities which is her dominant side.

Impression: Recurrent carcinoma left lower lobe of lung

Plan: Pneumonectomy of left lung. The patient is agreeable to general endotracheal anesthesia or the use of epidural narcotic. She is agreeable to postoperative ventilation if necessary.

Progress Notes

1/3   **Attending Physician:** Admit for recurrent lung carcinoma, s/p radiation therapy. Consent signed for pneumonectomy. Epidural morphine usage postop explained to and discussed with the patient. She is agreeable.

Anesthesia Preop: Patient evaluated and examined. General anesthesia chosen. Patient agrees. Will provide postop epidural morphine for pain management s/p thoracotomy.

Procedure Note:

Preop Dx: Local recurrence of carcinoma of the lung

Postop Dx: Same

Procedure: Pneumonectomy with muscle flap coverage of bronchial stump

Complications: R/O intraop MI

Anesthesia Postop: Patient in stable condition following GEA with possible intraoperative MI due to hypotension. CPK to be evaluated as available. Patient comfortable with epidural morphine. No adverse effects of anesthesia experienced.

1/4   **Attending Physician:** Path report confirms recurrent adenocarcinoma. Patient stable but with persistent hypotension resolving slowly—will consult cardiology. CPK MB positive. Incision clean and dry. COPD stable, arthritis stable.

       Cardiology Consult: The patient has resolving intraoperative myocardial infarction. Will continue to monitor.

1/5   **Attending Physician:** Looks and feels well, weaning off morphine. Blood pressure stable. Left pleural space expanding and filling space. Chest tube removed, epidural cath removed.

       Cardiology Consult: The patient looking and feeling better.

1/6   **Attending Physician:** Patient stable for discharge in a.m. Cardiology to follow.

Operative Report

Date: 1/3

Operation: Pneumonectomy

Preoperative Diagnosis: Recurrent carcinoma of left lung

Postoperative Diagnosis: Same

Anesthesia: General endotracheal anesthesia

Operative Findings: There was a large mass in the left lower lobe.

The patient was prepped and draped in the usual fashion. Following thoracotomy the left lung was completely removed. A muscle flap coverage was used for the bronchial stump. During the procedure the patient experienced an episode of hypotension, watch for resulting MI. The patient was fluid resuscitated and sent to the recovery room in good condition.

Pathology Report

Date: 1/3

Specimen: Left lung, resected

Clinical Data: This is a 63-year-old female with recurrent disease on CT scan

Diagnosis: Adenocarcinoma of the apical portion of the lung, bronchial margin is free of disease

Radiology Reports

Date: 1/3

Chest X-Ray: Reveals mass in the left lower lobe. There are surgical clips in the thorax from apparent previous surgery. The thoracic organs are midline and the vasculature is normal.

Impression: Carcinoma LLL, no congestive heart failure

Date: 1/4

Chest X-Ray: Reveals absence of left lung. Other architecture is normal other than post-operative changes. The thoracic organs are midline and the vasculature is normal.

Impression: Postop changes consistent with lobectomy, no congestive heart failure.

EKG Report

Date: 1/3

Normal sinus rhythm

Date: 1/4

There are nonspecific ST changes consistent with possible evolving myocardial infarction.

Date: 1/5

Possible acute myocardial infarction, please correlate with other clinical findings.

Code Assignment Including POA Indicator

ICD-9-CM Principal Diagnosis: _____

ICD-9-CM Additional Diagnoses: _____

ICD-9-CM Procedure Code(s): _____

ICD-10-CM Code(s): _____

7.35.   The following documentation is from the health record of a 50-year-old female patient.

Discharge Summary: The patient is a 50-year-old female with known carcinoma of the right breast with widespread pulmonary and bone metastases. She recently completed the third of six outpatient chemotherapy treatments for the metastases. The patient also has a history of a right mastectomy for the breast carcinoma two years ago and is no longer receiving any treatment for this carcinoma. The patient was now admitted for treatment of lumps of the lower-outer quadrant of the left breast. A left mastectomy with bilateral insertion of tissue expanders has been recommended as treatment for the lumps of the left breast due to the patient's history of right breast carcinoma with metastases. The patient has agreed to the recommended treatment.

The patient was taken to surgery, and a left simple mastectomy was performed. Via an open approach, tissue expanders were inserted under both pectoral muscles bilaterally, to start the reconstruction process.

Pathology report revealed benign fibroadenoma.

The patient was discharged in satisfactory condition to see me in the office in 10 days.

Code Assignment Including POA Indicator

ICD-9-CM Principal Diagnosis: _____

ICD-9-CM Additional Diagnoses: _____

ICD-9-CM Procedure Code(s): _____

ICD-10-CM Code(s): _____

ICD-10-PCS Code(s): _____

7.36. The following documentation is from the health record of a 72-year-old male patient.

Discharge Summary

History of Present Illness: The patient is a 72-year-old male with a history of abdominal perineal resection for colon cancer in 1985 and left hemicolectomy in 1995 for splenic flexure recurrence of cancer. Subsequent right nephrectomy, right adrenalectomy, right posterior hepatic wedge resection in February for metastatic colon carcinoma. The patient is admitted with complaints of lower back pain and bilateral thigh pain for 2 months, increasing in intensity.

Physical Examination: Examination on admission: Temperature 99°F, pulse 72, respirations 24, blood pressure 150/90. The examination was remarkable for left lower quadrant colostomy from previous operation, mildly tender lumbar spine, and the patient was barely able to stand. It was also noted that the patient had decreased sharp/dull discrimination on the neural examination of the lateral thighs.

Laboratory Data: On admission the laboratory values were: Urinalysis: Specific gravity 1.021, pH 5; chem. tests were negative; nitrite negative; blood negative, 12 white cells, moderate bacteria. The clinical chemistry results were: Serum sodium 141, BUN 42, potassium 4.9, chloride 104, CO_2 28, glucose 99, creatinine 1.8, SGOT 12, SGPT 16, alkaline phosphatase 68, total protein 6.6, albumin 3.8, total bilirubin 0.7, direct bilirubin 0.0, GGT 87, calcium 10.3, magnesium 2.0, phosphorus 3.2, uric acid 5.7, PT 12.9, PTT 28.4, white blood cell count 8.0, hemoglobin 15.0, hematocrit 43.8, platelets 223,000. The CEA level was noted to be 508 nanograms per mL on admission. Metastatic workup for the colon carcinoma revealed no evidence of metastatic disease to the head or the thoracic and cervical spine.

Radiologic Studies: CT and MRI revealed left celiac ganglion node plexus enlarged, diagnosed as metastasis. Multiple small lung nodules, bilaterally, suspicious for metastasis. Pathological fractures of L2 and L4, with compression of L2, effacement of the spinal canal space and apparent cord compression at the L2 level. Subsequent urine culture grew out greater than 10 to the 5th *Pseudomonas aeruginosa*, which was sensitive to ciprofloxacin. The patient was treated for this UTI with ciprofloxacin 500 mg p.o. q. 8 hours and subsequent urine culture showed no growth.

Hospital Course: The patient went to the operating room for L2 laminectomy with decompression and anterior allograft bone fusion. The patient fell 3 days after surgery while ambulating without significant injuries. Further physical therapy was marked by continued improvement in ambulation with walker and no further setbacks. Clinically, the patient is afebrile without signs and symptoms of infection, no CVA tenderness, and no dysuria. The patient will be discharged home today. Condition on discharge fairly good.

Treatment: The patient will go home on Vicodin p.o. q 4 to 6 hours for pain, and Capoten. He will resume Capoten b.i.d. dosing per his internist's recommendations for his hypertension, 25 p.o. b.i.d. Prognosis: The long-term prognosis is poor as the patient has extensive metastatic colon CA; short-term prognosis is fairly good with improvement in ambulation. Ambulation is with walker assistance. Follow-up: The patient will return to see me next Wednesday.

Final Diagnoses: Metastatic colon cancer to lung and bone
Pathologic fracture of L2 secondary to metastasis, with cord compression

Code Assignment Including POA Indicator

ICD-9-CM Principal Diagnosis: _____

ICD-9-CM Additional Diagnoses: _____

ICD-9-CM Procedure Code(s): _____

ICD-10-CM Code(s): _____

ICD-10-PCS Code(s): _____

7.37.   The following documentation is from the health record of a 59-year-old cancer patient.

History and Physical Examination

Present Illness: The patient is a 59-year-old female admitted with a diagnosis of seizure disorder and acute seizure. This patient's illness began last year when she was diagnosed with a metastatic lesion in her brain, which was a metastatic hypernephroma from her right kidney. She had the isolated metastasis removed surgically, had been on Tegretol since then, but she has only been taking her nighttime dosages. The dosages she felt kind of wiped her out a little bit. She then was scheduled for renal surgery but developed chest pain, and a coronary angiogram revealed severe three-vessel disease, inoperable and not a candidate for any kind of surgical procedure. Since then her treatment has been expectant with treatment of chemotherapy per usual protocols. She did not have any radiation to the brain previously. Her CT scan in the ER last night was showing some questionable areas.

Past Medical History: She has had the metastatic lesion to the head, renal carcinoma, and severe coronary artery disease. She had no prior surgeries or illnesses.

Review of Systems: Was doing well until yesterday, but she was taking the treatment and taking her Tegretol mainly at night. Her level was 5.9 where 8 or 9 is therapeutic.

Family History: She is adopted but has a brother. She is divorced with two children. She is living with her daughter. She is on disability from work. She was employed actively.

Physical Examination: She is a well-developed, well-nourished white female.

HEENT: Negative

Neck: No bruits

Chest: Clear

Heart: Regular sinus rhythm

Abdomen: Soft; no masses

Pelvic/Rectal: Deferred at this time

Extremities: Negative

Neurologic: Negative. At this time, the daughter states that her right leg and arm stiffened out during her seizure.

Impression(s): Seizure disorder secondary to metastatic renal to brain. She is to get an MRI done today, and we are going to increase dosage to the Tegretol. I think she can go home and if she does have metastatic lesion, she will probably need to have radiation done and will be set up through a radiation oncologist whom I think has been consulted previously on her condition.

Discharge Summary

Admission Date: 06/01/XX

Discharge Date: 06/03/XX

Consultants: 1. Oncologist
                       2. Neurosurgeon

Discharge Diagnosis

1. Convulsion, secondary to malignant neoplasm of the brain secondary to a hypernephroma

Hospital Course: The patient was seen by the neurosurgeon, who felt conservative management was needed. She is going to begin radiation treatment to her head. This will be done as an outpatient in order to control the metastatic disease to the brain.

Discharge Medications/Instructions: She was discharged home on:

1. Lopressor 50 mg each morning
2. Decadron 4 mg twice a day
3. Tegretol 200 t.i.d. Her Tegretol level was a little low at the time of admission.

So, she will be followed then to begin radiation treatment on Monday for follow-up there.

Consultation

Physical Examination: She is a well-developed, well-nourished white female with partial baldness to the right side of her head. Her neck exam reveals turbulence transmitted from the thorax bilaterally to both carotids. On lung exam there were no crackles or wheezes and her respiratory effort is normal. Cardiac exam reveals S1 and

S2 to be physiologic with no S3 or S4 gallop. There is a murmur at the left ventricular apex most compatible with a flow murmur. The apex is not well palpated. She has no gallop or rub appreciated. Abdominal exam is supple without organomegaly. The back exam is normal. Her extremity exam reveals no clubbing, cyanosis, or edema. HEENT exam reveals partial baldness of the right side of the scalp. There is a well healed craniotomy scar. She has no xanthelasma nor is there any gum bleeding. Her musculature and gait are relatively normal without any obvious lateralizing signs.

Final Assessment: This is a lady who has incredibly severe coronary disease and a poor prognosis with regard to her heart. She tolerated a craniotomy 6 months ago before knowledge of her coronary artery disease. She could probably tolerate another craniotomy but would be at increased risk for a perioperative infarction during general anesthesia. This would be obviously magnified if she had hemodynamic instability. The anticipated surgery would not involve a vascular challenge as would the nephrectomy. Nonetheless, the general anesthetic would pose a cardiovascular risk that seems to be unpreventable. The plan is to proceed with radiation and reserve surgery for nonavoidable indication. I have discussed this with the radiation oncologist, and the patient is most agreeable with this sort of approach as well. I hope this information can be of some help to you. Thanks again.

History of Present Illness: This 59-year-old woman is well known to me, undergoing craniotomy for resection of a metastatic renal cell carcinoma in January of 20XX. At that time she presented with weakness of her left upper and lower extremity. She was continued on a daily Tegretol dose as she did not tolerate Dilantin. She was doing well until she presented with a generalized tonic clonic seizure yesterday and postictal Todd's paralysis which is now resolving. She was brought to the hospital, underwent a CT scan and subsequent MRI scan that does show a solitary lesion in the postoperative bed consistent with recurrence of her metastatic disease. She has never received whole brain radiation postoperatively. Currently she tells me her right kidney was never resected as she has significant cardiovascular disease and was thought by the cardiologist not to be able to tolerate a nephrectomy. Currently treatment options include:

1. Whole brain radiation
2. Surgical removal of the lesion followed by whole brain radiation if she can obtain surgical clearance
3. Possibility of doing stereotactic radiosurgery on the lesion, again followed by whole brain radiation

Recommendations: Currently, I have placed the patient on Decadron 400 mg twice daily and will ask the neurosurgeon and his associates to evaluate the possibility of a craniotomy on the patient.

Which of the following is the correct code assignment?

ICD-9-CM Code(s):

a. 198.3, 189.0, 780.39, 414.01
b. 780.39, 198.3, 189.0, 414.01
c. 189.0, 198.3, 780.39, 414.01
d. 198.3, 189.0, 414.01

ICD-10-CM Code(s): _____

Optional MS-DRG Exercise (for users with access to MS-DRG software or tables)

What is the correct MS-DRG for this case? _____

Which MDC does this MS-DRG belong to? _____

Disorders of the Nervous System and Sense Organs

7.38.   The following documentation is from the health record of a 62-year-old male patient.

Discharge Summary

Admission Diagnosis: Transient ischemic attack, possible stroke

Final Diagnoses

1. Transient vertigo versus posterior circulation transient ischemic attack
2. Non-insulin-dependent diabetes
3. Coronary artery disease status post coronary bypass grafting
4. Hyperlipidemia

Consultants: Neurology

History

This is a 62-year-old white male who was admitted through the Emergency Department with a variety of symptoms, somewhat vague, describing components of dizziness, double vision, slightly slurred speech, vague numbness and tingling of the upper extremities for two or possibly three days. He has had intermittent different episodes off and on over the last two to three months. The patient has several risk factors including coronary disease, hyperlipidemia, and he is a smoker. He was admitted with possible TIAs or CVA.

Hospital Course: After being admitted to the Intermediate Care Unit and Stepdown Unit for monitoring and being started on Heparin, his symptoms resolved very rapidly.

Diagnostics: A CT of the brain indicated a possible ischemic event in the right frontoparietal region and an old lacunar infarct to the basal ganglia on the right. The chest x-ray showed mild congestive heart failure, although this was not clinically apparent. Carotid studies showed minimal abnormalities with approximately 30% disease on the left internal carotid. The right side was normal.

An echocardiogram of the heart indicated minor valvular abnormalities of no significance and an ejection fraction of 35–40%, and no embolic clots were noted. A routine cardiogram showed some old findings of left anterior hemiblock.

As mentioned, the patient's symptoms rapidly resolved. He was seen in consultation by Dr. G. the following morning who felt that he did not need IV heparin for the current event and that aspirin should be sufficient. Some consideration was given that if he had future episodes, of starting either Plavix or possible long-term Coumadin. Arrangements were made for discharge, as the patient's basic clinical status has returned to baseline.

Discharge Medications

1. Glucophage 500 mg b.i.d.
2. Glyburide 5 mg b.i.d.
3. Lipitor 20 mg daily
4. Ecotrin 325 mg daily

Discharge Instructions

Diet—ADA diet, low fat. He was advised at length about smoking cessation. Activity—As tolerated, but no heavy exertion. It was suggested that at some point the patient have an MRI and an MRA as an outpatient and consideration be given to stronger anticoagulation if he has further episodes. Follow-up in the office in approximately one to two weeks.

Emergency Department

History of Present Illness: This is a 62-year-old male who complains of five days of dizziness and three days of weakness, decreasing ambulation, and unsteadiness. He complains of no pain or numbness of the lower extremities, chest pain, fever, or headache. He does complain of having mild vision blurring with turning when he turns his head. The patient has also had slurring of his speech. He was seen yesterday by his private physician who noticed his ataxia and has him scheduled for a magnetic resonance imaging today.

Past Medical History

1. Diabetes mellitus
2. Myocardial infarction times three in the past
3. Coronary artery bypass graft done in the last five years
4. Hypertension
5. Mild neuropathy secondary to his diabetes mellitus

Social History: The patient lives in a private home by himself. He smokes two packs of cigarettes a day. He denies any drinking.

Medications

1. Glucophage
2. Talacen

Allergies: No known allergies.

Review of Systems: Negative except for the pertinent positives and negatives noted in the history of present illness.

Physical Examination

Vital Signs: Temperature is 97. Pulse of 84. Respirations 20. Blood pressure 132/73. General: The patient is mildly sleepy but very alert and cooperative with the examination. HEENT: He is normocephalic. Atraumatic. He has some mild preauricular swelling on the right as compared to the left. His tympanic membranes were normal bilaterally. Extraocular muscles intact. Pupils equal, round, reactive to light and accommodation. Oral pharynx is normal. He did have some staining consistent with tobacco.

Neck: Supple. No adenopathy.

Heart: Regular rate and rhythm without any murmurs, thrills, or rubs. He has 2+ pulses radial and brachial bilaterally.

Lungs: Breath sounds are clear bilaterally with no tachypnea or retraction.

Abdomen: Mildly tender at the left upper quadrant over the rib area. Otherwise the abdomen was soft and nondistended.

Extremities: He had upper and lower extremity strength of +5.

Neurology: There is 212 and grossly intact. He had no pitting edema or other lesions noted. The patient was ataxic.

Laboratory and Diagnostics: Labs were obtained. Basic metabolic profile showed a sodium of 138, potassium 4.0, chloride of 107, bicarbonate of 22, glucose of 106, blood urea nitrogen of 21, and creatinine of 0.8. Calcium is 9.4. PT and partial prothrombin time were 13.2 and 29.8. White blood cell count was 11.4. H&H is 15.4 and 45.7. He had 222,000 platelets, 62 segs, 29 lymphs, 4 monocytes, 3 eosinopllils, and no basophils. CT scan of the head showed a new infarction of the brain and old lacunar infarct.

Emergency Room Course: We talked to the primary care doctor who agreed with the admission of this patient.

Plan: The patient was admitted to a monitored bed. Assisting physician helped coordinate the care, management, and treatment of this patient with myself. The patient is being admitted to the primary care doctor's service.

Neurologic Consultation

History: This is a 62-year-old white male whom we were asked to evaluate regarding dizziness and a possible new stroke.

The patient's neurologic history recently appears to date back to approximately one month ago when he developed what he described as some double vision. He was seeing things side by side. He did see his primary care physician who felt this may have been due to a diabetic extraocular movement palsy, and the patient was given a patch. After three weeks, his symptoms resolved. Around that same time, about a month ago, he noticed some numbness and tingling in his fingertips which at times is still bothersome. He was doing fine until this past Saturday when he had the onset of what sounds like dysequilibrium or vertigo where he had difficulty walking. This was transient and then seemed to resolve. This is not currently a problem for him now, and he is much better. The patient tells me that his son told him he may have had some slurred speech, but he is not aware of it. He reported no other specific symptoms. Specifically, he reported no headache. He denies any new change in his vision in the last week. He reported no other areas of focal numbness or tingling.

He reported no trouble with focal weakness. He felt like his balance was only off for a short period of time but then resolved. His bowel and bladder function had been fine. He has had no nausea or vomiting. He denies any chest pain, palpitations, or shortness of breath. He did see his primary care physician who told him that some of his problems may have been related to recent medication change and felt that otherwise he would be okay. However, when seeing the physician the day of admission, he was noted to be somewhat ataxic and was admitted to rule out a new stroke.

Laboratory Data: Current blood work on admission showed normal electrolytes. Digoxin level was less than 0.3. CPK levels have been normal. White count was 11.4 with the remainder of his CBC normal. INR was normal at 1.3. He has remained neurologically stable since admission.

Diagnostics: MRI and MRA are pending. Echocardiogram was grossly suboptimal with an ejection fraction of 35% to 40%. Carotid ultrasound preliminarily showed no stenosis. Heparin is on hold at this time pending our evaluation and the results of the MRI and MRA.

Current Medications

1. Glucophage
2. Insulin coverage
3. Lasix
4. DiaBeta
5. Lipitor

Neurologic Examination: On exam, the patient is awake and alert. He is fully oriented. He is able to name and repeat. Attention, concentration, and memory are okay. Cranial nerves II–XII are grossly intact. Neck is supple with no bruits. Motor exam appears symmetric with no significant focal weakness. He has fairly good bulk and tone. There is no tremor. Sensory exam is remarkable for stocking glove sensory loss. Reflexes are symmetric and somewhat diminished in the lower extremities. Gait is only minimally wide based and he is able to ambulate on his own without any clear ataxia noted at this time. Coordination testing is symmetric. Romberg is negative. He does have difficulty with heel-to-toe walk.

Impression: The patient presents now with transient vertigo along with some slurred speech. This combined with the recent history of double vision certainly warrants a workup for vertebrobasilar insufficiency.

Recommendations

Echocardiogram as done

Carotid ultrasound as done

MRI and MRA as done

IF MRI and MRA are negative, along with the other studies, then treatment with antiplatelet therapy is certainly reasonable.

Physical therapy

Blood pressure and blood sugar control while avoiding relative hypotension

We will likely need to stop heparin or discontinue its use even while being held, as long as studies appear normal. If all of this is okay, and the patient is stable on his feet, discharge then could be shortly.

Code Assignment Including POA Indicator

ICD-9-CM Principal Diagnosis: _____

ICD-9-CM Additional Diagnoses: _____

ICD-10-CM Code(s): _____

7.39.   The following documentation is from the health record of a 67-year-old female patient.

Discharge Summary

This is a 67-year-old lady with complaints of low back pain, with radiation down her right leg to her foot. This pain has been progressively worse over the past 6 months. She had an MRI scan that showed degenerative disc disease at L2–L3, L3–L4, and L4–L5; L3–L4 with mild central canal stenosis; and facet arthropathy at L3–L4 and L4–L5. She has a past medical history of coronary artery disease, hypertension, and lumbar osteoarthritis. Her current medications include Lipitor, Avapro, Ecotrin, Imdur, Lasix, K-Dur, calcium, and Vioxx. She had a CABG 2 years ago. She also had PTCA with cardiac stents placed 3 years ago. Patient is admitted for lumbar epidural steroid injections for her lumbar radiculopathy—as noted on MRI results.

Which of the following is the correct code assignment?

ICD-9-CM Code(s):

a. 722.52, 721.3, 724.02, 724.4, 414.00, 401.9, V45.81, V45.82, 03.92, 99.23, 88.93
b. 724.4, 414.00, 401.9, V45.81, V45.82, 03.92, 99.23, 88.93
c. 722.52, 721.3, 414.00, 401.9, V45.81, V45.82, 03.92, 99.23, 88.93
d. 722.52, 721.3, 414.00, 401.9, V45.81, V45.82, 03.91, 88.93

ICD-10-CM Code(s): _____

ICD-10-PCS Code(s): _____

Optional MS-DRG Exercise (for users with access to MS-DRG software or tables)

Which of the following statements is true regarding the MS-DRG assignment for this case?

a. This case is assigned to a medical MS-DRG.
b. This case is assigned to a surgical MS-DRG.
c. MS-DRG assignment is changed based on the procedure code (03.92).
d. The MS-DRG assigned to this case falls into MDC 1, diseases and disorders of the nervous system.

Newborn/Congenital Disorders

7.40. The following documentation is from the health record of an 18-day-old baby boy.

Discharge Summary

This is an 18-day-old male infant who was admitted after he was noticed to be developing omphalitis. He was immediately placed on intravenous cefotaxime and ampicillin, later changed to cefotaxime and clindamycin. A culture taken from the umbilical stump grew *Staphylococcus aureus* and group H *Streptococcus*.

After the first day, there was great improvement, and the patient continued to improve completely. Now there is no redness or swelling whatsoever. The child has remained afebrile and has continued to eat very well. He shows no sign of abdominal tenderness or peritonitis. I feel that we have treated this well. He has had 5 days of intravenous antibiotics. I will finish the treatment with Keflex by mouth seeing that both *Streptococcus pyogenes* and *Staphylococcus aureus* are sensitive. The mother will watch the child closely and let me know if any problems occur. I have instructed her to watch for any more redevelopment of the redness, swelling, or discharge. We will recheck this in 2 weeks at his 1-month checkup.

Which of the following answers contains the correct diagnostic code(s) for this admission?

ICD-9-CM Code(s):

a. 771.2, 041.09
b. 686.9, 041.11, 041.09
c. 771.4
d. 771.4, 041.11, 041.09

ICD-10-CM Code(s): _____

7.41. The following documentation is from the health record of a three-day-old baby boy.

Discharge Summary

The patient is a 3-day-old male infant. He was born at home after approximately 38 weeks' gestation and brought to the Emergency Room shortly thereafter with difficulty breathing. The baby's respirations were very quick and shallow. This was the mother's fourth child, all of whom have been born at home. This was the first child born with complications.

The newborn was resuscitated and placed in the NICU under continuous oxygen therapy.

Admission history and physical examination were otherwise unremarkable. Chest x-ray showed wet lungs. Repeat chest x-ray 24 hours later showed the lungs had cleared. PKU specimen was taken and sent to the state laboratory, as required.

By the second day of hospitalization, the patient was able to be weaned off the oxygen and discharged from the NICU to a bassinet.

The mother requested that the baby be circumcised. This was accomplished without incident.

The infant is discharged to be seen in the clinic at 1 month for a well-baby visit.

Which of the following answers is correct to code this admission?

ICD-9-CM Code(s):

a. 770.6, V30.10, V50.2, 96.04
b. V30.1, 770.6, V50.2, 64.0, 93.93, 93.96
c. V30.1, 769, V50.2, 64.0, 96.04
d. V30.10, 768.6, V50.2, 64.0, 96.05, 93.96

ICD-10-CM Code(s): _____

ICD-10-PCS Code(s): _____

Optional MS-DRG Exercise (for users with access to MS-DRG software or tables)

In addition to the principal diagnosis, the MS-DRG for this admission is based upon which of the following factors listed below?

a. Complication or comorbid condition
b. Major complication or comorbid condition
c. Procedure code
d. Other significant problems

7.42.   The patient is a 3-year-old child with congenital patent ductus arteriosus. The patient has had several open-heart surgeries attempting to correct the defect. The patient was born prematurely at 34 weeks' gestation. The patient continues to be below average on standard growth charts in size and weight, and the mother states the child is not very active.

Recent echocardiogram revealed an area of the aorta leaking blood into the pulmonary artery. The child is now admitted for further corrective surgery.

On the day after admission, the child was taken to the OR. Open-chest surgery was performed through the existing scar, and the ribs were spread to gain access to the operative field. Several areas of communication between the aorta and the left pulmonary artery were identified and closed. The chest was then closed. Throughout the procedure, the patient's vital signs were monitored and remained at satisfactory levels. The patient tolerated the procedure well.

The day after surgery, the patient was allowed to be up and walking. The child appeared to have increased energy and was a healthy pink color. The child was eating and asking for more.

The patient was discharged on the third postop day to be followed as an outpatient in the cardiac education center.

Final Diagnosis: Patent ductus arteriosus

Which of the following answers is correct to code this admission?

ICD-9-CM Code(s):

a. 747.0, 765.10, 765.27, 38.85
b. 745.9, 35.39
c. 747.0, 38.85
d. 745.0, 38.85

ICD-10-CM Code(s): _____

ICD-10-PCS Code(s): _____

7.43. The following documentation is from the health record of a five-year-old girl.

Discharge Summary

The patient is a 5-year-old female child born with myelomeningocele spina bifida. The patient has previously undergone several procedures to cover the defect at the bottom of her spine, including the insertion of a ventriculoperitoneal (VP) shunt to drain the cerebrospinal fluid (CSF) accumulation from her hydrocephalus.

The patient was admitted this morning through the emergency department with a plugged shunt. The child was rushed to the OR for emergent irrigation of the shunt. Irrigation was attempted several times but was unsuccessful. Therefore, the shunt was removed and replaced with another VP shunt.

The patient tolerated the procedure, although she was very anxious about having surgery and being in the hospital. Her parents were very caring and present to calm her at all times.

The patient was discharged on the second day postop to be followed in the office.

Final Diagnoses: Congenital myelomeningocele spina bifida
Plugged VP shunt

Operative Report

Preoperative Diagnosis: Plugged VP Shunt

Postoperative Diagnosis: Plugged VP Shunt

Procedure: Ventriculoperitoneal shunt revision

Description of Procedure: After informed consent was obtained from the parents, the patient was taken to the operating room. General anesthesia was induced. The patient's head was turned to the left side and the posterior scalp was prepped and draped in usual fashion. Sutures from previous surgery were removed.

A new bur hole site was identified posterior and lateral to the previous entry site to approach the lateral ventricle. Cautery dissection was carried out to establish the subgaleal plane and a pocket was created. The previous incision was opened and the shunt valve was encountered and dismantled. The shunt was found to be plugged. Attempts were made to connect a new valve system from the new pocket to the old pocket. This was not successful therefore the entire old shunt system was removed.

The abdominal incision was again explored before removing the old shunt. A new valve with a new distal catheter was tunneled from the new pocket. The catheter was guided into the frontal horn and connected to the distal system and the distal catheter was then placed into the peritoneal cavity without difficulty.

All wounds were copiously irrigated. The skull defect at the previous site was filled with cranioplasty material and all wounds were sutured closed. Sterile dressings were applied and the patient was taken to the recovery room in good condition.

Which of the following answers is correct to code this admission?

ICD-9-CM Code(s):

a. 996.75, 741.03, 02.42
b. 996.2, 741.03, 02.41, 02.42
c. 741.03, V45.2, 02.42, 02.43
d. 996.75, 742.3, 741.00, 02.42

ICD-10-CM Code(s): _____

ICD-10-PCS Code(s): _____

Pediatric Conditions

7.44.   The following documentation is from the health record of a 13-year-old boy.

Preoperative Diagnosis: Right inguinal hernia, hypospadias

Postoperative Diagnosis: Same

Operation: Right inguinal herniorrhaphy, repair of hypospadias

Indications: The patient is a 13-year-old male with reducible right inguinal hernia and hypospadias who now presents for definitive care.

Procedure: The patient was brought to the operating room and placed in the supine position. After the adequate general endotracheal anesthesia, a 4-cm incision was made in the right inguinal region. The subcutaneous tissues were divided, and hemostasis achieved with electrocautery. The external oblique fascia was identified and cleaned using Metzenbaum scissors. An incision was made in the external oblique and carried down to the external ring using Metzenbaum scissors. The external oblique was freed from the underlying cord using two pairs of forceps. The cremasteric fibers were divided and the hernia sac grasped. Pulling the hernia sac up on some tension, we were then able to tease off the cremasteric fibers, as well as the vas and vessels. At this point, we were able to control the hernia sac between the two hemostats. We then teased off the vas and vessels as we dissected proximally toward the internal ring. At this point, the sac was twisted, sutured ligated, × 2, amputated, and then the sac was allowed to fall back into the peritoneal cavity. We continued the dissection distally. The anterior wall was opened using electrocautery. At this point, we placed the cord back into the inguinal canal. The external oblique fascia was closed using interrupted 4-0 silk sutures. The external oblique fascia and the structures below it were infiltrated using .05 percent Marcaine. The Scarpa's fascia was closed using 5-0 VICRYL. The skin was closed using interrupted 5-0 subcuticular stitches. Steri-Strips were applied.

With this completed, attention was then turned to repairing the hypospadias. Procedure commenced by placing a 4-0 Prolene stay suture through the glans for traction and observing the distal shaft penile hypospadias without chordee and with a dorsal hooded foreskin.

The urethroplasty was begun by making parallel lines with a marking pen on either side of the urethral meatus, going out to the tip of the glans, connecting these proximally from the meatus for a distance of about 2.5 cm. With a tourniquet used intermittently, an incision was made in these lines to create two rectangular flaps connected at the urethral meatus. On the left side of the meatus there was a small nevus just lateral to the incision line, and the incision was extended around this to excise a small nevus, less than 0.6 cm in diameter, which will be sent for pathology. After mobilization of both skin flaps, the proximal one off of the shaft and the ventral one off of the underlying tissue of the glans, optical magnification was used to convert these two flaps into a neourethral tube using 6-0 PDS sutures. The neourethral tube came together quite well.

Next, an incision was made in the midline, out to the tip of the glans, through the incision point at the previous site of the distal flap, to accomplish mobilization of the urethra and advance this urethra out to the tip of the glans. Wedge-shaped areas of glandular tissue were excised to make a smooth passageway for the neourethra. Then the neourethra was sutured into position at the tip of the glans with 6-0 and 5-0 PDS sutures.

Next, a second layer was created by approximating the subcutaneous tissue, adventitial tissue, and elements of the corpus spongiosum over the neourethral reconstruction at the corona, and carrying this with a running 6-0 PDS suture proximally to provide a second layer of coverage.

When this was done, the glans itself was approximated with 4-0 PDS sutures, placing about three sutures into position to firmly reconnect the wings of the glans and to keep them from pulling apart. This left an aperture for the neourethra, which was then sutured into position with 4-0 and 5-0 PDS sutures. When this was done, a #11 French Silastic catheter was used, and a portion of its wall was cut out to turn it into a splint. It was positioned into the urethra and sutured into place at the meatus with a 4-0 Prolene suture to hold it into position. The next step was to close the skin defect on the ventral shaft with interrupted 3-0 chromic catgut suture.

The next part of the operation involved performing circumcision of the redundant dorsal and lateral preputial tissue. First, this was marked with a marking pen, and then an incision was made in the pen lines to allow excision of the redundant foreskin. Hemostasis was obtained with electrocautery, and 3-0 chromic catgut suture was used to complete the circumcision.

The next step was to consider the ability of this patient to void. Because of his hernial repair and this operation on the prepuce, I was afraid he would be in urinary retention. I therefore inserted a #8 French feeding tube through the #11 French Silastic catheter, passed it all the way into the bladder, and allowed it to drain urine freely. Then a light sterile dressing of 1-inch Adaptic roller gauze soaked in tincture of benzoin was loosely wrapped around the shaft for mild compression and hemostasis. The last few wraps of this incorporated the catheter.

The patient was taken to the recovery room in satisfactory condition.

Which of the following code sets is correct for reporting this operative episode?

ICD-9-CM Code(s):

a. 752.61, 550.91, 752.69, 58.49, 53.02, 64.0, 57.94
b. 752.61, 605, 550.90, 239.5, 58.47, 53.01, 64.2, 57.94
c. 752.61, 550.91, 752.69, 58.49, 53.00, 57.94
d. 752.61, 605, 550.90, 222.1, 58.45, 53.02, 64.0, 64.2, 57.94

ICD-10-CM Code(s): _____

ICD-10-PCS Code(s): _____

7.45. The following documentation is from the health record of an 11-year-old boy.

Preoperative Diagnoses: 1. Ewing sarcoma, left scapula
                              2. Down syndrome

Postoperative Diagnosis: Same

Findings: This is an 11-year-old boy with Down syndrome who presented 4 days ago with a large mass in the left scapular region. Outpatient x-ray and CT scan showed laminated new bone with a large, expansile, permeative lesion in the scapular body. It did not appear to involve the glenohumeral joint. Outpatient bone scan showed marked increased uptake and questionable area of uptake in the right seventh rib and left first vertebral body. CT of the lungs was reportedly normal. At the time of biopsy, there was obvious stretching of the posterior trapezius and deltoid musculature over the mass and a very soft calcific mass noted within the central area of the substance. Frozen pathology sections showed many small cells, but definitive diagnosis could not be made off the frozen section. Final pathologic diagnosis was malignant bone tumor consistent with Ewing sarcoma. He will be started on a chemotherapy program, and definitive surgery will be planned.

Procedure: Following an adequate level of general endotracheal anesthesia, the patient was turned to the right lateral decubitus position with the left side up. The left shoulder region was prepped and draped in routine sterile fashion. Before beginning the biopsy, a venous access device was inserted into the subcutaneous tissue of the abdominal wall on the right side using an open approach.

A 3-cm incision was then made over the spine of the scapula. Electrocautery was used for hemostasis and the incision deepened with electrocautery. When we were in the area of the soft-tissue mass noted on the CT scan, biopsies were taken. The initial biopsies showed primarily muscle fibers, so we deepened the incision at this point and obtained some of the obvious calcific soft-tissue mass. These cultures were more consistent with tumor, and, at this point, hemostasis was achieved with a combination of bone wax, packing, and electrocautery. Meticulous hemostasis was achieved prior to closure, and then a two-layer interrupted closure was performed, closing the skin with a running subcuticular suture of 4-0 VICRYL. Bulky dry sterile dressing was applied, and the patient was awakened and returned to the recovery room in good condition.

Which of the following is the correct code set to report this procedure?

ICD-9-CM Code(s):

a. 170.4, 758.0, 77.41
b. 170.4, 170.3, 170.2, 77.81

c. 170.4, 758.0, 77.61, 86.07

d. 170.4, 758.0, 77.41, 86.07

ICD-10-CM Code(s): _____

ICD-10-PCS Code(s): _____

Optional MS-DRG Exercise (for users with access to MS-DRG software or tables)

What is the correct MS-DRG assignment for this admission?

a. 517, Other musculoskeletal system and connective tissue OR procedure without CC/MCC

b. 497, Local excision and removal internal fixation devices except hip and femur without CC/MCC

c. 479, Biopsies of musculoskeletal system and connective tissue without CC/MCC

d. 477, Biopsies of musculoskeletal system and connective tissue with MCC

Conditions of Pregnancy, Childbirth, and the Puerperium

7.46.   The following documentation is from the health record of a 19-year-old female patient.

Discharge Diagnosis:
1. Term pregnancy
2. Previous cesarean section
3. Failed attempt at vaginal birth after cesarean delivery
4. Arrest of descent, secondary to occiput posterior position

Procedures Performed: Repeat low transverse cesarean delivery

History of Present Illness: The patient is a 19-year-old, gravida 3, para 1 with an estimated date of delivery in two weeks. She is with a 37-week pregnancy. She has prior beta strep culture, positive. She underwent spontaneous rupture of membranes. Shortly after the rupture of the membranes the patient went to the hospital. Upon admission, the patient's membranes were ruptured.

Hospital Course: The patient was started on intravenous Clindamycin for positive group B strep. Further, she was started on Pitocin for induction of labor because of the premature rupture of membranes. The patient had a slow labor course, eventually establishing a good labor curve. She dilated completely to a zero station but failed to descend with pushing. Then the decision was made to perform a low transverse cesarean delivery because of arrest of descent resulting in obstruction. She underwent a cesarean delivery without complications. Estimated blood loss was 600 cc. This resulted in delivery of a live male infant weighing 7 pounds 4 ounces having Apgars of 9 at one minute and 9 at five minutes.

Postoperatively, the patient did well. She was ambulating and tolerating her diet. She was afebrile and her incision looked clear so the patient was discharged home on the third postoperative day.

Medications/Aftercare Plan

1. The patient is to limit her activity around the home for a one-week period.
2. She will be followed up in the office in one to two weeks.
3. Birth control method was discussed and the patient is considering Depo-Provera. She will finalize her decision on this and let us know in the office.

The patient's discharge medications consist of:

1. Motrin 800 mg one every eight hours p.r.n.
2. Tylenol #3 1–2 every four hours p.r.n.
3. The patient should continue her prenatal vitamins and irons.
4. Colace 100 mg b.i.d.
5. There are no diet restrictions.

Assign the correct codes:

ICD-9-CM Principal Diagnosis: _____

ICD-9-CM Additional Diagnoses: _____

ICD-9-CM Procedure Code(s): _____

ICD-10-CM Code(s): _____

ICD-10-PCS Code(s): _____

7.47. Discharge Summary

Date of Admission: 2/3

Date of Discharge: 2/5

Discharge Diagnosis: Full-term pregnancy (39 weeks)—delivered male infant

Patient started labor spontaneously three days before her due date. She was brought to the hospital by automobile. Labor progressed for a while but then contractions became fewer and she delivered soon after. A midline episiotomy was done. Membranes and placenta were complete. There was some bleeding but not excessive. Patient made an uneventful recovery.

History and Physical

Admitted: 2/3

Reason for Admission: Full-term pregnancy

Past Medical History: Previous deliveries normal and mitral valve prolapse

Allergies: None known

Chronic Medications: None

Family History: Heart disease—father

Social History: The patient is married and has one other child living with her.

Review of Systems

  Skin: Normal

  Head/Scalp: Normal

Eyes: Normal

ENT: Normal

Neck: Normal

Breasts: Normal

Thorax: Normal

Lungs: Normal

Heart: Slight midsystolic click with late systolic murmur II/VI

Abdomen: Normal

Impression: Good health with term pregnancy. History of mitral valve prolapse—asymptomatic

Progress Notes

2/3:   Admit to Labor and Delivery. MVP stable. Patient progressing well. Delivered at 1:15 p.m. one full-term male infant.

2/4:   Patient doing well. MVP prolapse stable. The perineum is clean and dry, incision intact.

2/5:   Will discharge to home.

Delivery Record

Date: 2/3

The patient was 3 cm dilated when admitted. The duration of the first stage of labor was 6 hours, second stage was 14 minutes, third stage was 5 minutes. She was given local anesthesia. An episiotomy was performed with episiorrhaphy repair. The cord was wrapped once around the baby's neck, but did not cause compression. The mother and liveborn baby were discharged from the delivery room in good condition.

Code Assignment Including POA Indicator

ICD-9-CM Principal Diagnosis: _____

ICD-9-CM Additional Diagnoses: _____

ICD-9-CM Procedure Code(s): _____

ICD-10-CM Code(s): _____

ICD-10-PCS Code(s): _____

7.48.   The following documentation is from the health record of a 32-year-old female patient.

Inpatient admission: The patient, gravida II, para 1, was admitted at approximately 33 weeks gestation with mild contractions. She was contracting every 7-8 minutes. An ultrasound showed twins of approximately 4 pounds each. The patient was given magnesium sulfate to stop the contractions, but she contracted through the drug. After developing a fever with suspected chorioamnionitis, a low cervical cesarean section was performed. The umbilical cord was wrapped tightly around the neck of twin 1.

Discharge diagnoses: Cesarean delivery of liveborn twins prematurely at 33 weeks gestation; chorioamnionitis; umbilical cord compression.

Code Assignment Including POA Indicator

ICD-9-CM Principal Diagnosis: _____

ICD-9-CM Additional Diagnoses: _____

ICD-9-CM Procedure Code(s): _____

ICD-10-CM Code(s): _____

ICD-10-PCS Code(s): _____

7.49. ## Discharge Summary

Admission Diagnosis: A 38-week intrauterine pregnancy with leaking amniotic fluid

Discharge Diagnosis: Postpartum female—status post classical cesarean section secondary to prolonged second stage of labor; endomyometritis, postoperative ileus, persistent fever—suspected septic pelvic thrombophlebitis; wound seroma

Operative Procedure: Classical cesarean section

Admission History: This is a 26-year-old gravida 1, para 0 female who presented at 38 weeks gestation complaining of leaking fluid in the morning. She had very mild leaking noted. She had positive nitrazine. She had no gush of fluid at that time and good fetal movement. She had some mild cramping and minimal contractions. No nausea, vomiting, headache, or shortness of breath. No chest pain. Her pregnancy had been uncomplicated. She has had mildly elevated blood pressures over the past couple of weeks, but otherwise nothing significant.

Past medical and social history is negative.

Ob-Gyn History: She is gravida 1

OB Laboratory Data: Blood type is O positive. Antibody screen negative. HIV negative. GBS negative. Rubella nonimmune. RPR nonreactive. Hepatitis B negative.

Objective

Vital Signs: Stable; BP: Elevated at 152/102; it did come down between the 130 to 140s/70 to 80

Lungs: Clear to auscultation

Heart: Regular rate and rhythm

Abdomen: Soft and nontender

Pelvic: Cervix is 1 cm, 70% effaced, and –2 station. The amniotic bag could still be palpated, but it was thought that the patient might be leaking fluid; therefore, artificial rupture of membranes was performed with clear fluid. Tocol showed irregular contractions.

Assessment and Plan: Term intrauterine pregnancy at 38 weeks with mild leaking of fluid. The patient is admitted, and she is given an IV Hep-lock with expectant management.

Hospital Course: The patient did require Pitocin augmentation, as after several hours, she was not contracting adequately. She progressed slowly but adequately over the next 24 hours. She was completely dilated at approximately 7:00 in the morning. She began pushing. She pushed for 3 hours. The baby progressed from a +1 to a +2–3 station. She had no further progression. She was counseled on the risks regarding cesarean section versus forceps delivery. The patient did elect for a cesarean section. She is, therefore, taken for a C-section; see operative report for details. The patient did undergo a classical cesarean section due to the fact that the fetal head could not be reduced from the vagina, and a classical was performed in order to grab the fetal feet and deliver in a breech fashion.

Postoperatively the patient did become febrile within a few hours, and this was felt to be caused by endomyometritis due to the prolonged rupture, prolonged labor, and the significant manipulation of the uterus with cesarean section. The patient was started on Ancef during the procedure and was started on gentamicin within 12 hours of the surgery. The patient continued on IV antibiotics. Her temperature continued to spike on a fairly regular basis over the next 2 postoperative days. She was tolerating a regular diet and ambulating, in addition to passing minimal flatus. On postoperative day 1 she did have a fever as high as 103°F with a tachycardic episode in the 160s. She was somewhat lightheaded when she was out of bed to go to the restroom, but improved with rest. Her heart rate did decrease at that point. An EKG was done and this showed sinus tachycardia. She denied any shortness of breath or chest pain. No nausea or vomiting. Her laboratory studies showed her hemoglobin to be 8.9, white count 12, with a morning repeat of 8.8 and a white count of 9. Blood cultures also were done at that time.

On postoperative day 2, the patient was beginning to feel distended. Her pain was getting worse secondary to the descent. She denied any shortness of breath or chest pain. She was still passing some flatus, but minimal. No nausea or vomiting. On examination her temperature was 103.3°F, which was the maximum. Her abdomen is soft; however, she did have moderate to severe distention at that time. She had good bowel sounds in all the quadrants. Her incision was intact. The extremities showed no calf tenderness. A chest x-ray was done because of the continued elevated temperature; there was bowel distension and suspected ileus. Abdominal x-rays were then done which did confirm an ileus, but no signs of bowel obstruction. Her hemoglobin was repeated and showed 7.4 with stable platelets. Blood cultures were negative, as well as her urine. BUN and creatinine were normal. The patient was made n.p.o. and given an NG tube for the postoperative ileus. She did note some relief to her abdominal discomfort and pain. She was afebrile throughout most of the day at that time. The NG tube had 250 cc out initially.

On postoperative day 3, the NG tube was continued, and her belly was somewhat less distended. She continued to pass flatus and her pain was otherwise controlled. Her temperature was 101.6°F, and clindamycin was added to the antibiotic regimen to treat the persistent fevers. On examination, her distention was improved. She was still having some bowel sounds, although hypoactive. The incision showed no significant erythema. Blood cultures remained negative, and the NG tube was continued with intermittent suction.

On postoperative day 4, the patient was feeling better and producing stools. No nausea or vomiting or shortness of breath, chest pain, dizziness, or lightheadedness. She was having normal lochia and pain was controlled. The NG tube had collected a minimal amount overnight, and her temperature was 101.6°F. She was then started on a clear diet and, if tolerated, the NG tube was to be discontinued. Her hemoglobin level was

6.9, with a decreased potassium level of 3.2. All other lab work was essentially normal. The NG tube was discontinued, and she was given KCl to replace her potassium.

On postoperative day 5, she continued to be febrile with a temperature of 101.5°F. The abdomen was soft and nondistended. She was appropriately tender, more on the left side than the right. The incision still appeared well. Laboratory studies showed the hemoglobin to be 6.8 and stable. Her potassium continued to decrease to 3.1. At that time a CT of the abdomen and pelvis was ordered to rule out a pelvic abscess. *C. difficile* was ordered due to continued diarrhea. Another physician was consulted. A suspicion of septic pelvic thrombophlebitis was then entertained as her fever continued despite adequate antibiotic therapy. The patient was started on Lovenox, and the CT scan showed normal postoperative changes, but no evidence of an abscess.

On postoperative day 6, she was feeling better and had no further diarrhea. *C. difficile* was negative and she was tolerating a regular diet. Her incision did show some erythema, and it was probed with some serosanguineous drainage from the left side, but no purulent drainage. Her laboratory studies were stable, and she was continued on Lovenox and antibiotics. The incision was to be cleaned twice daily.

Postoperative day 7, the patient continued to improve and was feeling well. She was tolerating a regular diet and remained afebrile in which she remained for 27 hours and therefore was discharged home.

Consultation Report: The patient is a 26-year-old female who is gravida 1, now para 1. The patient required a C-section because of prolonged labor and maternal exhaustion. The patient was ruptured for a little over 24 hours prior to delivery. The C-section was complicated by the inability to reduce the fetal head from the vaginal canal and was converted to a breech extraction; therefore, the patient had a primary low transverse C-section that had to be converted to a classical C-section. The patient had some tachycardia on the date of delivery. Ancef was continued and gentamicin was started. On postoperative day 1, she developed a temperature up to 103°F. Urinalysis was unremarkable, along with blood cultures. A chest x-ray revealed some atelectasis at the bases, which the radiologist ultimately felt was possibly consistent with bibasilar pneumonia. At that point the patient was switched from Ancef to ceftriaxone; clindamycin was added on postoperative day 2.

It was noted on the chest x-ray that she had a probable ileus, which was confirmed on the abdominal films. She was placed n.p.o. and an NG tube to intermittent suction was started. The fevers persisted with concomitant chills through today, postoperative day 5; however, now her temperature spikes are more in the 101°F range. The patient's ileus has resolved, and she is tolerating a normal diet. The patient clinically had endometritis after the delivery with a tender lower abdomen. However, this has gradually improved even though her fevers are persisting.

Review of systems performed in addition to physical examination.

Data Interpretation: Laboratory data reviewed; chest x-ray also reviewed by myself revealed some atelectatic changes in the lung bases with bibasilar patchy infiltrates read as possible hypostatic pneumonia. Follow-up x-ray 3 days later revealed definite improvement with less bibasilar infiltrated, now with just some minimal atelectatic changes in the left lung base. CT scan today revealed an enlarged uterus with prominent endometrial stripes, felt to be probably iatrogenic from the surgery. There was some pelvic cobwebbing, but no obvious abscess and some subcutaneous edema anterior in the abdomen with some pockets of gas, also felt to be iatrogenic. With all of these factors, infection could not be entirely excluded. No obvious evidence of thrombophlebitis was seen.

Assessment: Persistent postpartum fever with clinical evidence of endometritis initially that has improved. The patient has had good broad-spectrum antibiotic coverage and with persistent fever, the possibility of a pelvic septic thrombophlebitis must be entertained.

Diarrhea with negative *C. difficile*, possibly still related to antibiotics; also Prevacid has been shown to cause diarrhea.

Postoperative anemia—stable.

Heart murmur—likely secondary to her anemia and being immediately postpartum.

Hypokalemia, which has been difficult to normalize—likely related to GI losses.

Plan: She has received appropriate IV antibiotic coverage for her endomyometritis and no other source of infection is identified; would recommend that anticoagulation be initiated for the possibility of pelvic septic thrombophlebitis or ovarian vein thrombosis.

Would recommend continuing the patient's current antibiotic coverage; however, because the most recent x-ray did not show significant evidence of pneumonia, the ceftriaxone could be discontinued.

Would recommend adding potassium to her IV fluids to try to correct her hypokalemia. The hypokalemia could add to her ileus.

If the patient does not improve in the next couple of days, other considerations would be to add amp or Unasyn to her regimen for possible resistant organism, such as *Enterococcus*. Also agree with continued intermittent blood cultures if she continues to spike.

Her anemia is stable, would recommend continuing to watch for now; however, if it drops or she becomes symptomatic, transfuse.

Consider echo if fever persists to rule out endocarditis.

Operative Report

Preoperative Diagnosis: Gravida 1 para 0 female at 38 weeks' gestation; prolonged rupture of membranes; prolonged second stage of labor with failure to descend

Postoperative Diagnosis: Same

Operation: Primary cesarean section, classical

Anesthesia: Epidural

Complications: Classical extension of initially low transverse incision

Findings: Viable female infant; complete placenta with three-vessel cord; normal uterus, tubes, and ovaries

Indications: This is a 26-year-old female gravida 1 para 0 who presented at 38 weeks' gestation with complaints of leaking fluid. The patient was approximately 1 cm dilated and 80% effaced at that time. She was felt to be having some leaking, although membranes could still be palpated. Therefore, artificial rupture of membranes was performed. The patient progressed very slowly in labor and required Pitocin augmentation. Over the next 24 hours, she progressed to finally complete dilation and began pushing for 3 hours. She started at approximately 0 to +1 station and progressed to + 2 or 3 station. Fetal head was seen with separation of the labia; however, after 3 hours and maternal exhaustion, she made no further progression of the fetal head over the last hour of pushing. The patient was counseled regarding the need for assistance, and forceps assistance versus cesarean section were offered. The risk and benefits of both were explained, and the patient opted for a cesarean section.

Technique: The patient was taken to the operating room and placed under epidural anesthesia. She was prepped and draped in the normal sterile fashion in dorsal supine position with leftward tilt. Pfannenstiel skin incision was made two fingerbreadths above the symphysis pubis in the midline and carried through to the underlying fascia. The fascia was incised in the midline and extended laterally with Mayo scissors. The rectus muscles were dissected off the fascia using both blunt and sharp dissection. Rectus muscles were then separated in the midline. The peritoneum was entered bluntly and extended superiorly and inferiorly. The bladder blade was inserted. The vesicouterine peritoneum was grasped with pickups and entered with Metzenbaum scissors. This was extended laterally, and the bladder flap was created digitally. The bladder blade was reinserted. The lower uterine segment was incised in a transverse fashion with a scalpel and extended laterally with blunt dissection. The infant's head was very low in the pelvis. Attempt to deliver the fetal head was difficult, and we were unable to reduce the fetal head from the vaginal canal. Nursing staff did apply pressure to the fetal head from the vaginal canal, but still was unable to be dislodged. An attempt was made to retract on the shoulders of the infant in order to dislodge the fetal head from the vaginal canal, but again this was unsuccessful. For this reason, the uterine incision was extended vertically in a classical fashion, and the feet were grasped and pulled to the uterine incision. The feet were then delivered, and the infant was delivered in a breech fashion. Nose and mouth were suctioned and cord was clamped and cut. The infant was then handed off to the waiting pediatrician.

Cord gas was obtained. The cord blood was inadvertently not obtained. The placenta was removed. The uterus was cleared of clots and debris. The uterus was exteriorized for better visualization; 0 VICRYL sutures were used to close the vertical incision in the uterus in several layers. Two layers were done initially, then the transverse portion of the incision was closed. There was a cervical extension distally, and this was also closed with 0 VICRYL sutures. Once the transverse portion of the incision was closed, attention was again turned back to the vertical incision. The uterus was returned to the abdomen and inspection of the incision appeared to be hemostatic. With all the layers being closed, the sponge, lap, and needle counts were correct $\times$ 2. The patient tolerated the procedure well and was taken to the recovery room in stable condition.

Progress Notes

Postop day 1: Patient with episode of tachycardia consistent with endomyometritis

Postop day 2: Abdomen feels distended endomyometritis, suspect ileus

Postop day 3: Endomyometritis, ileus

Postop day 4: Ileus resolved, temperature improving

Postop day 5: Continued fever, endomyometritis, internal med consult

Postop day 6: Prolonged postpartum fever with initial endometritis, probable pelvic septic thrombophlebitis—on Lovenox, postop anemia, stable; hypokalemia—improved

Postop day 7: Patient improved; will discharge home

Code Assignment Including POA Indicator

ICD-9-CM Principal Diagnosis: _____

ICD-9-CM Additional Diagnoses: _____

ICD-9-CM Procedure Code(s): _____

ICD-10-CM Code(s): _____

ICD-10-PCS Code(s): _____

Disorders of the Respiratory System

7.50. The following documentation is from the health record of a 57-year-old male patient.

Preoperative Diagnosis: Chronic right calf skin ulcer with necrosis of the bone; *E. coli* sepsis with acute respiratory failure and disseminated intravascular coagulation (DIC)

Postoperative Diagnosis: Same

Procedure: Right below-the-knee amputation

Description of Procedure: The patient was brought to the operating room and placed supine on the operating room table. The patient was placed under general endotracheal anesthesia. A tourniquet was placed on the right proximal thigh and the right lower extremity was prepped and draped in a standard sterile fashion.

A below-the-knee amputation was carried out directly below the tibial tubercle with a posteriorly based flap. The skin and soft tissue were cut sharply to bone along the line of the skin incision. Once the soft tissue was incised the tibia and fibula were provisionally cut with an oscillating saw and the remainder of the right lower extremity was removed and sent to pathology. Next, the tibia and fibula were dissected out subperiosteally proximal to the anterior portion of the skin incision and re-cut with the oscillating saw. The anterior portion of the tibia was beveled again with the oscillating saw and smoothed with a rasp. The fibular cut was beveled in a lateral to medial direction while extending posteriorly.

The nerves and blood vessels were then addressed. The anterior tibial and posterior tibial arteries, as well as the peroneal artery and attendant veins, were suture ligated with #1 Vicryl suture. The anterior and posterior tibial nerves and peroneal nerve were also identified, pulled out of the wound, cut short, and allowed to retract back into the soft tissue. In addition, large veins were identified and ligated. The tourniquet was then released for a total tourniquet time of 32 minutes and minimal bleeding was encountered. Several smaller bleeders were ligated. There was some clotting observed, which was important as the blood clotting was of significant concern preceding this operation. The wound was closed over a medium Hemovac drain with 2 limbs, with the posterior flap brought anteriorly. The fascia was closed using interrupted 1 Vicryl suture, and the subcutaneous tissue was closed using interrupted 3-0 Monocryl suture in a simple buried fashion. Staples were placed at the level of the skin in the interest of time.

After a sterile compressive dressing was placed and Hemovac drain extension and reservoir were attached and activated, the patient was awoken from anesthesia and sent to the ICU in unchanged condition.

Code Assignment Including POA Indicator

ICD-9-CM Principal Diagnosis: _____

ICD-9-CM Additional Diagnoses: _____

ICD-9-CM Procedure Code(s): _____

ICD-10-CM Code(s): _____

ICD-10-PCS Code(s): _____

Optional MS-DRG Exercise (for users with access to MS-DRG software or tables)

What is the MS-DRG assignment on this case? _____

7.51.   The following documentation is from the health record of an 80-year-old male patient.

Discharge Summary

History: The patient is an 80-year-old male with a 4- to 5-week history of pulmonary disease, apparently developing out of an acute influenza-like illness. He was admitted to his local hospital approximately 22 days ago with right middle lobe and right lower lobe alveolar filling infiltrates. Initial cultures were negative. Treatment with intravenous Ancef was not effective. The patient's hospital course was manifested by progressive pulmonary infiltrates unresponsive to erythromycin, Claforan, and Primaxin. Complications of nasogastric feeding tube placement in the right pleural space and administration of 1 L of Osmolite into the pleural space apparently occurred during hospitalization. The patient had a chest tube placed with effective removal of the Osmolite. Because of fatigue, the patient was twice placed on a ventilator but has been off the ventilator for approximately 1 week. He has become severely malnourished and was placed on TPN. Diarrhea has intervened with tube feedings. Cultures and ova and parasite findings showed *Trichomonas*. Because of failure to resolve pneumonia, malnutrition, and persistent fever, he was transferred here.

Physical Examination: The patient is a chronically-ill-appearing, thin man, responsive but unable to talk secondary to a very dry mouth. Blood pressure 144/70, pulse rate 110 per minute and regular, temperature 99.4°F, respirations 28. He is on nasal oxygen. Skin is dry. Lymph nodes are negative. Head: No deformity. Eyes: Increased bilateral purulent drainage. Sclerae are not red. Pupils round and equal. Throat very dry with caked secretions on teeth and palate. Neck is supple. Jugular venous pulse flat, carotids equal. Chest nontender. He ventilates with the left chest fairly well with scattered rhonchi. The right chest, however, showed decreased breath sounds with a line of consolidation about halfway up. Scattered rhonchi were noted above the area of consolidation. No friction rub was heard. The patient had evidence of a right pleural effusion versus right pleural thickening. Heart: PMI was at the midclavicular line. A regular rhythm was noted, no significant murmur, gallop, or rub. Abdomen: Soft and scaphoid, no organomegaly or tenderness, bowel sounds active. The patient passed a green watery stool during examination. Rectal: Slightly decreased sphincter tone, no masses were felt. Prostate was +2 enlarged, no nodules. Extremities showed no edema, clubbing, or cyanosis.

Initial Laboratory and X-Ray Findings: Blood gas on 4 L of nasal oxygen showed pH 7.48, pCO_2 37, pO_2 65. Initial chest x-ray showed bilateral mixed infiltrate and consolidation throughout both lungs, most prominently in the right midlung and right lung base. A left subclavian venous catheter was seen. Initial hematocrit level was 40. Within 2 days after hydration, this was noted to be 27. Sed rate 96 mm per hour. White blood cell count 16,000 with 5 bands, 73 segs, 15 lymphs, 5 monos, 2 eosinophils. Platelets 464,000. PT and PTT negative. SMA profile: Cholesterol 113, triglycerides 110, electrolytes normal except chloride of 96, CO_2 34. Blood sugar 120. BUN 20, creatinine 0.8. Serum osmolality was 338. Urine osmolality was 456. Creatinine clearance was 81 mL per minute. Urinalysis was negative, except for an initial elevated specific gravity of 1.032. The patient was malnourished by low albumin and transferrin levels. IV albumin was ordered. Cryptococcal antigen of spinal fluid positive at a titer of 1:32.

Hospital Course: The day after admission on 1/9, the patient was submitted to bronchoscopy for bronchoalveolar lavage. His culture showed beta hemolytic streptococcus A, *Proteus mirabilis*, and a gram-negative bacillus that was not further identified. Legionella culture was negative. Stool showed no pathogens. Spinal tap was done with the finding of cryptococcal antigen of 1:32 in spinal fluid, the patient was started on amphotericin B for his meningitis, but he could not tolerate this and was thus switched to fluconazole. On 1/12, it became evident that the large volume of sputum he was required to mobilize and his generally weakened state resulted in increasing fatigue resulting in acute respiratory failure, such that it was necessary to transfer the patient to the ICU, intubate, and place him on ventilatory assistance. Because of continued deterioration, antibiotics were modified to include vancomycin and imipenem. Because of the inability to obtain a fully established diagnosis, the patient was submitted to right open-lung biopsy. The open-lung biopsy showed advanced fibrosis and scarring. Despite therapy with aggressive pulmonary toilet and ventilatory support, his condition continued to deteriorate. The patient experienced cardiac arrest on 1/16. The patient remained on the ventilator up until the time of expiration for a total of 94 consecutive hours of ventilation.

Final Diagnosis:	Pneumonia, apparently due to gram-negative bacteria
Additional Diagnoses:	Acute respiratory failure Cardiac arrest Cryptococcal meningitis Severely malnourished
Procedures:	Open-lung biopsy Ventilatory assistance

Code Assignment Including POA Indicator

ICD-9-CM Principal Diagnoses: _____

ICD-9-CM Additional Diagnoses: _____

ICD-9-CM Procedure Code(s): _____

ICD-10-CM Code(s): _____

ICD-10-PCS Code(s): _____

Optional MS-DRG Exercise (for users with access to MS-DRG software or tables)

Which of the following is the correct MS-DRG for this case? _____

a. 163, Major Chest Procedures with MCC
b. 853, Infectious and Parasitic Diseases with OR Procedure with MCC
c. 178, Respiratory Infections and Inflammations with CC
d. 003, ECMO or Tracheostomy with Mechanical Ventilation 96+ Hours or Principal Diagnosis Except Face, Mouth and Neck with Major OR

7.52. Discharge Summary

Date of Admission: 1/31

Date of Discharge: 2/3

Discharge Diagnosis: Right lower lobe pneumonia due to gram-negative bacteria, resistant to erythromycin

Admission History: This is a 56-year-old type 1 diabetic female whose diabetes is out of control whom we have been following for hypertension, degenerative joint disease of both knees, aortic stenosis, and diabetic retinopathy. Over the past three days she has noted increased cough and chest congestion with a fever of approximately 102 degrees. She was found to have a right lower lobe infiltrate and was started on therapy with erythromycin. Despite initial therapy, the patient's clinical status has worsened over the past 24 hours.

Course in Hospital: Patient was admitted with the diagnosis of right lower lobe pneumonia. She was begun on intravenous ceftriaxone. Because of difficulties with venous access, patient was switched to intramuscular ceftriaxone on her third hospital day.

By 2/3 the patient was afebrile and her cough had diminished. Her blood pressure was well controlled at 140/74.

Instructions on Discharge: Follow up with me by phone in three days and in my office in two weeks. Repeat chest x-ray to be done then.

Medications

1. Calan SR 180 mg b.i.d.

2. Zestril 20 mg PO q. a.m.

3. NPH Insulin, 30 units, sub q., a.m.

4. Levoquin 500 mg PO daily × 10 days

5. Celebrex 100 mg PO b.i.d.

History and Physical

Admitted: 1/31

Reason for Admission: Physical examination on admission revealed a well-developed, acutely ill appearing black female.

History of Present Illness: A 56-year-old diabetic followed for hypertension and diabetic retinopathy. Over the past three days she has noted increased cough and chest congestion with a fever of approximately 102 degrees. She was found to have a right lower lobe infiltrate and was begun on therapy with erythromycin. Despite initial therapy, the patient's clinical status worsened over the past 24 hours and hospitalization was recommended.

Past Medical History: Hypertension, degenerative joint disease in both knees, and moderate aortic stenosis

Allergies: Dust

Chronic Medications: CalanSR 180 mg PO b.i.d., Insulin (NPH), Zestril 20 mg PO daily, Celebrex 100 mg PO b.i.d.

Family History: Notable for hypertension in mother

Social History: Noncontributory

Physical Examination

   General Appearance: The patient is a well-developed black female in moderate distress.

   Vital Signs: T 102, P 80, R 16, BP 150/80

   Skin: Warm and dry

   HEENT: Significant for mildly inflamed mucous membranes. Retinopathy evident in both eyes.

   Neck: Supple. Symmetrical with no bruits.

   Lungs: Coarse rhonchi bilaterally, right greater than left

   Heart: Regular rate and rhythm, positive S1, positive III/VI SEM

   Abdomen: Soft, nontender, no mass

   Genitalia: Deferred

   Rectal: Deferred

   Extremities: No edema

   Neurologic: Normal

Laboratory Data

   1. EKG: NSR, widespread ST-T wave abnormalities, LV hypertrophy
   2. CBC: Hgb 13, Hct 38, WBC 12.8
   3. Glucose: 281
   4. Urinalysis: Unremarkable
   5. Sputum: Gram stain—a few WBCs, moderate gram-negative rods

Impression

   1. Right lower lobe pneumonia possibly due to gram-negative bacteria
   2. Diabetes mellitus on insulin—Uncontrolled
   3. Hypertension—Stable
   4. Degenerative joint disease—Stable
   5. Moderate aortic stenosis

Plan: Admit, IV antibiotics for pneumonia. Monitor blood sugars.

Progress Notes

1/31   Patient admitted for cough associated with increased temperature with chest x-ray indicative of pneumonia. Will obtain sputum culture and begin on ceftriaxone. Will monitor blood pressure and blood sugars. Will use sliding scale to bring blood sugar into control. Patient with recent echocardiogram as outpatient that showed stable aortic stenosis.

2/1   The patient is responding well. Will request diabetic education nurse to meet with her and set up an appointment for classes following this admission.

2/2   Sputum culture reveals gram-negative bacteria as suspected. Patient's temperature is down. Patient resting comfortably. Blood sugar better.

2/3   Blood sugar with increasing control today. The importance of appropriate diet emphasized. Will discharge with p.o. antibiotics.

Code Assignment Including POA Indicator

ICD-9-CM Principal Diagnoses: _____

ICD-9-CM Additional Diagnoses: _____

ICD-9-CM Procedure Code(s): _____

ICD-10-CM Code(s): _____

ICD-10-PCS Code(s): _____

7.53.   The following documentation is from the health record of a 65-year-old male patient.

Hospital Course: This unfortunate gentleman was discharged from the hospital yesterday after being treated for several days for congestive heart failure. He presented back to the hospital within 24 hours after he developed significant respiratory discomfort and shortness of breath. He was found to be in respiratory failure and have pneumonia. The patient required intubation with subsequent mechanical ventilation in the emergency room. His x-ray showed diffuse infiltrates bilaterally, a condition also consistent with possible congestive heart failure. The patient did not have an elevated BNP. He was taken to the intensive care unit for further evaluation and treatment. It was explained to his wife and family that he was critically ill, and his survival was very guarded. The patient required blood pressure support. He was treated for pneumonia and his sputum cultures grew methicillin-resistant *Staphylococcus aureus*. He was treated with vancomycin. He had a stroke while admitted and had right-sided hemiparesis. He was found to have a left-sided internal carotid artery stenosis. He was felt not to be a surgical candidate because he was critically ill. He was placed on Bumex infusion for his congestive heart failure. His respiratory status remained very tenuous despite maximum medical management. He was placed on TPN via peripheral vein. His condition never improved despite all efforts. He remained poorly responsive, and he developed acute renal failure, as well. On day 15, it was clear that his survival was unlikely. His family asked that his ventilator support be discontinued. Shortly after, the ventilator was discontinued.

Discharge Diagnoses

Acute respiratory failure secondary to pneumonia and congestive heart failure

Cerebrovascular accident with infarction

Methicillin-resistant *S. aureus* infection

Acute renal failure

Lung mass

Chronic obstructive pulmonary disease

Diabetes mellitus

Hemiplegia secondary to stroke

Operative Procedures

Mechanical ventilation greater than 96 hours

Packed red blood cell transfusion $\times$ 2 (via peripheral vein)

Code Assignment Including POA Indicator

ICD-9-CM Principal Diagnoses: _____

ICD-9-CM Additional Diagnoses: _____

ICD-9-CM Procedure Code(s): _____

ICD-10-CM Code(s): _____

ICD-10-PCS Code(s): _____

Optional MS-DRG Exercise (for users with access to MS-DRG software or tables)

Which of the following is the correct MS-DRG for this case?

a. 189, Pulmonary Edema and Respiratory Failure
b. 291, Heart Failure and Shock with MMC
c. 207, Respiratory System Diagnosis with Ventilator Support 96+ Hours
d. 064, Intracranial Hemorrhage or Cerebral Infarction with MCC

7.54. History and Physical Exam

Present Illness: This 74-year-old male presented to the emergency room last night with complaints of increased weakness and shortness of breath. In the emergency room, he was found to be hypotensive. Blood pressure 83/42 apparently—actually that was the recording at home. In the emergency room, it was 130/80. He was afebrile, tachypneic per usual, respiratory rate of 32, and admitted with acute pneumonia. He was started on Levaquin. He has a history of purulent sputum for several days. Since admission, he feels better; tachypnea and weakness have improved. His blood pressure readings have somewhat improved. His peripheral edema improved with a diuretic.

Past Medical History: End-stage pulmonary disease, atherosclerotic heart disease and congestive heart failure, gastroesophageal reflux disease, gout, and hypothyroidism

Family History: Unremarkable

Social History: Has six children and is a widower

Physical Exam: On physical examination, blood pressure 102/70, pulse 90, respirations 28. He is pleasant, alert. Color is good. No JVD.

Chest: He has bilateral rales, which are chronic.

Heart: There is a systolic ejection murmur, grade 3, with an S4 gallop.

Abdomen: The abdomen is soft, nontender. No palpable organomegaly.

Extremities: Extremities reveal trace to +1 peripheral edema. He does have some stasis pigmentary changes. He does have clubbing of his fingers.

Musculoskeletal: No atrophic changes

Skin: Unremarkable except as noted

Neurological: He has no focal sensory or motor deficits and reflexes are physiologic.

Impressions: I suspect he probably just has purulent bronchitis and that is the cause of his deterioration. He is on Levaquin and seems to be improving. We will observe until tomorrow. If still doing reasonably well, we will let him go.

Discharge Summary

History of Present Illness: This 74-year-old male with end-stage pulmonary fibrosis was admitted via the emergency room with increased breathlessness. The admitting diagnosis was pneumonia. While here, he did not develop any significant fever.

Laboratory Studies: On admission PO_2 58, PCO_2 37, pH 7.45 on 3.5 L, his electrolytes were normal with the exception of BUN 28, creatinine 1.3, white blood cell count 8.6, hemoglobin 11.4, platelet count slightly low 117, urinalysis fairly unremarkable with trace protein, rare red and white blood cells.

Hospital Course: The patient was continued on Levaquin, which had been started 1 day previously. His chest x-ray showed decreased cardiac size from the previous examination, chronic infiltrates bilaterally, no acute infiltrates; pneumonia ruled out. Electrocardiogram showed sinus rhythm, right bundle branch block, left anterior hemiblock. He did receive intravenous diuretic and with this did achieve significant diuresis. My concern at the time of admission was the possible hypotension, which was recorded at home, but all blood pressure recordings here varied from the 100 to 130 systolic range.

Discharge Diagnosis: Probably acute bronchitis with possible mild congestive heart failure.

What are the correct code sets for this admission?

ICD-9-CM Code(s):

a. 466.0, 515, 428.0
b. 491.22, 428.0
c. 491.22, 466.0, 515, 428.0
d. 428.0, 466.0, 515

ICD-10-CM Code(s): _____

7.55. **Admission Diagnosis:** Pneumonia, hypoxemia

Discharge Diagnosis: Bilateral pneumonia, respiratory failure, dehydration, quadriplegia with old C5–C6 fracture, atonic bladder, tobacco use (2 packs of cigarettes for the past 30 years)

Disposition: The patient is being discharged to home. Her daughter stays with her full-time to care for her. She is to come to our office in one week to get a repeat chest x-ray and then further treatment with her pending results.

Hospital Course: The patient is a 50-year-old female who is a quadriplegic after a motor vehicle accident in which she suffered a C5–C6 fracture. She had a fever two days prior to admission, so we called her in a prescription for Keflex. She did not improve on this medication, and she came to the emergency room on the day of admission complaining of shortness of breath and cough. She reported a two day history of shortness of breath, fever, and cough productive of green and yellow sputum. There was no elevation in her temperature. A chest x-ray in the emergency room showed bilateral lower lobe infiltrates. She was admitted to the hospital for intravenous antibiotics for her pneumonia and treatment of her hypoxemia. Her pO_2 in the emergency room was 50 on room air. Her temperature was 102.6°F.

After admission to the hospital, the patient was placed on Biaxin, and she did become afebrile and started to feel better. Her caretaker, who is her daughter, felt that she could care for her at home. The patient is being discharged to the daughter's care.

Work-up during this admission included a glucose of 81, a BUN of 6, a creatinine of 0.5. Electrolytes were normal. Her arterial blood gases show a pH of 7.482, a pCO_2 of 33, a pO_2 low at 50, HCO_3 324, and total CO_2 was 55. Her O_2 saturation was only 88 percent on room air. She was started on handheld nebulizer treatments, and she rapidly improved.

At the time of discharge, she was breathing easy on room air. She was benefiting from her handheld nebulizer treatments, and she wants to return home.

The work-up during admission, in addition to that above, included serum electrolytes, which were normal except for a potassium level of 3.3. This was corrected with additional potassium. Her hemoglobin level on admission was 13.5. Hematocrit was 40.1, RBC was 4.40. Her MCV was 91. Her MCH was 33.6. RDW was 12.7. The urinalysis showed a moderate amount of hemoglobin but no red cells. Her chest x-ray did show a definite infiltrate in her left lower lobe and a questionable infiltrate in her right lower lobe. There is question that possibly her paraplegia may affect her ability to breathe, necessitating her seeing us for respiratory infections. The patient is discharged to home. She will be seeing Dr. Jones in two weeks after repeat chest x-ray.

Code Assignment Including POA Indicator

ICD-9-CM Principal Diagnoses: _____

ICD-9-CM Secondary Diagnoses: _____

ICD-10-CM Code(s): _____

7.56.   Discharge Summary

Admit Date: 3/19/20XX

Discharge Date: 3/25/20XX

Admitting Diagnoses: Acute exacerbation of asthma, chronic obstructive pulmonary disease with acute exacerbation, acute bronchitis, hormonal replacement therapy

Discharge Diagnoses: Acute exacerbation of asthma, chronic obstructive pulmonary disease with acute exacerbation, acute bronchitis, hormonal replacement therapy

Discharge Instructions: Patient is to follow up in the office in 1 week.

Discharge Medications: Spiriva as directed daily, Pulmicort inhaler two puffs p.o. every 12 hours, Serevent Diskus one puff p.o. every 12 hours, Augmentin 500 mg p.o. 3 times a day for 6 days, prednisone 35 mg to decrease by 5 mg every day until gone.

Brief History: The patient is a 57-year-old white female who presents with an approximate 1-day history of increasing dyspnea to the point where any ambulation required increasing effort as she could not catch her breath. The patient also had mild complaints of sore throat, neck pain, and headache. She denied any fever, although a low-grade one was present on admission. The patient also admitted to a nonproductive cough.

The patient had an acute exacerbation of asthma and was admitted to observation. However, this did not clear with IV steroids, nebulizer treatments, or supportive therapy, so she was admitted for inpatient treatment of acute exacerbation of asthma with possible bronchitis and respiratory distress. During her initial 2-day stay, Z-Pak, Decadron, and albuterol and Atrovent treatments were continued because her respiratory distress did not significantly improve. The patient had increased anxiety secondary to her nebulized treatments and her medication was changed to Xopenex with some improvement.

Chest x-ray was checked on the second hospital day, and a two-dimensional echocardiogram was ordered in addition to a pulmonary consult. The patient's Zithromax was changed to Augmentin to better cover *Haemophilus influenzae* as a possibility. Inhaled steroids were added as the bronchodilators were continued. The patient's respiratory distress subsequently improved with less agitation with continued high-dose Xopenex. The two-dimensional echocardiogram was normal. The patient's respiratory condition improved with less dyspnea with her lung exam overall cleared. The patient was discharged in stable condition.

History and Physical: This is a 57-year-old female who presents with an approximate 1-day history of increasing dyspnea to the point where any ambulation required increasing effort, and she could not catch her breath. The patient stated that approximately 1 month ago some cold medication was phoned in for her, which cleared up her congestion but did not feel she totally got well. She was admitted from the emergency room to observation, but her symptoms did not resolve so she is being admitted for inpatient treatment. Patient smokes approximately one pack of cigarettes a day and denies any alcohol use.

Physical Exam

General: The patient is alert and oriented, appearing in mild to moderate respiratory distress

Lungs: Showed decreased breath sounds throughout with no wheezing present

Abdomen: Soft and nontender, with good bowel sounds present

Extremities: No cyanosis or edema

The patient is currently on 2 L of nasal cannula with O_2 saturations at approximately 92 percent. Her chest x-ray is unremarkable.

Assessment and Plan: Acute exacerbation of asthma/chronic obstructive pulmonary disease/acute bronchitis. The patient will continue with Zithromax given at 500 mg p.o. q. 24 hours. Continued on 10 mg of Decadron q. 8 hours, given albuterol as well as Atrovent treatments on a daily basis.

Hormone replacement therapy on Premarin 0.625 mg/day

Consultant Report

Reason for Consultation: Acute bronchitis

Impression: Acute bronchitis either representing acute exacerbation of chronic bronchitis and/or asthma. Cigarette use greater than 40-pack-years.

Recommendations: Change Zithromax to Augmentin because she has had antibiotics in the past 90 days, and there is a high incidence of resistant *H. influenzae* and streptococcal pneumonia.

Handheld steroids

Prophylactic H_2 blockers and low molecular with heparin

Check sputum for eosinophils

Cigarette cessation

Discussion: The patient has purulent bronchitis and wheezing on top of chronic daily shortness of breath and wheezing. This is compounded by at least 40-pack-years of smoking history. It is difficult to tell if this is just chronic obstructive pulmonary disease exacerbation due to infection or whether or not she has a large component of asthma. Whatever the initial diagnosis is, she would benefit with albuterol and Atrovent, inhaled steroids, and antibiotics.

On the long-term basis, she will need PFTs and a long-acting bronchodilator, Spiriva or Advair depending on the way she responds on her pulmonary function test abnormalities. Advair is recommended if the FEV1 is less than 50 percent; Spiriva would be a better choice if this is all chronic obstructive pulmonary disease.

Emergency Room Report: Chief Complaint: Shortness of breath

History of Present Illness: The patient is a 57-year-old female complaining of shortness of breath since yesterday evening. She states that breathing difficulty became very severe to the point that she felt like she could not catch her breath. She could not walk across the room without becoming severely dyspneic. Also complaining of soreness in her neck bilaterally and of a headache.

Impression/Management Plan: Breathing difficulty with marked bronchospasm, possible fever with chills present. Rule out superimposed pneumonia. Symptoms consistent with exacerbation of asthma. Initial oxygen saturation on presentation to the emergency department 89 percent on room air.

Course in the Emergency Department: The patient received intravenous fluids, Decadron, magnesium. The patient did develop a fever in the emergency department with temperature up to 100.7°F, for which she received Tylenol. The patient received multiple nebulizer treatments in the emergency department and has persistent expiratory wheezes with somewhat labored respirations. Chest x-ray read negative for acute changes by my reading. The patient received initial dose of Zithromax in the emergency department. Decision for further treatment was made with an admission to the observation unit.

Final Diagnosis: Asthma with acute exacerbation.

What is the correct code assignment for this admission?

ICD-9-CM Code(s):

a. 493.91, 305.1, V07.4
b. 466.0, 493.22, 305.1, V07.4
c. 493.22, 305.1, V07.4
d. 493.21

ICD-10-CM Code(s): _____

7.57.   Discharge Summary

Date of Admission:	12/18/XX
Date of Discharge:	12/22/XX

Admitting Diagnoses:
1. Right lung mass
2. Postobstructive pneumonia
3. COPD
4. Respiratory acidosis

Procedure: Fiberoptic bronchoscopy on 12/20/XX

History of Present Illness: This 80-year-old white male was admitted with a 4-day history of increasing dyspnea, fever, and productive cough. Initial evaluation suggested a right lower lobe pneumonia based on ER data. He was known to have underlying chronic obstructive pulmonary disease, and labs verified the presence of respiratory acidosis.

Physical Examination: He presented with a temperature of 97.9, respiratory rate of 28, pulse 127, blood pressure 162/80. There were coarse crackles heard in the right base with poor air flow throughout.

Hospital Course: The patient was admitted for treatment of right lower lobe pneumonia and acute exacerbating COPD. He was initially placed on Zinacef one gram q8 hours and Solumedrol 60 mg q6 hours. He was also provided supplemental oxygen as required and supervised inhalation therapy. On the 20th, the Solumedrol was changed to Prednisone 50 mg per day and the Zinacef changed to Ceftin 500 mg po b.i.d. With that, the cough, etc., began to improve.

Further investigation in the right lower lobe abnormality via a CT scan of the chest showed a 2-cm inferior hilar mass obstructing the right lower lobe bronchi associated with post productive infiltrate and/or atelectasis. This was suspicious for right inferior hilar neoplasm. Biapical scarring was also suggested. On 12/20/XX, fiberoptic bronchoscopy was performed. Fortunately, this showed no distinct endobronchial lesion. Any obstruction was peripheral to the area visible. Washings were negative for acid-fast bacilli. Brushings showed only atypical cells. Perioperatively, the patient had some worsening of his CO_2 retention, which was transiently benefited by Bi-PAP for his sleep. He had not required this prior to this admission and his sedation has not resolved. It was felt that this was a long-term need.

Laboratory Data: During this stay, an SMA7 was done on the 18th, showing glucose 126, BUN 26, and creatinine 1. Sodium 145, Potassium 3.8, Chloride 96, CO_2 32. The most recent blood gas was on the 22nd, showing a pH 7.4, pCO_2 67, pO_2 43, on 2 L nasal cannula. Theophylline level was 15.9. Hemoglobin of 14.4 and hematocrit of 42.4. White blood cell count 14,600 with 9 percent Bands.

Discharge Summary

Disposition/Recommendations: The patient is being discharged home with plans for continued antibiotics therapy and steroid taper, and arrangements for an outpatient fine-needle aspirate of the lung abnormality.

Discharge Medications:
1. Atrovent 2 puffs inhalation q6 hours
2. Albuterol 2 puffs q4 hours while awake prn
3. Ceftin 500 mg po q12 hours for 10 more days
4. Prednisone 30 mg per day for 6 days and then decrease by 5 mg every other day until weaned

Activity and Diet: As tolerated.

As mentioned, request will be made for Radiology to arrange for an outpatient fine-needle aspiration of the lung abnormality. The patient understands that there is a risk of pneumothorax and if such occurs, he may return to the hospital for treatment of same.

Condition on Discharge: Improved.

History and Physical Exam

Date of Admission: 12/18/XX

History of Present Illness: This is an 80-year-old gentleman who presented to the emergency room last night. He had called me earlier in the evening with complaints of increasing breathlessness of about 4 days' duration. His evaluation in the emergency room suggested a right lower lung zone pneumonic infiltrate, and he did have a leukocytosis. He was admitted.

I have known this patient for approximately 3 years. For many years he has been treated for chronic obstructive pulmonary disease secondary to a long history of tobacco use. He has been oxygen-dependent for at least 3 years. In this interval, he has had 1 admission that I am aware of for exacerbation of COPD. His recent history is that of 4 days of increasing cough, purulent sputum production, and probably fever. He does describe chills and diaphoretic episodes.

Past Medical History: His past medical history is relatively unremarkable with the exception of his chronic obstructive pulmonary disease. As far as I know, he has no prior history of cardiovascular disease, stroke, or myocardial infarction.

Physical Examination: He is pleasant, alert, feels a bit more comfortable this morning. His blood pressure is 162/80, pulse 100, respirations 26. HEENT: Mouth and oropharynx are adequately hydrated. He does have a scar on his left lip at the site of corrective surgery for a harelip. Neck: Supple. There is no jugular venous distention. Chest: He does have somewhat of a pectus excavatum deformity with slight sternal retraction. He has coarse rales over his right chest laterally and posteriorly with a congested cough. Breath sounds are diminished on the left side. Heart: Regular rhythm without murmur or gallop. Abdomen: Soft, nontender. No masses. No organomegaly. Back and extremities: No clubbing, cyanosis, or peripheral edema. Distal pulses are easily palpable. Neurological: There are no focal neurological deficits.

Impression: 1. COPD. Plan: IV steroids and inhaled beta agonists.

   2. Pneumonia. Plan: IV Zinacef. We will add Zithromax for community-acquired organisms.

EKG

Impression: Sinus tachycardia with premature ventricular contractions. Cannot exclude old inferior myocardial infarction, stable pattern.

Progress Notes

12/18   80 y/o admitted with 4 day hx of SOB, fever, and productive cough. #1 Pneumonia #2 COPD

12/19   CXR mass of lung neoplasm

12/19   Plan bronchoscopy

12/20   Bronchoscopy note dictated. No lesions noted. Pt. tolerated procedure well.

12/20   House Doctor: Pt. apparently very sedated after bronchoscopy –Demerol 12.5 mg and Phenergen 12.5 mg. Has now gotten 3 doses of Narcan with noticeable alertness with each dose but then drifts off to deep sleep again. V: BP 130/70, P 70 to 80s. SaO$_2$ now 95 to 97 on 2 L. Pt. opens eyes briefly with prompting but not enough to answer ?'s or follow commands. CV: RRR, Lungs: occ rales B Extremities: edema. A/P: Excessive sedation is what I suspect. Continue Narcan as needed. Will discuss with Dr. X.

12/21   S: No complaints

   O: Afebrile, VSS, Lungs: poor air flow, bronchial washings neg.

   A: Lung mass, post obstructive pneumonia, respiratory acidosis

   P: D/C home for outpatient for FNA, scenario discussed with family

12/22   Discharged home with family.

Operative Report

Operation Performed: Bronchoscopy.

Premedication: 12.5 mg Demerol, 12.5 mg Phenergan, and 0.4 mg Atropine

Description of Procedure: The patient was taken to the endoscopy room. The nasopharynx and upper airway were anesthetized with 1 percent Xylocaine. The Olympus fiberoptic bronchoscope was introduced into the left nostril without difficulty. The nasopharynx and upper airway appeared normal. The vocal cords moved anatomically to the midline. The trachea was then entered. The carina was sharp. The right main stem bronchus was entered. There were inflammatory changes.

The bronchoscope was advanced into the right middle lobe. The mucosa was somewhat friable, but no endobronchial lesions were identified. The bronchoscope was then introduced further into the right lower lobe and brushings were obtained. The area was then irrigated with saline, and washings were recovered. The bronchoscope was then passed quickly to the left side and no endobronchial lesions were present.

The patient was monitored via blood pressure, pulse, and oximetry throughout, maintaining oximetry in the 85 to 92 range, and other vital signs were normal.

Following the procedure, the patient was given an amp of Narcan.

Impression: Bronchoscopy suggestive of inflammatory process in the right lower lobe.

Code Assignment Including POA Indicator

ICD-9-CM Principal Diagnoses: _____

ICD-9-CM Additional Diagnoses: _____

ICD-9-CM Procedure Code(s): _____

ICD-10-CM Code(s): _____

ICD-10-PCS Code(s): _____

Optional MS-DRG Exercise (for users with access to MS-DRG software or tables)

What is the MS-DRG assignment for this admission? _____

Trauma and Poisoning

7.58.   The following documentation is from the health record of a four-year-old male patient.

Case Summary: The patient is a 4-year-old male child who, at the age of 2 years, swallowed some Drano while playing in the bathroom. He was found at that time with acid burns of the mouth, throat, trachea, and esophagus. Plastic repair has been performed on the mouth and throat. He is now being admitted by a plastic surgeon for plastic reconstruction and removal of scar tissue to the trachea. The patient was admitted, prepped, and taken to surgery where the scar tissue of the trachea was removed, and plastic repair was accomplished. The patient's recovery was uneventful, and the patient was discharged in satisfactory condition 3 days postsurgery.

Which of the following code sets is correct for reporting the diagnoses of the most recent admission?

ICD-9-CM Code(s):

a. 709.2, 909.1, E929.2
b. 478.9, 909.1, 906.8, E929.2
c. 709.2, 909.5, 906.8, E864.2
d. 478.9, 909.5, E864.2

ICD-10-CM Code(s): _____

Optional MS-DRG Exercise (for users with access to MS-DRG software or tables)

What is the MS-DRG assignment for this admission? _____

7.59.   The following documentation is from the health record of a 22-year-old male patient.

Case Summary: The patient is a 22-year-old male, admitted through the Emergency Department after the motorcycle he was driving collided with an elk while driving in the mountains. It was noted that when the accident occurred the patient was driving in the mountains and not on the road. The patient was not wearing a helmet and sustained a skull fracture over the left temporal and orbital roof areas with depressed zygomatic arch on the left side. The patient was unconscious at the scene and upon examination in the ED, with a GCS score of 3: eyes, never open; no verbal response; no motor response. Left pupil was blown (fixed and dilated), indicating intracranial injury. Hypoxemia, hypotension, and cerebral edema were noted. The patient was admitted to the ICU with continuous monitoring of intracranial pressure (percutaneous). The patient experienced increasing periods of apnea and was placed on a ventilator following endotracheal intubation. The patient's family (in another state) was notified and arrived two days later. There was no improvement in the patient's status over the following five days. The patient continued to be monitored and was unconscious. Attempts to wean from ventilation were unsuccessful. Brain wave measurement showed no brain wave electrical activity. The family made the decision to discontinue life support and the life-sustaining efforts were discontinued.

Code Assignment Including POA Indicator

ICD-9-CM Principal Diagnoses: _____

ICD-9-CM Additional Diagnoses: _____

ICD-9-CM Procedure Code(s): _____

ICD-10-CM Code(s): _____

ICD-10-PCS Code(s): _____

7.60. The following documentation is from the health record of a 28-year-old female patient.

Case Summary: The patient is a 28-year-old female passenger in a motor vehicle accident involving the car passenger was in being involved in a collision with another car while traveling at high speed on the freeway. Upon arrival in the ED the patient was complaining of severe abdominal pain. CT scan revealed laceration of the liver and increasing hematoma. The patient was taken immediately to the OR, where exploratory laparotomy revealed a traumatic rupture approximately 2 cm deep. It was felt that the parenchyma could not be adequately repaired, so a right lobectomy was carried out with evacuation of the hematoma. The patient's postoperative course was stormy. The patient developed infection and dehiscence of the operative wound, necessitating return to the OR for opening and drainage of the abdominal wound. The patient was also given a 10-day course of IV gentamicin. The patient was finally able to be discharged on the 12th day postop in satisfactory condition.

Code Assignment Including POA Indicator

ICD-9-CM Principal Diagnoses: _____

ICD-9-CM Additional Diagnoses: _____

ICD-9-CM Procedure Code(s): _____

ICD-10-CM Code(s): _____

ICD-10-PCS Code(s): _____

7.61. The following documentation is from the health record of a 32-year-old male patient.

History of Present Illness: A 32-year-old male was brought to the ED via ambulance. He was the unrestrained front-seat passenger in a single-vehicle crash that occurred because of a tire blow-out at high speed; the car collided with a barricade off the highway. The patient was ejected from the vehicle and had brief loss of consciousness witnessed at the scene. Paramedics reported the following vital signs en route: BP 110/palp; heart rate 90, respiratory rate 20. A large-bore intravenous access was established, and fluids were begun.

Physical Examination
Vital signs: Unchanged
HEENT: 2-cm superficial laceration over left eyebrow
Lungs: Clear to auscultation
CV: Regular rate, S1/S2; NSR on EKG monitor
Abdomen: Mild epigastric tenderness without rebound
Pelvis: Stable, no crepitans
Extremities: No deformities
Neuro: GCS 13, nonfocal exam

Radiology: Chest x-ray, lateral C-spine, and pelvis film all are reviewed by the chief resident on call and noted to be normal. CT scan of the patient's abdomen demonstrated free intra-abdominal fluid, perisplenic hematoma, and splenic laceration. Patient remained hemodynamically stable during the scan.

Because of the patient's young age and hemodynamic stability, nonoperative management of his splenic injury was begun. The patient was admitted to the ICU for hemodynamic monitoring, serial measurement of hematocrit, and serial abdominal examinations. He was transferred to the floor on hospital day 2 and made an uneventful recovery.

Diagnoses: 1. Minor concussion with 10 minutes of loss of consciousness
2. Perisplenic hematoma and splenic laceration of capsule

Which of the following code sets for the diagnoses would be correct?

ICD-9-CM Code(s):

a. 865.11
b. 865.02, 850.9, E816.1, E849.5
c. 865.02, 850.11, E816.1, E849.5
d. 865.01, 865.02, 850.11, E816.1, E849.5

ICD-10-CM Code(s): _____

Chapter 8

Case Studies from Ambulatory Health Records

Note: Even though the specific cases are divided by setting, most of the information pertaining to the diagnosis is applicable to most settings. Even the CPT codes in the ambulatory and physician sections may be reported in the same manner. The differences in coding in these two settings may involve modifier reporting, evaluation and management CPT code reporting, and other health plan reporting guidelines unique to settings. If you practice or apply codes in a particular type of setting, you may find additional information in other sections of this publication that may be pertinent to you.

Every effort has been made to follow current recognized coding guidelines and principles, as well as nationally recognized reporting guidelines. The material presented may differ from some health plan requirements for reporting. The ICD-9-CM codes used are effective October 1, 2012, through September 30, 2013, and the HCPCS (CPT and HCPCS Level II) codes are in effect January 1, 2013, through December 31, 2013. The current standard transactions and code sets named in HIPAA have been utilized. The 2013 draft edition of ICD-10-CM was utilized.

Instructions: Assign all applicable ICD-9-CM diagnosis codes including V codes and E codes. Assign all applicable ICD-10-CM diagnosis codes including Z codes and external cause codes. Assign all CPT Level I procedure codes and HCPCS Level II codes. Assign Level I (CPT) and Level II (HCPCS) modifiers as appropriate. Outpatient healthcare settings represented in the case examples include emergency room (ER), urgent care, outpatient surgery, observation, ancillary outpatient, wound care, interventional radiology, radiation therapy, or other outpatient department. Final codes for billing occur after codes are passed through payer edits. Medicare utilizes the National Correct Coding Initiative (NCCI) edits. CMS developed the NCCI edit list to promote national correct coding methodologies and to control improper coding leading to improper payments for Medicare Part B. The purpose of the NCCI edits is to ensure the most comprehensive code is assigned and billed rather than the component codes. In addition, NCCI edits check for mutually exclusive pairs.

Cases are presented as either multiple choice or fill in the blank.

- For multiple-choice cases:
  - Select the letter of the appropriate code set.

- For the fill-in-the-blank cases:
  - Assign up to three reasons for visit ICD-9-CM codes to describe the reason for unscheduled visits such as emergency room. Reason for visit coding is required on the UB-04 for all "unscheduled" outpatient visits.
  - Sequence the primary diagnosis first followed by the secondary diagnoses including any appropriate V codes and E codes (both cause of injury and place of occurrence).
  - Sequence the CPT procedure code first followed by additional procedure codes including modifiers as appropriate (both CPT Level I and HCPCS Level II modifiers).
  - Assign HCPCS Level II codes only if instructed (case specific).
  - Assign evaluation and management (E/M) codes only if instructed (case specific).
    - Medicare Type A Emergency Department visits are reported with CPT Level I codes 99281–99285 and critical care codes 99291 and 99292.
    - Medicare Type B Emergency Department visits are reported with Level II HCPCS codes G0380–G0384.

The scenarios are based on selected excerpts from health records. In practice, the coding professional should have access to and refer to the entire health record. Health records are analyzed and codes assigned based on physician documentation. Documentation for coding purposes must be assigned based on medical record documentation. A physician may be queried when documentation is ambiguous, incomplete, or conflicting. The queried documentation must be a permanent part of the medical record.

The objective of the cases and scenarios reproduced in this publication is to provide practice in assigning correct codes, not necessarily to emulate complete coding that can be achieved only with the complete medical record. For example, the reader may be asked to assign codes based on only an operative report; in real practice, a coder has access to documentation in the entire medical record.

The *ICD-9-CM Official Guidelines for Coding and Reporting of Outpatient Services*, published by the National Center for Health Statistics (NCHS), supplements the official conventions and instructions provided within ICD-9-CM. Adherence to these guidelines when assigning ICD-9-CM diagnosis codes is required under the Health Insurance Portability and Accountability Act (HIPAA) of 1996. Additional official coding guidance can be found in the American Hospital Association (AHA)'s *Coding Clinic* publication.

Disorders of the Blood and Blood-Forming Organs

8.1.   The following documentation is from the health record of a 39-year-old male.

Emergency Department Services

History of Present Illness: The patient is a 39-year-old African-American male who has a known history of sickle cell anemia and who presented to the emergency department with diffuse extremity pain and pain along the right inguinal area. The pains started on Friday, became a little bit better on Saturday; then improved, and again started in the past 24 hours. He denies any problems with cough or sputum production. He denies any problems with fever.

Past Medical History: See recent medical records in charts. He does have a new onset of diabetes, probably related to his hemochromatosis. He does have evidence of iron overload with high ferritins.

Review of Systems: Otherwise unremarkable except for those related to his pain. He denies any problems with fever or night sweats. No cough or sputum production. Denies any changes in gastrointestinal or genitourinary habits. No blood per rectum or urine.

Physical Examination: This is a 39-year-old African-American male who is conscious and cooperative. He is oriented × 3 and appears in no acute distress. Vital signs are stable. HEENT is unremarkable. The neck is supple. No evidence of any gross lymphadenopathy. The heart is irregular in rate without any murmurs heard. Lungs are clear to auscultation and percussion. The abdomen is soft and benign. Extremities reveal no edema. No palpable cords. He does have some tenderness along the inner aspects of his right lower extremity near the inguinal area; however, no masses were palpable and no point tenderness is noted.

He had a problem with his right inguinal area. He had evidence of pain. There was some pain on abduction of his right lower extremity. The rest was unremarkable. There was no evidence of any Holman, no palpable cords, and no masses were palpable.

Because of his sickle cell anemia, rule out the possibility of osteonecrosis of the femur. Complete x-rays of his femur and hip were carried out. However, these were both negative.

Patient is being transferred to a larger facility for treatment of his sickle cell crisis. Doppler studies should also be carried out to rule out any venous thrombosis.

Diagnoses: 1. Painful sickle cell crisis
2. Type II diabetes mellitus
3. Chronic atrial fibrillation

Condition on Discharge: Stable on pain meds

What codes would the facility report for this Medicare service? The patient met the fourth acuity level in the facility's criteria for evaluation and management in the ED.

ICD-9-CM and CPT Code(s):

a. 282.61, 789.09, 427.31, 250.00, 99285
b. 282.62, 733.42, 99284, 73550, 73510
c. 282.62, 427.31, 250.00, 73550, 73510
d. 282.62, 427.31, 250.00, 99284-25, 73550, 73510

ICD-10-CM Code(s): _____

8.2. The following documentation is from the health record of a 66-year-old male patient.

Outpatient Hospital Department Services

History: This is a 66-year-old male who had coronary artery bypass graft in February. He did well. He was discharged home. Some time after that when he was home, he had 2 days of black stools. He mentioned it to the nurse, but I'm not sure anything was done about it. He has not had any other evidence of hematesis, melena, or hematochezia but was feeling rather weak and fatigued. He had blood work done that showed a hemoglobin of 5.7, hematocrit of 20.9, and MCV of 80. Serum iron of 8.2 percent saturation. No indigestion or heartburn. No abdominal pain of any kind. No past history of anemia or GI bleed.

Past Medical History: General health has been good.

Allergies: None known

Previous Surgeries: Coronary artery bypass graft

Medications: At the time of admission include Glucotrol, Lasix, potassium, and aspirin

Review of Systems: Endocrine: He does have diabetes controlled with medication. Cardiovascular: History of coronary artery disease with coronary artery bypass graft. No recent symptoms of chest pain or shortness of breath. Respiratory: No chronic cough or sputum production. GU: No dysuria, hematuria, history of stones, or infections. Musculoskeletal: No arthritic complains or muscle weakness. Neuropsychiatric: No syncope, seizures, weakness, paralysis, depression.

Family History: Is positive for cardiovascular disease and diabetes in his mother. No history of cancer.

Social History: The patient is married. Never smoked. Does not drink any alcohol. Works in a factory.

On physical examination, a well-developed, well-nourished, alert male in no acute distress. Blood pressure: 146/82. Respirations: 18. Heart rate: 78. Skin: Good turgor and texture. Eyes: No scleral icterus. Pupils are round, regular, equal, and react to light. Neck: No jugular venous distention. No carotid bruits. Thyroid is not enlarged. Trachea in the midline. Lungs are clear. Heart: No murmur noted. Abdomen is soft. Bowel sounds present. No masses, no tenderness. Liver and spleen are not palpably enlarged. Extremities: Good pulses. Trace edema of the feet.

Laboratory values show severe anemia with a hemoglobin of 5.7. Hemoccult is also positive. His iron studies showed low iron and low ferritin, consistent with chronic blood loss anemia. His B12 and folate levels were normal. His SMA-12 was essentially unremarkable.

Impression:
1. Anemia. Probably he is anemic after bypass and then had stress gastritis with a little bit of bleeding and has never recovered from that. No evidence of acute or active bleeding at this time. The patient is stable. Possibility of occult malignancy or active peptic ulcer disease does exist.
2. Arteriosclerotic heart disease of native vessel, stable

Recommendations: Admit patient as an outpatient for blood transfusion. Patient is being transfused. He should have an esophagogastroduodenoscopy and colonoscopy, possible biopsy, or polypectomy, which has been explained to the patient along with potential risks and complications including bleeding, transfusion, perforation, and surgery. These tests will be scheduled as soon as possible.

Discharge Note

Final Diagnoses:
1. Severe blood loss anemia; weakness
2. Type II diabetes mellitus
3. History of coronary artery disease status post coronary artery bypass graft

The patient received three units of packed red blood cells, leukoreduced, CMV negative. He felt better, with subsidence of his shortness of breath, and his weakness improved. His last hemoglobin was 8.4, with a hematocrit of 27.7.

The patient was scheduled for EGD to rule out peptic ulcer disease and colonoscopy to rule out occult malignancy in 1 week. The patient will be discharged home, and he will have a clear liquid diet. He is to call for any problems. He will continue with his home medications, and he was placed on ferrous sulfate, one tablet twice a day.

What codes are reported for this outpatient encounter? The facility purchases its blood from the blood bank.

ICD-9-CM, CPT, and/or HCPCS Code(s):

a. 280.0, 792.1, 414.01, 250.00, V45.81, V17.49, 36430, P9051 (3 units)
b. 285.9, 780.79, 36430, P9051 (3 units)
c. 280.0, 578.1, 414.01, 250.00, V45.81, V17.49, 36430
d. 285.9, 792.1, 414.01, 250.00, V45.81, V17.49, P9051 (3 units)

ICD-10-CM Code(s): _____

8.3.   The following documentation is from the health record of an 87-year-old female patient.

Emergency Department Services

History: The patient is an 87-year-old white female brought to the ED because of pleural effusion, urinary tract infection, and dehydration. She had been taking medication. She lives at the nursing home and has been doing fairly well. Today she was found to be weak and not eating well. Then she was sent to the emergency room for evaluation and found to have pleural effusion and dehydration, urinary tract infection, also thrombocytopenia with petechial hemorrhage. She was found to have a platelet count of 77,000.

Past History: She has a history of cholecystectomy.

Social History: She is a retired woman. No smoking, no drinking, no allergies.

Family History: Noncontributory

Systemic Review: Otherwise normal

Physical Examination: Today reveals blood pressure is 163/62. Pulse of 80. Respirations of 15. Temperature of 98.6°F. General condition of the patient showed chronically ill, confused, disoriented. No jaundice, no cyanosis. No pallor, no edema. The patient has dehydration +3. Scalp and skull are normal. There was a bluish color around the eyes and petechial hemorrhage at the eyelid and conjunctiva. Ears, nose, and throat are normal. Neck showed normal cervical spine. The neck veins are flat. No bruits of the carotid arteries. The trachea is midline. Thyroid gland cannot be palpated. Lymph glands cannot be palpated. Chest shows normal contour. The breasts are normal. Movement of the chest equal on both sides. There is dullness of the chest with some rales and rhonchi. Heart shows apex beat is at the fifth intercostal space, left midclavicular line. No diffuse precordial pulsation, no thrill. Heart rate is 80, regular, with premature ventricular contraction, no murmur. Back is normal. Abdomen showed normal contour, soft, nontender, no guarding, no rigidity. Liver, spleen, and kidneys cannot be palpated; no mass is palpable. Bowel sounds are positive. No fluid thrill. No shifting dullness. No bruits of the abdominal vessels. Extremities show no clubbing of the fingers. No varicose veins. No phlebitis. Hematoma of the right hand. Peripheral pulses are normal. The deep tendon reflexes are normal. Babinski sign is negative.

Laboratory Studies: Hematocrit was 43, white count 9,000 with 82 percent neutrophils, and the platelet count 77,000. The MCV was 102. Creatinine was 1.7. Bilirubin was 1.7. The alkaline phosphatase was 122. AST 498, ALT 493, and albumin 3.6. The prothrombin time was 18 seconds; the PTT was 25 seconds. The chest x-ray showed a right pleural effusion.

Impression: 1. Urinary tract infection
2. Dehydration
3. Pleural effusion from congestive heart failure
4. Primary thrombocytopenia with petechial hemorrhage
5. Type II diabetes mellitus

Plan of Treatment: The patient will be stabilized and started on IV fluids. Also will start IV antibiotic for urinary tract infection. Patient will be transferred at the family's request to a larger facility. A consultation with hematology will be arranged, and a transfusion of platelets may be indicated.

What are the appropriate diagnosis codes for this service?

ICD-9-CM Code(s):

a. 599.0, 276.51, 428.0, 287.5, 250.00
b. 599.0, 276.51, 428.0, 511.9, 287.5, 250.00
c. 599.0, 276.51, 428.0, 287.30, 250.00
d. 599.0, 276.51, 428.0, 511.9, 287.30, 782.7, 250.00

ICD-10-CM Code(s): _____

8.4.   The following documentation is from the health record of a 39-year-old female patient.

Hospital Outpatient Department Services

This 39-year-old female was diagnosed with breast cancer 2 years ago. At that time she had a mastectomy performed, with no evidence of metastases to the lymph nodes. About 8 months ago, metastases were discovered in her liver. The patient was given chemotherapy. She has been losing weight and developing increased fatigue. Patient was referred to hospice care program, with a life expectancy of 4 to 6 months. Progressive weight loss due to loss of appetite led to cachexia and program of home intravenous hyperalimentation. Progressive, unrelenting abdominal pain led to chronic use of analgesics. Patient is awake, alert, and desires to spend more time with family. Progressive weakness and dropping hemoglobin led to the decision to transfuse the patient every 2 weeks with 2 units of packed cells. Patient is stable and more comfortable on this regimen.

She is coming into the outpatient department now for transfusion.

Diagnosis: History of breast cancer, current liver metastases, anemia in neoplastic disease and due to chemotherapy.

What are the correct diagnosis codes assigned in this case?

ICD-9-CM Code(s):

a. 285.22, 285.3, 197.7, V10.3, E933.1
b. 285.9, 197.7, V10.3, E933.1
c. 197.7, 285.22, V10.3, E933.1
d. 285.9, 197.7, V10.3

ICD-10-CM Code(s): _____

Disorders of the Cardiovascular System

8.5. The following documentation is from the health record of a 60-year-old male patient.

Outpatient Hospital Diagnostic Services

A 60-year-old man was given a stress test for recent left arm pain that occurred with exercise the day before. His only medication was Dyazide 1 daily. He was exercised by the Bruce protocol for a duration of 6 minutes, 2 seconds using the treadmill. Maximum heart rate achieved was 137; 85 percent maximum predicted was 136. His blood pressure during the stress test went up to 182/80. He denied any arm pain with the exercise. He did have 2 mm of ST depression at a point of maximum exercise in 2, 3, AVF, but these were all upsloping. Also in V5, V6, he had 1.4-mm ST depression, also upsloping.

Following exercise he was placed at rest. At about 1 minute, 45 seconds post exercise, his STT waves changed. He had STT wave depression with T-wave inversion in the interior and V5 and V6 leads. The patient remained asymptomatic throughout, with no arrhythmias. His blood pressure dropped to a low of 38 systolic over 0 at 6 minutes post exercise and remained low for several minutes. During this time period, an IV was started and D5 1/2 normal saline at 200 cc/hour was given to elevate the blood pressure. IV started at 12:30 and stopped at 13:20. The patient remained pain-free during this episode and felt fine during the entire episode. At the 10-minute mark, the T-wave inversion started resolving, and the STT waves returned to normal.

Upon consultation with Dr. Jones at Magic Memorial, the patient was advised to report for a cardiac catheterization to rule out ischemic heart disease.

Which codes are reported by the hospital for this outpatient service?

Note: The cardiologist is not employed by the hospital reporting the test.

In addition to the IV infusion codes, which codes are reported by the hospital for this outpatient service?

ICD-9-CM and CPT Code(s):

a. 786.50, 796.3, 93015
b. 729.5, 796.3, 93015
c. 414.8, 458.29, 93017
d. 729.5, 458.9, 93017

ICD-10-CM Code(s): _____

8.6.   The following documentation is from the health record of a patient who received hospital outpatient surgical services.

Preoperative Diagnosis:	Hypertensive cardiovascular disease with end-stage renal disease and congestive heart failure
Postoperative Diagnosis:	Same
Procedure:	Placement of AV fistula with Gore-Tex graft of the right forearm for dialysis access

Description: After placement on the operating table, the patient was premedicated with .05 mg of Versed. The right arm was prepped and draped in the usual sterile fashion. Following the infiltration of 1 percent lidocaine, a transverse incision was made just beyond the antecubital fossa. Dissection was carried down, the basilic vein and artery were identified and mobilized, and Silastic loops were placed. Another incision was then made, just above the wrist. After the area was infiltrated with lidocaine, a 6-mm Gore-Tex graft was tunneled through the loop. Anastomosis to the artery was accomplished after the patient received 2,000 units of IV heparin. End-to-side anastomosis was accomplished with 6-0 and 7-0 Prolene sutures. The end areas were interrupted and the edges approximated with running sutures. On removal of the clamps, excellent blood flow was evident. Anastomosis was deemed satisfactory. Venous anastomosis was then accomplished with 6-0 and 7-0 Prolene sutures. Flushing and back-bleeding were allowed prior to completion of the anastomosis. Upon completion, excellent flow was evident through the vein. After a period of observation with no bleeding, both wounds were closed with subcutaneous 3-0 VICRYL in a running fashion, and the skin was closed with 4-0 Prolene sutures. Dressings were applied and the patient returned to the outpatient recovery area in stable condition.

Which of the following is the correct code set?

ICD-9-CM and CPT Code(s):

a. 404.92, 36830
b. 404.93, 585.6, 428.0, 36830
c. 585.6, 428.0, 401.9, 36821
d. 404.93, 36821

ICD-10-CM Code(s): _____

8.7.   The following documentation is from the health record of a patient who received hospital outpatient diagnostic services.

Preoperative Diagnosis:	Angina
Postoperative Diagnosis:	Patent coronary arteries and grafts, ASHD present
Procedure:	Right and left heart cath with coronary angiography

The patient was brought to the cath lab in a fasting state. The right groin was prepped and draped in the usual sterile fashion. After local anesthesia was administered, sheaths were placed percutaneously into the right femoral artery and vein. IV heparin 3,000 units were given.

Using a thermodilution catheter, right heart pressures were measured, and thermo-dilution cardiac outputs and AV oxygen differences were obtained. A pigtail catheter was inserted into the left ventricular cavity, and simultaneous left ventricular pressures were measured. A pullback was obtained across the aortic valve.

Using a 7R4 catheter, angiography was performed of the right coronary artery and both vein grafts. A 7L4 was used for angiography of the left coronary artery. Additional attempts were made to image the vein graft to the right coronary artery with a right coronary artery bypass catheter. The pigtail catheter was reinserted, and left ventricular angiography and aortic root angiography were performed. The patient tolerated the procedure well and returned to the recovery room in good condition.

Which codes are assigned for this service?

ICD-9-CM and CPT Code(s):

a. 414.00, 413.9, V45.81, 93461
b. 414.01, 414.02, 93453, 93460
c. 414.00, 413.9, V45.81, 93453, 93462
d. 414.01, 414.02, 413.9, V45.81, 93461

ICD-10-CM Code(s): _____

8.8. This 21-month-old male presents to the Emergency Department with nausea and vomiting since 10 pm last night, at least 8 times, which is nonbloody but bilious. Temp of 39.8 since last night. He has a history of Tetralogy of Fallot, s/p repair 2 months ago. He has known immunodeficiency, laryngomalacia, and a gastrostomy tube. After examination, working differential diagnoses are acute gastroenteritis, bacteremia, or possible septicemia. Symptoms similar to episode about 1 month ago that was determined to be bacteremia with G-tube site infection. The patient is treated with Zofran 2 mg IV, followed by Ceftriaxone 600 mg IV. The patient is discharged after resolution of vomiting and fever. Diagnosis listed as acute gastroenteritis.

Assign the correct codes for the facility services provided today.

ICD-9-CM Code(s):

a. 558.9, 279.3, 748.3, V13.69, V15.1, V44.1
b. 558.9, 790.7, V15.1, V44.1
c. 787.01, 558.9, V44.1
d. 787.03, 780.60, 558.9, 745.2, V15.1, V44.1

ICD-10-CM Code(s): _____

8.9. A 69-year-old patient was hit by a car, causing intra-thoracic trauma and hemorrhage. The patient was taken directly from the Emergency Department to the operative suite where the chest was opened and hemorrhage was controlled, but the patient's heart stopped. Open heart massage was performed but the patient expired before the patient could be admitted.

Assign the appropriate CPT code(s) and any required modifier(s) to report this service.

a. 32110-CA
b. 32110, 32160
c. 32160-CA
d. 32110-CA, 32160-CA

8.10. This 63-year-old male patient presents to the ED by ambulance after collapsing while mowing the lawn at home. He has a diminished level of consciousness but says that he had palpitations and lightheadedness followed by apparent syncope. His wife saw him fall and immediately called 9-1-1. He has a prior history of MI 3 years ago and coronary atherosclerosis of the native vessels. His vital signs on presentation show hypotension with a heart rate of 110. His EKG shows arrhythmia. While on the heart monitor the patient's rhythm changes to ventricular fibrillation. 150-J biphasic cardioversion shock is performed, following standard advanced cardiac life-support protocols. Arrhythmia continues following cardioversion, and the patient arrests. CPR is performed, and the patient is resuscitated.

The physician documents: 35 minutes of critical care provided, exclusive of the time spent performing cardioversion, for a patient with acute ventricular tachycardia, ventricular fibrillation, prior MI, coronary atherosclerosis of native vessels, and cardiac arrest, successfully resuscitated.

What are the correct diagnosis and procedure codes for this patient?

ICD-9-CM and CPT Code(s): _____

ICD-10-CM Code(s): _____

8.11. The following documentation is from the health record of a patient who received hospital outpatient radiology department services.

Preoperative Diagnosis: Left carotid aneurysm, internal extracranial portion

Postoperative Diagnosis: Same

Procedure: Left carotid artery test occlusion

Procedure Description: With the patient properly prepared and draped in sterile fashion, a 6-French sheath was inserted in antegrade fashion into the right femoral artery. A diagnostic catheter was inserted coaxially through the sheath and used to select the left internal carotid artery. An exchange 018 wire was placed through the catheter and then the catheter was removed. A 6 mm × 2 cm balloon catheter was threaded over the wire and positioned with the balloon across the lumen of the proximal left internal carotid artery. The balloon was inflated to 0.5 atmosphere while slowly injecting contrast through the end of the balloon around the wire. Complete stasis of the carotid artery was documented. Neurologic testing was performed for 5 minutes. The patient was placed on heparin prior to this procedure, and a 5,000-unit bolus was administered in the left carotid artery just prior to balloon inflation. Another 1,000 units of heparin were slowly administered through the tip of the balloon over a 5-minute period, along with saline. Only a small amount of total fluid was administered, and contrast was found to be static in the carotid artery during the entire period. After 5 minutes, the balloon was deflated and the patient was sent to the recovery area in good condition.

What is the correct code assignment?

ICD-9-CM and CPT Code(s):

a. 437.3, 36100, 37204, 75894
b. 442.81, 36620
c. 442.81, 36100, 37204, 75894
d. 442.81, 61626, 36100, 75894

ICD-10-CM Code(s): _____

8.12. The following documentation is from the health record of a cardiac catheterization patient.

Procedures Performed: Left heart catheterization.
Coronary angiography.
Right coronary artery mid in-stent restenotic lesion.
Percutaneous transluminal coronary balloon angioplasty.
Placement of intracoronary stent.
Right coronary artery-distal stent edge lesion.
Percutaneous transluminal coronary balloon angioplasty.
Placement of intracoronary stent.
Adjunct use of intravenous Aggrastat infusion.

Complications: None.

Indication: This is a 70-year-old white male with known history of hyperlipidemia, TIA, and coronary artery disease status, post PTCA with stent placement of the mid right coronary artery on July 27, 20XX, who presented with recurrence of chest pain. The stress MIBI cardiac scan performed on January 29, 20XX, revealed proximal inferior wall perfusion defects extending to the LV apex.

Diagnostic Angiography: After obtaining informed consent, the patient was brought to the cardiac catheterization laboratory in a fasting state. The bilateral femoral areas were prepped sterilely in the standard fashion, and ECG monitoring was established. Using the modified Seldinger technique, arterial access was obtained in the right femoral artery.

The #7 French Cordis JL-4 HF and JR-4 HF catheters were used to perform the diagnostic coronary angiography. The left main artery was large and essentially normal. The left anterior descending artery was moderate-sized, long, and wrapped around the apex without significant lesion. The first diagonal branch artery was large, bifurcated, and essentially normal. The second diagonal branch artery was small-sized and normal. The left circumflex artery was large and had 40 to 50 percent ostial stenosis. The first and second obtuse marginal arteries were small and normal. The right coronary artery was dominant and had 90 to 95 percent multifocal in-stent restenosis in the mid artery. There was also 60 to 70 percent distal stent edge stenosis in the early distal right coronary artery. The PDA and PLB arteries were normal.

Procedure: Mid right coronary artery (RCA) in-stent restenosis and distal stent edge lesions: Following the diagnostic coronary angiography, Aggrastat 16.1 cc IV bolus was then given to the patient with continuous infusion at rate of 14 cc/hour for 50 minutes. Heparin, 5,400-unit IV bolus, was also given to the patient to control ACT around 200 to 300 seconds. After this, a #8 French Cordis JR-4/side hole guiding catheter was used to engage into the ostium of the right coronary artery. After baseline angiography was performed, a Guidant 0.014 inch Hi-Torque floppy extra support guidewire was then advanced out of the guide into the RCA. The guidewire was then advanced across the mid RCA in-stent restenotic lesion and positioned in the distal PLB artery without difficulty. After this, an NC Ranger balloon, 2.75 mm in diameter by 22 mm in length, was advanced over the guidewire into the mid RCA in-stent restenotic lesion. The balloon was positioned across the lesion and inflated twice at 18 atmospheres and 20 atmospheres for 60 seconds, respectively. The patient had transient chest pain and ST-T wave elevation in the inferior leads.

Following this, the balloon was then advanced further to cross the distal stent edge lesion in the early distal right coronary artery and inflated at 10 atmospheres for 60 seconds. Repeat angiogram still revealed some residual narrowing at the distal stent edge lesion. After this, the balloon was then exchanged out for a BX Velocity, 2.75 mm × 8 mm, coronary stent that was advanced to deploy cover in the distal stent edge lesion at 12 atmospheres for 15 seconds; however, the stent did not overlap with the mid RCA previously stented segment. Repeat angiogram revealed a small dissection at the distal RCA in the gap between the old and the new coronary stent. The operator then elected to deploy another short stent to cover the dissection. The second BX Velocity, 2.75 mm × 8 mm, coronary stent was then advanced to position to cover the dissection, overlapping with the mid RCA and distal RCA stented segment. The stent was then successfully deployed at 12 atmospheres for 30 seconds. Follow-up angiogram revealed good luminal dilatation in the distal RCA stented segment; however, there was increased renarrowing within the mid RCA in-stent restenotic lesion with irregular border. The operator decided to deploy another stent to cover within the mid RCA in-stent restenotic lesion. The third BX Velocity, 2.75 mm × 18 mm, coronary stent was then advanced to position within the mid RCA in-stent restenotic lesion and successfully deployed at 14 atmospheres for 30 seconds. After this, the stent balloon was used to post dilate sequentially within the entire mid RCA and distal RCA stented segment at 10 atmospheres and 12 atmospheres for 3 minutes of total duration.

Final orthogonal angiogram revealed no residual stenosis in the overlapping stented mid- and distal RCA in-stent restenotic lesion and distal stent edge lesion. There was no angiographic evidence of dissection or thrombus. Flow to the distal vessel was TIMI grade 3. Plavix, 375 mg, was given to the patient after the stent deployment. At this point, it was elected to conclude the procedure. Balloon, wires, and catheters were removed. The hemostatic sheaths were sewn in place. The patient was transferred back to the ward in stable condition.

Conclusions: 1. Significant multifocal in-stent restenotic lesion in the mid RCA with distal stent edge lesion in the distal RCA.
2. Successful percutaneous transluminal coronary balloon angioplasty and placement of three overlapping coronary stents (BX Velocity 2.75 mm × 18 mm, 2.75 mm × 8 mm, and 2.75 mm × 8 mm) in the mid RCA in-stent restenotic lesion and distal stent edge lesion in the early distal right coronary artery.

What are the correct diagnosis and procedure codes for this patient?

ICD-9-CM First-Listed Diagnosis: _____

ICD-9-CM Additional Diagnoses: _____

CPT Code(s): _____

ICD-10-CM First-Listed Diagnosis: _____

ICD-10-CM Additional Diagnoses: _____

8.13. **Emergency Services:**

Chief Complaint: Cardiac Arrest

HPI: The 37-year-old female was found on the floor of her bathroom by her husband. She was in full arrest and he started CPR immediately. She could have been down as long as 20 minutes prior to him finding her. The EMTs took over CPR when they arrived some 20 minutes later and applied AED. They intubated her with a 7.5 ET—the cords were visualized and taped at 24 cm. Good breath sounds bilaterally after intubation.

The EMTs administered 1 mg EPI and 1 mg Atropine—no response and ECG was still in asystole.

Physical Exam upon Arrival: The patient was unconscious and apneic and pulseless. Skin: Purple from just above the clavicle and skin was cool and dry. HEENT: Pupils fixed and dilated. Neck: No JVD or trachea deviation. Chest: clear and equal bilateral sounds with intubation. Abdomen: Distended and tight. Extremities: Flaccid and cool.

Emergency Physician's Note: This 37 y/o white female arrived by ambulance in full arrest. Epi and bicarb were given on the way to the hospital. Two leads showed agonal asystole rhythm.

A high dose of epi 5 mg was given IV and shock with 360 joules $\times$ 2—no response. A total of 4 amp of bicarb and 4 high dose epi given with intervening defib at 360 joules. No response. Her pupils were fixed and dilated on arrival—has full neck and chest venous stasis. The endo tube was aerating both lungs. Blood gases revealed:

Ph 6.909, PO_2 57, HCO_3 9.9, Base 22.4, O_2 sat 64%, PCO_2 49

The patient arrived at 11:10 and the code was called at 11:45. Patient never had any pulse or spontaneous electrical activity.

Which of the following codes represent the services provided for this patient?

ICD-9-CM and CPT Code(s):

a. 427.5, 782.5, 92950, 92960, 99291, J0171
b. 427.5, 92950, 92960, 99291, J0171
c. 427.5, 782.5, 92950, 92960, 99291
d. 427.5, 99291, J0171

ICD-10-CM Code(s): _____

Disorders of the Digestive System

8.14. The following documentation is from the health record of a 86-year-old female patient.

Preoperative Diagnosis: Paraesophageal hernia

Postoperative Diagnosis: Paraesophageal hernia

Procedure: Laparoscopic reduction of paraesophageal hernia

Indication: The patient is a pleasant, 86-year-old female who presented with an acute onset of hematemesis. Endoscopy was performed, which revealed a large portion of the patient's stomach in her chest. The condition was discussed with the patient and her family. The options of open versus laparoscopic repair of her hernia were discussed. The patient and her family understood the risks versus benefits, as well as potential complications of both procedures, and elected to undergo the laparoscopic procedure. Based on the presence of multiple other chronic illnesses, the patient and family have signed a Do Not Resuscitate order as of today.

Procedure Description: After consent was obtained, the patient was taken to the operating room and placed supine on the operating table. After adequate general endotracheal anesthesia, the patient's abdomen was prepped and draped in the usual surgical fashion. Initial entry was gained through an infraumbilical elliptical incision. Cut down technique was used. A 5-mm trocars was inserted. A pneumoperitoneum was then obtained. Two additional 5.0 mm trocars were placed—one in the left epigastric region and another in the left upper quadrant. The initial 5.0-mm infraumbilical trocar was replaced with a 12-mm trocar. A 10-mm 30 degree scope was used throughout the procedure for visualization.

The stomach was then grasped with the soft bowel grasper and reduced from the chest in a hand-over-hand fashion. There were dense attachments of the stomach to the superior portion of the hernia sac in the chest. These were carefully taken down with the harmonics shearers. This allowed for good mobilization of the stomach and return of the stomach to the abdomen. The hernia sac was resected and sent to Pathology. The 1.0 cm defect of the diaphragm around the esophagus was repaired with mesh implantation.

The abdomen was then inspected for hemostasis which was noted to be pristine. The laparoscopic trocars were removed and the CO_2 insufflation was released. The skin incisions were closed with Monocryl, benzoin, and Steri-strips and followed by sterile Band-Aids. The patient tolerated the procedure well. She was awakened, extubated, and taken to the recovery room in satisfactory condition.

What codes will be reported for the outpatient care of this Medicare patient?

ICD-9-CM and CPT Code(s):

a. 578.0, 553.3, V49.86, 43281
b. 553.3, 49652
c. 553.3, V49.86, 43282
d. 578.0, 553.3, 43659

ICD-10-CM Code(s): _____

8.15. A patient reported to the ambulatory surgery department at the request of her general surgeon.

Operative Report:	Hospital Outpatient Surgery Department
Preoperative Diagnoses:	1. Inguinal hernia 2. Postcolorectal resection for CA
Postoperative Diagnosis:	Same
Procedure:	Right inguinal herniorrhaphy

Description of Procedure: Under general anesthetic, an incision was made over the anterior wall of the inguinal canal, which was opened. The cord was isolated, taking care to protect the nerve. The hernia sac was seen, which has direct hernia on the medial aspect of the wound. This was reduced and held in place using mesh that was stapled into place with a hole being made for the cord. The anterior wall of the inguinal canal was then closed with VICRYL, a hemostasis was achieved, and the wound closed with skin clips. Following this, the attention was turned to a screening colonoscopy, which was performed to the ileocecal valve without difficulty. Ascending, transverse, and descending colon were normal. There was no true evidence of diverticula. The sigmoid was normal, and a retroflex view of the rectosigmoid anastomosis in the rectum shows no gross abnormalities. The patient tolerated the procedure well and will be followed up in the office.

Which code set is reported by the facility for this outpatient surgery?

ICD-9-CM and CPT Code(s):

a. 550.90, 562.10, V10.05, 49505-RT, G0105
b. 550.90, V76.51, V10.06, 49505-RT, 45378
c. 550.91, V76.51, V10.05, 49505-RT, 49568-RT
d. 550.90, V10.06, 49520-RT, 45330

ICD-10-CM Code(s): _____

8.16. The following documentation is from the health record of a 70-year-old Medicare patient who received hospital outpatient services.

Operative Report

History and Indications: The patient is a 70-year-old female who previously underwent a cholecystectomy but presents again with similar pain in the right upper quadrant in the presence of disturbed liver function studies.

Procedure: ERCP sphincterotomy and stone extraction. The Olympus Video side-viewing duodenoscope was atraumatically introduced into esophagus and advanced with slide-by technique into the stomach. The gastric mucosa was normal. The pyloric channel was normal and easily intubated. The first and second parts of the duodenum were visualized. The ampulla appeared normal. Initial cannulation with a precurved catheter revealed a normal pancreatic duct. A single injection was made into the pancreas. Repositioning was accomplished with the assistance of a straight 0.035 guidewire, and free cannulation and injection of the papilla of Vater was accomplished. Full visualization of the common duct was obtained, revealing a large multifaceted free-floating stone within the proximal duct. The intrahepatic biliary system appeared normal. The extrahepatic biliary system appeared dilated. An exchange was made with the 20-millimeter sphincterotome and a sphincterotomy was performed with perfect hemostasis. The duct was then swept with a 15-millimeter stone extraction balloon, and the stone was pulled into the duodenal lumen. The duct was "swept" two more times with negative results. Additional spot and overhead films were obtained to confirm clearance of all stone material. The procedure was terminated with the patient in satisfactory condition, and she was returned to the recovery area.

Assessment: Choledocholithiasis associated with obstruction.

Which code set will be submitted for this Medicare patient for the services described?

ICD-9-CM and CPT Code(s):

a. 574.50, 43262, 43273
b. 574.50, 43262, 43264
c. 574.51, 43262, 43264, 43273
d. 574.51, 43262

ICD-10-CM Code(s): _____

8.17. The following documentation is from the health record of a 65-year-old male who received hospital outpatient GI laboratory services.

Endoscopy Record

Preoperative Diagnosis:	Guaiac positive stools
Postoperative Diagnosis:	Multiple colon polyps, diverticulosis
Procedure:	Total colonoscopy with biopsy and polypectomy

Indications: This is a 65-year-old male who was found to have guaiac positive stools on a routine exam; no change in bowel habits or appreciable weight loss.

The patient was brought to the endoscopy suite and placed in the left lateral decubitus position. 50 mg of Demerol and 2 mg Versed were administered. Digital rectal exam was performed, which was normal. Olympus colonoscope was inserted and passed under direct vision. A large polyp was seen immediately at 20 cm. This appeared to be pedunculated and approximately 1.5 cm long. Scope was passed all the way to the cecum and then slowly withdrawn. Cecum, ascending colon, hepatic flexure, transverse colon all appeared normal except for fairly extensive diverticula in the cecum and scattered throughout the rest of the sets. At the splenic flexure at 80 cm, there was a lesion, which was biopsied with a hot biopsy probe. At 60 cm, there was another small polyp, which was cauterized at the base with the probe and excised. At 20 cm, the pedunculated rectal polyp was snared and removed. The exam of the base revealed complete excision. The rest of the sigmoid and the rectum were unremarkable.

The pathology report showed mucus polypoid tissue at 80 cm and adenomatous polyps at 60 cm and 20 cm.

Which of the following code sets should be reported?

ICD-9-CM and CPT Code(s):

a. 211.3, 211.4, 562.10, 45385, 45384-59, 45380-59
b. 211.3, 569.0, 45384
c. 211.3, 569.0, 45385, 45384-59, 45380-59
d. 792.1, 211.3, 569.0, 562.10, 45385, 45384

ICD-10-CM Code(s): _____

8.18. This is the health record of a patient treated in Ambulatory Surgery

Significant Findings: This patient is an 84-year-old male with complaint of recurrent left inguinal hernia with associated discomfort. The original surgery on this patient was 2 years ago and the patient wraps his abdomen without physician's order. This in fact is increasing the discomfort in his abdominal. He currently denies any urological or GI problems. The physical examination revealed a very pleasant senior citizen in minimal distress. HEENT were normal. Chest/heat revealed no rales or rhonchi. Skin: warm and dry to the touch although he does have an eczematous rash on the upper chest which has not been diagnosed previously. He admits to using some type of OTC cream for this. His inguinal area is significant for a healed scar in the left groin area which today shows a significant and reducible bulge. There was a smaller hernia on the right side.

Laboratory Findings: Electrolyte panel was within normal limits. Bleeding time acceptable at 2 minutes. His white count was 12,500. HB was 14 and HCT 43 with a normal differential. Urinalysis showed the following results: Dark yellow, cloudy urine with evidence of pyuria. RBCs 2; WBC 10; pH6 Potassium 15. Findings suggest early UTI.

Two view chest x-ray was normal with some moderate cardiomegaly and healed rib fractures.

Admitting Diagnosis: Recurrent left inguinal hernia and initial right inguinal hernia

Postoperative diagnosis was the same.

Procedure: Laparoscopic repair of recurrent left inguinal hernia and right inguinal hernia

Description of Procedure: The patient was taken to the Ambulatory Surgery suite where he was prepped and draped in the usual manner and placed in the supine position on the table. Monitoring equipment was attached and he was given general anesthesia for a laparoscopic repair of a recurrent left inguinal hernia and an initial right inguinal hernia.

Trocars were inserted for laparoscopy and the hernias repaired. A piece of 3 × 5 mesh was trimmed to fit the defect in the left inguinal hernia and was placed down in the inguinal canal. It was tacked down using interrupted sutures. A unilateral repair of the initial right hernia was done.

The procedures were performed without any complications. The patient was sent to PACU where he was monitored for several hours. The incisions remained dry and there was no evidence of any unusual swelling in the inguinal areas. The IV was discontinued and the patient was discharged to home. He was given a Lortab prescription and advised to return to the hospital if any complications should occur. The patient was given 1,000 mg of Ampicillin Sodium IM for UTI.

Which codes will be reported for this ambulatory surgery service?

ICD-9-CM and CPT Code(s):

a. 550.93, 49650, 49651, J0290 × 2
b. 550.92, 49650, 49651, 49568
c. 550.93, 49650, 49651
d. 550.91, 550.90, 49650-50, J0290 × 2

ICD-10-CM Code(s): _____

8.19. The following documentation is from the health record of a 40-year-old female patient.

Emergency Department Services

HPI: This is a 40-year-old female with a 3-year history of diarrhea and a 1-year history of epigastric discomfort. She had a CT scan with a mass on the tail of the pancreas, as well as gastrin level greater than 1,000 while taking Prilosec. She has been amenorrheic for the past 4 months.

The patient presents to the ED with severe diarrhea and dehydration after discontinuing medications to allow for a repeat gastrin level off medications to eliminate the compounding effect of Prilosec on gastrin levels. Unfortunately, she was unable to stay off medication long enough, and she developed severe diarrhea with dehydration and a creatinine greater than 3, and she was admitted to observation services. Gastrin level is 1,023 with VIP of 290.

Patient was rehydrated and orally treated with 200 mEq of potassium. The patient had significantly elevated calcium, which normalized with rehydration. Vitamin D level is pending, and PTH level also has returned elevated, concurrent with a calcium of 9.9. MRI of the abdomen has revealed multiple lesions in the liver with a density consistent with metastatic malignancy. Additionally on the MRI, a 6-cm pancreatic mass was noted at the tail of the pancreas.

This scenario is most consistent with multiple endocrine neoplasia syndrome (MEN-1) with parathyroid hyperplasia leading to hypercalcemia when dehydrated. Most likely, the recent normal calcium is due to a concurrent hypovitaminosis D, which is, in turn, secondary to chronic diarrhea. Dostinex has been initiated today at 0.25 mg 2 times a week. Most likely she has MEN-1 given the current pancreatic and pituitary evidence of adenoma.

She is transferred to Memorial Hospital for CT-guided biopsy of a possible adenocarcinoma and to rule out the possibility of MEN-1.

Discharge Diagnoses:
1. Pancreatic and pituitary adenomas with multiple lesions on the liver with questionable metastasis
2. Probable carcinoid syndrome (MEN-1)
3. Hypercalcemia while dehydrated with normalization on rehydration
4. Severe chronic diarrhea with hypokalemia and hypomagnesemia
5. Amenorrhea

Discharge Medications:
Prevacid 30 mg, one p.o. b.i.d.
Magnesium oxide 400 mg, one p.o. t.i.d.
Sandostatin ampules 0.5 amp of 1 mg per amp every 8 hours
Trazodone 50 p.o. q. h.s. p.r.n. insomnia
Darvocet N 100 mg p.o. q. 4–6 hours p.r.n.
Dostinex 0.5 mg 1/2 tab every Wednesday and Saturday

Which of the following is the correct code set for this observation service?

ICD-9-CM Code(s):

a. 237.4, 573.8, 275.42, 276.51, 787.91, 276.8, 275.2, 626.0
b. 211.6, 227.3, 197.7, 275.42, 276.51, 787.91, 276.8, 275.2, 626.0
c. 235.5, 237.0, 197.7, 275.42, 276.51, 787.91, 276.8, 275.2, 626.0
d. 237.4, 573.8, 259.2, 275.42, 276.51, 787.91, 276.8, 275.2, 626.0

ICD-10-CM Code(s): _____

8.20. The following documentation is from the health record of a 57-year-old male patient.

Hospital Outpatient Department Services

Diagnoses: 1. Lung cancer
2. Chemotherapy with Taxol and carboplatin with dexamethasone
3. Type 1 diabetes with neuropathy and nephropathy, uncontrolled
4. Hyperlipidemia
5. Hepatomegaly

This patient is a 57-year-old male who presents to the outpatient department for chemotherapy, which has been complicated by his diabetes because it has been difficult to control. He had surgery for lung cancer in September and has now undergone chemotherapy with Taxol and carboplatin, including dexamethasone as part of his chemo and prophylaxis for nausea. He has done very well with the chemotherapy. His diabetes is complicated by neuropathy and nephropathy. Dr. Johnson consulted with the patient to manage his diabetes. He has been on 70/30 insulin, 25 units in the morning and 15 units in the evening, for over 1 year. His hepatomegaly has enlarged from the last time that I saw him. I question whether this is fatty infiltration due to poor diabetes control, or whether there is now some involvement with metastatic carcinoma.

Taxol and carboplatin were infused today, followed by dexamethasone; see infusion sheet. The patient appears to have tolerated the chemotherapy well.

Laboratory Data: Sodium 128, potassium 5.5, chloride 89, CO_2 34, BUN 13, creatinine 0.8, glucose 210, calcium 9.4, WBC 9.8, hemoglobin 11.6, hematocrit 34.3, platelets 277,000

Plan: One difficulty here is the cyclic nature of his treatment regimen, likely to produce major shifts in his glucose, which is already difficult to control. The patient will need to monitor his glucose levels closely and follow up with Dr. Johnson. The patient has instructions to call in to Dr. Johnson's nurse on a daily basis for the next week. He is to follow up with me for further chemotherapy next week.

Which of the following is the correct code set combination for this outpatient visit?

ICD-9-CM Code(s):

a. 162.9, 250.63, 357.2, 250.43, 583.81, 272.4, 789.1
b. V58.11, 250.63, 250.43, 272.4, 789.1
c. V58.11, 162.9, 250.63, 357.2, 250.43, 583.81, 272.4, 789.1
d. 162.9, 250.03, 272.4, 789.1

ICD-10-CM Code(s): _____

Disorders of the Genitourinary System

8.21.   The following documentation is from the health record of a 22-year-old male patient who received hospital outpatient surgery services.

A patient with chronic benign hypertension and stage V chronic kidney disease requiring chronic dialysis, replacement of a permanent Quinton catheter, and the formation of an arteriovenous graft in the left forearm. Following heparinization, the anastomosis was performed, which resulted in a good pulse, but no thrill. The vein was then explored where an area of stenosis was found. This was opened and a dilator passed, but no more than 2-mm diameter was possible. Therefore, the anastomosis was taken down, a tunnel formed, and a 4 × 7 Impra graft used. The graft originated at the antecubital fossa, which was opened transversely. The vein here was about 4 mm, so there were no problems passing a dilator. The graft was then anastomosed over a distance of approximately 5 mm, resulting in good flow. Wounds were closed in layer fashion with 3-0 VICRYL for deep tissues and continuous suture of 6-0 Prolene.

Following completion of the graft, the patient was reprepped and draped for the changing of the Quinton catheter. Following administration of local anesthesia, an incision was made high in the neck close to the point of insertion in the internal jugular. A guidewire was then tunneled centrally through the existing catheter. The old Quinton catheter was removed and an obturator placed. Then a peel-away introducer was inserted easily. The wounds were then closed and a confirmatory x-ray obtained for placement. This showed the Quinton catheter extended well into the internal jugular. Dialysis was provided the same day.

Which of the following code sets will be assigned for this?

ICD-9-CM and CPT Code(s):

a. 585.6, 401.1, 36830, 90935
b. 403.90, 36825, 90935
c. 403.11, 585.5, 36830, 36581-59
d. 403.11, 585.6, 36830, 36581-59, 90935

ICD-10-CM Code(s): _____

8.22.   The following documentation is from the health record of a patient who received hospital radiology department services.

A patient who has had his bladder removed due to carcinoma without recurrence is ordered to have a radiology procedure to evaluate the patency of his ileal conduit, including a ureteropyelography using contrast media. The chief complaint and reason for service line in the progress note is blank. The entire procedure is performed in the radiology suite with the radiologist's impression of "normal functioning ileal conduit."

Which of the following procedure codes should be reported for the UB-04 in this case? Do not assign ICD-9-CM Volume III procedure codes.

ICD-9-CM and CPT Code(s):

a. V55.6, V45.74, V10.51, 50690, 74425
b. V55.2, V10.51, 74425
c. 596.8, 188.9, 74425
d. Contact the ordering physician to obtain a diagnosis before coding this encounter.

ICD-10-CM Code(s): _____

8.23. The following documentation is from the health record of a 47-year-old female.

Hospital Outpatient Surgery Services

Preoperative Diagnosis:	Menorrhagia, failure of conservative treatment
Postoperative Diagnosis:	Same
Procedure:	Hysteroscopy with biopsy, dilatation and curettage
Diagnosis:	Menorrhagia
Anesthesia:	General

Indications: The patient is a 47-year-old multigravida female with increasing irregular vaginal bleeding. The uterus is very tender, and ultrasound reveals no specific adnexal masses. A Pap smear shows some chronic inflammatory cells and cervicitis. Bleeding has not been controlled in the past month with conservative therapy; thus, the patient is admitted for dilatation and curettage, and a hysteroscopy and biopsy will be carried out.

Technique: Under general anesthesia, the patient was prepped and draped in the usual manner with Betadine, with her cervix retracted outward. Secondary uterine prolapse was noted with minimal cystocele, large rectocele, enterocele, and moderate cervical erosions. The vaginal vault appeared to be clear, as did both adnexa. However, the uterus was thought to be slightly enlarged. Sound was passed into the intrauterine cavity after the cervix was found to be 8 cm deep. The cervix was dilated with Hegar dilators up to #5. The 5-mm Wolff scope, with normal saline irrigation, was then inserted. An inspection of the endocervical canal showed no abnormalities.

Upon entering the uterine cavity, some irregular shedding of the endometrium was noted. Endometrial shedding was noted more to be the patient's left cornu area than the right. The contour of the cavity appeared to be normal; no bulging masses or septation were noted. The Wolff scope was removed, and the cervix was further dilated with Hegar dilators up to #12. A medium-sharp curette was inserted into the uterine cavity and the uterus was curettaged in a clockwise manner, with a moderate amount of what appeared to be irregular proliferative endometrium being obtained.

Again, the contour of the cavity appeared to be normal. Endometrial biopsies also were taken. The patient was transferred to the recovery room in good condition.

Pathology report reveals secretory proliferative endometrium without additional abnormalities noted.

Which of the following code sets will be reported?

ICD-9-CM and CPT Code(s):

a. 626.2, 618.4, 618.6, 616.0, 58558
b. 626.2, 58558
c. 626.2, 618.4, 618.6, 616.0, 58100, 58120
d. 618.4, 618.6, 616.0, 58558

ICD-10-CM Code(s): _____

8.24.   **Chief Complaint:**   Persistent hematuria

History of Present Illness: This is an 83-year-old white female with a 5-day history of gross hematuria. Patient contacted her family physician several days ago. He prescribed antibiotics but the problem is unresolved. The patient does not have a history of urinary tract infections and has never experienced hematuria prior to this episode. Patient had an IVP earlier today which disclosed relatively normal upper urinary tracts but some filling defects in the urinary bladder.

Her current medications include lanoxin for congestive heart failure, iron supplements, and one baby aspirin daily. She does have a history of long-standing CHF.

Allergies: NKA

Past Surgical/Medical History: Patient has had three normal pregnancies and 2 spontaneous abortions completed by dilation and curettage. The patient has a history of bunionectomy and comminuted wrist fracture following a fall several years ago. Generally, she is in good health.

Social/Personal History: Patient neither smokes nor drinks. She does consume several cups of caffeine each day in the form of coffee and hot tea.

Family History: Unremarkable from a urological standpoint.

Review of System: The ROS is unremarkable. The patient denies weight or gain, no shortness of breath or chest pain. No change in bowel habits, no nausea or vomiting. Patient has experienced no problems with gait or sensation and has no discernable pain.

Physical Examination: The patient is a well-nourished, slightly overweight, well-developed female. HEENT: Unremarkable. EOM are full and conjunctivae are normal. Neck: No lymphadenopathy, no enlargement of the thyroid. No bruits heard in the carotids bilaterally. Chest/lungs: Clear to A&P, no rales or rhonchi heard. Breasts: No lumps or adenopathy in the axillary area. Abdomen: No pain or tenderness. GU: External genitalia and pelvic examination do not reveal any obvious problems.

Procedure: Cystourethroscopy with resection of single bladder tumor

Anesthesia: General

Preoperative Diagnosis: Gross hematuria

Postoperative Diagnosis: Bladder tumor

Technique: The patient was placed in the modified dorsolithotomy position, prepped and draped in the usual manner. General anesthesia was attained. A urethroscopy was carried out with Foroblique lens. A 28-French resectoscope sheath with obturator was inserted into the bladder. Transurethral resection of the approximately 2.1-cm bladder tumor was performed and the specimen sent to pathology. Because of the suspicion for bladder carcinoma, fulguration of the surrounding bladder mucosa was performed. There did not appear to be any induration of the bladder mucosa with carcinoma. Instruments were withdrawn and a 20-French Foley catheter inserted. The patient was transported to PACU in stable condition.

Pathology Report

Tissue Submitted: Bladder tumor

Gross Findings: Received in formalin and labeled with the patient's name and "bladder tumor" are 2 irregular segments of soft, rubbery, pink-tan tissue ranging from $0.6 \times 0.3 \times 0.3$ to 1.2 cm $\times 0.9 \times 0.04$ cm.

Microscopic Findings: There appears to be evidence of a papillary lesion with thickened epithelium and nuclear pleomorphism. There may be a minimal degree of infiltration into the lamina propria but extensive infiltration is not noted and none of the muscularis is involved with tumor.

Pathological Findings: Papillary transitional cell carcinoma of the urinary bladder.

Which of the following would be reported for this encounter?

ICD-9-CM and CPT Code(s):

a. 188.9, 599.71, 52000, 52235
b. 233.7, 599.71, 52214
c. 188.9, 599.71, 52235
d. 188.9, 52214, 52235

ICD-10-CM Code(s): _____

8.25. Ambulatory Surgery Operative Report

Preoperative Diagnosis: Cervical dysplasia and right vaginal wall cyst.

Postoperative Diagnosis: Cervical intraepithelial dysplasia I and right vaginal wall cyst

Procedure: Cervical laser ablation; I&D of vaginal wall cyst; EUA.

History: The patient is a 28-year-old nulligravida who has had a history of PAP smears showing slight dysplasia. A colposcopy was done 2 weeks ago which showed a significant amount of erythematous, angry-looking areas. At that time it was noted that she had a sebaceous cyst of the right vaginal wall. Patient has type I diabetes mellitus but this seems to be under control with no significant complications. Preop lab work demonstrated sugar levels at 105, HGB 12.9, HCT 42, and BUN 12. Heart and lung exam were within normal limits.

Description of Procedure: The patient was taken to OP surgery where she was placed in the dorsal lithotomy position and prepped and draped in the usual manner. Induction of general anesthesia was successful. The perineum was cleansed with betadine. An EUA was performed and revealed a large right vaginal wall cyst measuring approximately 4 × 6 cm. There appeared to be significant cervical dysplasia although no masses were palpable. The uterus appeared within normal limits.

A speculum was placed into the vagina which allowed the cervix and vaginal wall to be well visualized. A 4-mm incision was made into the center of the vaginal cyst using electrocautery. A thick sebaceous substance oozed from the cyst. The contents of the cyst were thoroughly expressed.

Two areas of significant dysplasia around the cervical os were noted. The area of cervical dysplasia was ablated 8 cm deep using a CO2 laser at 40 watts. The surrounding area was brushed using a 20-watt laser. Good hemostasis was observed during the procedure. The speculum was removed from the vagina and the patient was sent to PACU in stable and good condition. Blood loss was minimal.

Pathological Findings: CIN 1 and sebaceous cyst of the right vaginal wall.

Which of the following represents correct coding for this service?

ICD-9-CM and CPT Code(s):

a. 233.1, 57420
b. 622.10, 57023, 57513
c. 622.11, 57420, 57513
d. 622.11, 623.8, 57513, 57010

ICD-10-CM Code(s): _____

Infectious Diseases/Disorders of the Skin and Subcutaneous Tissue

8.26.   The following documentation is from the health record of a 62-year-old female patient.

Hospital Outpatient Surgery Services

The patient is a 62-year-old female who has been in generally good health until last month, when she developed a crusty lesion inside the left naris. She initially treated it with Vicks ointment. When it failed to heal, she decided to seek medical attention. Her primary care physician biopsied this lesion, and the pathologic diagnosis was squamous cell carcinoma of the left internal nasal ala. She is posthysterectomy (10 years) for endometrial carcinoma. She has smoked $1\frac{1}{2}$ packs of cigarettes each day for the past 40 years.

The patient presented to the outpatient surgery center of the hospital for wide excision of the left internal nasal alar lesion, which is less than .5 cm in diameter. This procedure included a full-thickness resection in the middle and posterior thirds of the lateral cartilage, along with vestibular skin and mucous membrane. Nasal reconstruction was required to provide an acceptable cosmetic appearance following excision. A flap graft composite reconstruction was utilized for primary closure of the defect that was left following excision, using donor tissue from the right arm and requiring primary closure of a 2-cm graft.

Which of the following code sets is appropriate for this case?

ICD-9-CM and CPT Code(s):

a. 173.3. V10.42, 30118, 30400
b. 160.0, V10.42, 305.1, 30150, 15760
c. 160.0, 15760, 30150
d. 173.3, V10.42, 305.1, 14060

ICD-10-CM Code(s): _____

8.27. The following documentation is from the health record of a 44-year-old female patient.

Hospital Outpatient Surgery Services

Preoperative Diagnosis: Extensive superficial partial-thickness wounds to the abdomen, secondary to poor wound healing; status post abdominoplasty

Postoperative Diagnosis: Same

Operation: Split-thickness skin graft

History: This is a 44-year-old white female who underwent abdominoplasty for morbid obesity in October 20XX and had poor wound healing after the procedure. The patient underwent several debridement and presently has an extensive superficial, partial-thickness abdominal wound that is granulating well, but it was felt the patient would benefit significantly from split-thickness skin graft to decrease wound pain and decrease convalescence time.

Details of Procedure: The patient was taken to the operating room and prepared and draped in the usual sterile fashion, preparing the donor site of the right thigh as well as abdominal superficial partial-thickness wound. First, two donor grafts were taken with the Brown dermatome, adjusted to a #10 blade, 10:1000-of-an-inch size. The grafts were placed over the abdominal superficial partial-thickness wound in the abdomen after it was prepared by a sharp debridement with Bard-Parker #10 blade. The graft was scored with a #10 blade Bard-Parker in a meshing fashion. The graft was then sewn into place with multiple 5-0 VICRYL sutures. The wounds as well as the donor site were then covered with an Owens dressing. Sutures were placed, and the Owens was reinforced with wet saline cotton balls and with a fluff dressing. The stents were then tied in place and covered with a pressure dressing of Elastoplast, while the donor site received wet-to-dry dressing with ABD burn pad taped into place. The patient was extubated in the operating room. All needle and sponge counts were correct, and the patient was taken to the PAR in stable condition.

Pathology Report: None

Which of the following code sets is correct for this case?

ICD-9-CM and CPT Code(s):

a. 998.59, E878.8, 15100
b. 998.59, 15002, 15100
c. 998.83, E878.8, 15100, 15002
d. 998.83, 278.01, 15200

ICD-10-CM Code(s): _____

8.28. The following documentation is from the health record of a patient who received hospital outpatient surgery services.

Preoperative Diagnoses: 1. Biopsy-proven malignant melanoma, Clark Level I, right shoulder
2. Neoplasm on left heel

Postoperative Diagnosis: Same

Operations: 1. Wide excision of malignant melanoma, Clark Level I, right shoulder with wide undermining, rotation, and advancement flap reconstruction

2. Excision of left heel 2 cm × 1 cm × 0.5 cm giant pigmented neoplasm, rule out dysplasia vs. malignant melanoma, with wide undermining, rotation, and advancement flap reconstruction

Description of Procedure: The patient was placed on the operating table in the prone position with the back and left heel prepped and draped in sterile fashion. Utilizing 1 percent Xylocaine with epinephrine, a block of the two sites was performed.

The right shoulder lesion was outlined with Brilliant Green in the lines of relaxation, excised in full-thickness fashion down to the fascial level. Undermining over the fascial level was then performed with rotation flaps elevated into position and sutured deeply at the fascial level with #5-0 PDS interrupted, #6-0 PDS, superficial dermis, and #6-0 PDS running intracuticular on the skin. Total area slightly over 10.2 sq cm.

Attention was then turned to the left heel where the giant pigmented neoplasm was outlined with Brilliant Green, excised in full-thickness fashion, and closed at the fascial level with #4-0 PDS interrupted and 4-0 black nylon interrupted on the skin.

The patient tolerated the procedure quite well and was taken to the recovery room.

Pathology Report

Preoperative Diagnosis: Melanoma right shoulder and lesion left heel

Postoperative Diagnosis: Same

Macroscopic: Specimen 1: Received in formalin, labeled "melanoma right shoulder; biopsy proven Clark Level I" is one ellipse of tan skin, 5 × 1.3 × 1.8 cm. In the center is a healing pink ulcer, 0.6 × 0.4 cm.

The specimen is serially sectioned, and the central lesion is totally submitted in multiple cassettes.

Specimen 2: Received in formalin, labeled "lesion left heel" is one ellipse of tan skin, 1.8 × 0.9 × 0.4 cm. In the center is a brown macular lesion that covers much of the center of the specimen. The specimen is totally submitted in multiple cross sections.

Microscopic and Summary

Specimen 1: Right shoulder excision. Healing ulcer of skin overlying eschar. There is mild scarring and focal foreign body response.

Specimen 2: Left heel. Compatible with a giant pigmented dysplastic nevus.

Which of the following code sets would be reported for this ambulatory surgery?

ICD-9-CM and CPT Code(s):

a. 172.6, 216.7, 14001, 15002
b. 216.7, 216.6, 14000
c. 216.6, 238.2, 14001, 11606, 11423
d. 172.6, 238.2, 14001, 11423-59, 12041

ICD-10-CM Code(s): _____

8.29. The following documentation is from the health record of a patient who received hospital outpatient surgery services.

Preoperative Diagnosis: Nevus of the right auricle

Postoperative Diagnosis: Nevus of the right auricle

Operation: Excision of nevus, right auricle, with reconstruction with full-thickness skin graft, postauricular area

Description of Procedure: The patient was brought to the operating suite and placed under satisfactory general anesthetic using an indwelling endotracheal tube. The right ear and postauricular areas were prepped with Betadine.

A total of 6 cc of 1 percent Xylocaine with 1:200,000 adrenalin were utilized during the procedure. The lesion measured about 6 mm and was superficially infiltrating at its margins with some variegated color being present as well. The lesion was at a 2 o'clock position on the auricular helix. Margins of about 5 mm were made around the lesion. The tissues were submitted for permanent section.

The resulting defect could not be closed primarily. The postauricular incision was outlined for development of postauricular skin graft centered at the level of the cephaloauricular groove. The graft measured about 8 mm × 10 mm in its form and was elliptical in its orientation. The resulting defect postauricularly was closed in layers with 4-0 VICRYL to the subcutaneous layer and 4-0 nylon in an interrupted fashion to the skin.

The skin graft was placed and sutured in place with 4 sutures peripherally with 4-0 silk and then was tied over bolster sutures of 4-0 silk with a bacitracin-impregnated section of sponge rubber. The patient is to avoid contact sports and to keep a prescription for Duricef 250 mg twice a day for 10 days. A prescription for Cap elixir with codeine 1 to 2 tsp, 8 oz was also given. The patient is to be followed up in approximately 1 week in the office.

Pathology Report

Tissues/Specimen: Skin of external ear, nevus of right auricle

Clinical History: Right ear nevus

Gross Description: "Nevus right auricle" consists of small 4-mm fragment of skin. Entire specimen submitted.

Microscopic: Sections show the specimen to consist of an ellipse of skin showing a benign compound nevus. There is no evidence of malignancy.

Which of the following code sets will be reported for this service?

ICD-9-CM and CPT Code(s):

a. 216.8, 15240, 15004, 12051
b. 216.2, 15260, 11442
c. 173.2, 15260, 11442
d. 216.2, 14060

ICD-10-CM Code(s): _____

8.30.   The following documentation is from the health record of a male patient who received emergency department services (Type A provider-based emergency room).

ED Report

A patient who is a known heroin addict is brought in significant distress to the emergency room by friends. His genitalia are covered with many lesions. Due to his IV drug habit and sexual preference, he is at risk for HIV exposure and hepatitis. He has experienced febrile jaundice for 3 days. He is unable to provide a medical history, but the physician is able to get some information from his girlfriend. Although severely ill, he is not comatose. Medical decision making was stated to be of high complexity. The ER acuity system used by the hospital for medical visits indicated a Level IV service.

Physical examination reveals multiple excoriations covering the penis and scrotum with fluid-filled blisters. The patient is jaundiced and in significant distress. The last "fix" was 3 hours ago per the girlfriend, and the patient has been using heroin daily for the past 2 months. A number of laboratory tests were run, and it was determined that the patient should be transferred to a tertiary care center for definitive treatment and an infectious disease consultation and substance abuse rehabilitation when stable.

The physician's dictated report that details the test results shows the following diagnostic assessment:

1. Herpes simplex virus-2 infection, culture confirmed, severe outbreak
2. Hepatitis suspected, pending laboratory results for type, abnormal liver function studies confirmed; febrile jaundice × 3 days
3. HIV seropositive; recommend Western blot to confirm
4. High-risk lifestyle; sexual habits and drug dependence, continuous

Which of the following code sets will be reported in addition to chargemaster-reported codes?

ICD-9-CM and CPT Code(s):

a. 054.10, 782.4, 790.6, 042, 99284
b. 054.19, 573.3, 795.71, 305.51, V69.8, 99214
c. 054.13, 054.19, 070.1, 790.6, 795.71, 305.51, V69.2, 99284
d. 042, 305.51, 070.1, 99291

ICD-10-CM Code(s): _____

Behavioral Health Conditions

8.31. The following documentation is from the health record of a 26-year-old male.

Hospital Outpatient Services

On 1/15, a 26-year-old white male was admitted after being transferred from the outpatient evaluation service with severe homicidal and suicidal ideation. Admitting diagnosis was severe major depressive disorder with psychotic features. Pharmacological treatment was initiated, and suicide precautions were instituted. After a thorough diagnostic evaluation, the risks and benefits of ECT were reviewed. Due to the severity of the psychotic episode and the patient's delusional state, it was determined that ECT was warranted. Extensive efforts were made to secure informed consent from the patient, and a course of ECT was begun.

On 1/23, the psychiatrist reviewed the patient's status noting any changes in his physical condition and his response to the treatment. He performed a problem-focused interval history, a problem-focused examination, and medical decision making of low complexity. At this visit, the psychiatrist again reviewed the treatment options and confirmed the patient's continued consent for ECT. Subsequently on 1/23, the fourth treatment of ECT was administered via placement of a stimulus electrode frontotemporally. Sufficient electrical stimulus was applied to produce an adequate ictal response. A generalized seizure was monitored via EEG. EKG, blood pressure, and pulse remained acceptable throughout. Postictal observation was notable for cardiac arrhythmia, which subsided without sequelae. The patient tolerated the procedure well and was returned to his inpatient room in good condition.

He was discharged to a group home on 1/25 and returned to the hospital as an outpatient for his final planned ECT treatment. Again, sufficient electrical stimulus was applied to produce an adequate ictal response. A generalized seizure was monitored via EEG. EKG, blood pressure, and pulse remained acceptable throughout. Postictal observation was notable for cardiac arrhythmia, which subsided without sequelae. The patient tolerated the procedure well and was held in observation for 4 hours posttreatment, then discharged to the care of his group home supervisor in good condition.

Which of the following code sets is reported for the 1/25 outpatient hospital service?

ICD-9-CM and CPT Code(s):

a. 296.24, V62.85, V62.84, 90870
b. 296.24, V62.85, V62.84, 90870, 95812, 93040
c. 296.24, 298.9, V62.85, V62.84, 90870, 99211-25
d. 296.24, V62.85, V62.84, 90870, 95812, 93040, 99234-25

ICD-10-CM Code(s): _____

8.32.   The following documentation is from the health record of a 56-year-old man.

Emergency Department and Hospital Observation Services

Final Diagnosis: Subchronic schizophrenia, paranoid type with acute exacerbation; improved, compensated congestive heart failure

Pertinent Laboratory Results: Electrolyte panel within normal limits. Digoxin level was 0.6, hemoglobin A1C 6.5, triglycerides 138, CBC unremarkable. TSH 1.3, urinalysis negative. EKG showed normal sinus rhythm.

Assessment: This is a 56-year-old male who presented to the Emergency Room with his sister after decompensating at a hotel where he thought people were trying to get into his apartment, and he continued to decompensate with his paranoia and persecutory-type delusions, so that she felt he needed evaluation for hospitalization. Psychiatric consultation was initiated with Dr. Brown.

Recently, his personal physician has been switching his medications from Zyprexa to Seroquel to Risperdal, and then he started Prolixin. We requested and reviewed his records, and it appears he did quite well on Risperdal, so he went back to taking that, and he was titrated up to 30 mg q. h.s. of Risperdal and 100 mg of trazodone. These 2 medications helped significantly to eliminate his delusions and paranoid ideation. He was admitted to observation status and slept peacefully for 6 hours. His sister reported that he is doing the best that she has seen him in quite some time, and we were conversing at the time of discharge. After consultation with this psychiatrist about the change in medication, the patient was released in the custody of his sister to follow up with his personal physician next Tuesday.

Pertinent Findings on Mental Status at Discharge: Patient spent 45 minutes in the final examination. Behavior is cooperative, fair eye contact. Speech is of normal rate and volume. Not rapid or pressured. Mood euthymic, affect appropriate. Thought process is goal directed, decreased paranoid ideation. Negative for racing thoughts and flight of ideas. Thought content: He denies signs of active psychosis, denies current suicidal or homicidal intent. Insight and judgment improved. Impulse control is fair.

Prognosis: Fair. The main problem is that the patient did not respond well to medication changes. He did do well with the changes we made, but his mental illness may be exacerbated if his medical conditions are not well controlled or if he is noncompliant with dosages.

Aftercare Recommendations: The patient will be discharged to his sister's care and will be followed by his personal psychiatrist, Dr. X. Social services will follow the patient from his hometown.

The hospital acuity system used showed this to be a Level 4 ER service. Which of the following code sets is correct for reporting this service?

ICD-9-CM and CPT Code(s):

a. 295.34, 428.0, 99201
b. 295.32, 99283
c. 295.34, 428.0, 99284
d. 295.84, 99234

ICD-10-CM Code(s): _____

8.33. The following documentation is from the health record of a female patient who received psychiatrist treatment services in a hospital outpatient–based clinic.

XX/XX/XX 6:20 p.m. Dialectical behavior therapy (DBT), individual therapy—1:1 × 45 minutes at 5 p.m.

Subjective/Objective: Patient and I reviewed diary card and target hospitalizable behaviors and increased skills to stay out of the hospital and complete the outpatient program. Target goals 1 through 3 were reviewed today. Patient did not engage or act on urges for self-harm and urges for suicide after self-injurious behavior on XX/XX/XX. We focused on reinforcing skills of emotion regulation, highlighting times she used these while at work and with family members. Suicidal ideation today was minimal with sense of increased willingness to learn to apply skills. Discussed need to address ETOH dependence because patient notes increased risk of suicidal ideation with ETOH use. She identifies "fear" of "running in panic" will be what keeps her from staying with chemical dependency (CD) program. We addressed treatment plan (see below) to increase skills associated with CD treatment follow-through as well as structuring environment to "keep me in CD treatment."

Assessment: Major depressive disorder, recurrent; posttraumatic stress disorder, ETOH dependent; borderline personality disorder. Continued suicidal risk; patient has had some success over urges but is now coping well with the outpatient treatment where she receives therapy four times a week.

Plan: Patient and I identified targeting emotion regulation and distress tolerance in individual therapy to increase control over urges for suicidal thoughts, as well as follow-through with substance abuse treatment. Extended structuring continues with increased resources for managing son's behavior at home. Patient wants family meeting to orient family to DBT to increase chance they will be supportive of her treatment after discharge as opposed to disparaging, which, according to the patient, has increased her emotional vulnerability leading to increased suicidal urges. I gave times I would be available for a family meeting.

Addendum: Patient now has few suicidal urges and wants to do target behaviors. She reviewed skills with me to "get through" the rest of her week at home and at work. She notes that level of urges right now is manageable for her, and she believes she is improving.

Which of the following code sets is correct for reporting the outpatient services provided to this patient?

ICD-9-CM and CPT Code(s):

a. 296.20, 309.81, 303.92, 301.83, 300.9, 90819
b. 296.30, 309.81, 303.90, 301.83, 300.9, 90845
c. 296.30, 309.81, 303.90, 301.83, 90818
d. 296.30, 309.81, 303.90, 301.83, 300.9, 90818

ICD-10-CM Code(s): _____

8.34. The following documentation is from the health record of a 45-year-old female patient.

Mental Health Clinic Visit (Facility Services)

The 45-year-old patient is seen today for 20-minute medication review in the Community Mental Health Center. Patient continues to be somewhat elevated in her mood with some evidence of grandiosity but overall is goal directed and seems to be doing reasonably well with her chronic schizophrenia in the structured setting. Patient currently is now off Seroquel and will continue to transition from oral Prolixin to Prolixin Decanoate. She did receive Prolixin Decanoate 12.5 mg IM on XX/XX/XX. When I try to decrease her oral Prolixin dosage, we notice some more increased grandiosity as well as more impulsive behavior and more thought disorganization, so on XX/XX/XX we increased her Prolixin back to 5 mg q. h.s. orally. On seeing her today, she seems to be improving somewhat on that. Her appetite and sleep pattern were fine over the weekend. She had no evidence of aggressive behavior. I decided at this time to maybe increase her Prolixin Decanoate to 25 mg IM every 2 weeks, and that will start today. Will continue with the oral Prolixin for a period of time and then will be able to eliminate that. There is a meeting with her family this upcoming Wednesday, and we'll discuss patient's care and how they feel she is doing and also discuss discharge and aftercare planning if that's appropriate.

Mental Status Exam: Appearance: The patient is a female who looks her stated age. Behavior: Cooperative, fair eye contact. Speech: Normal rate and volume. Mood slightly elevated. Affect less labile. Thought process: More goal directed. Negative for racing thoughts, flight of ideas. Thought content: Has delusional belief system, but it has decreased in intensity. No evidence of auditory, visual, or olfactory hallucinations. Denies current suicide or homicide intent. Insight: Judgment remains impaired. Impulse control improving.

Impression: Axis I: Schizophrenia, catatonic type, acute exacerbation
Axis II: None known
Axis III: Combined hyperlipidemia; currently on Lipitor

Plan: At this time will continue on the Prolixin Decanoate but increase to 25 mg IM every 2 weeks. Will continue with the oral Prolixin at 5 mg q. h.s.

Which of the following is the correct code set for reporting this clinic service?

ICD-9-CM and CPT Code(s):

a. 295.24, 272.2, 90862
b. 295.20, 272.2, 90862
c. 295.20, 272.2, 90862, 99231
d. 295.24, 272.2, M0064, 99231

ICD-10-CM Code(s): _____

8.35. The following documentation is from the health record of a female patient who received services in a community mental health center.

Reason for Encounter: The patient has not had any self-injurious behavior or behavioral problems this past week except that she has used marijuana, which she endorses. Today we discussed her treatment, and overall she is happy with the DBT program and her chemical dependency program. She and I discussed future care and the need for her to get away from her current living arrangements.

Counseling/Coordination of Care: We reviewed how her DBT is going and what skills she could use when she has high urges to use marijuana. We also discussed that I would be doing periodic drug screenings.

Response to/Complications of Current Medications: None. The patient is happy with her medications as they are.

Examination:	WNL	Abnormal
General appearance	X	
Muscle strength/tone, gait		
Speech		
Thought process	X	
Associations/psychosis		
Suicidal/homicidal ideation	X	
Judgment and insight	X	
Attention span/concentration		
Orientation	X	
Recent and remote memory	X	
Fund of knowledge	X	
Mood and affect	X	

Assessment of Current Status: The patient appears to be stabilizing; however, she does appear to have a need for ongoing chemical dependency treatment and support, perhaps on an inpatient basis if the outpatient treatment plan fails to control relapses.

Diagnosis: Borderline personality disorder; major depression, recurrent; cannabis dependence

Plan: Continue DBT and chemical dependency treatment. The social worker and the patient should begin to work on alternative living arrangements because the patient is exposed to substance abuse in the current living arrangements and has conflicts with others living in the same apartment. We will not be changing any medications at this time.

Session Time: 25 minutes

Over 50 percent Counseling/Coordination of Care? __ Yes _x_ No

History: Problem focused

Examination: Problem focused

Decision Making: Straightforward

Which of the following code sets is correct for reporting this clinic visit with a psychiatrist?

ICD-9-CM and CPT Code(s):

a. 301.83, 296.30, 304.31, 99214
b. 301.83, 296.30, 304.30, 99212
c. 301.83, 296.30, 304.30, 90805
d. 301.83, 296.30, 304.31, 90805

ICD-10-CM Code(s): _____

Disorders of the Musculoskeletal System and Connective Tissue

8.36. The following documentation is from the health record of a 39-year-old male patient.

Hospital Outpatient Surgery Services

Operative Report

Preoperative Diagnosis: Right quadriceps tendon rupture

Postoperative Diagnoses: Right quadriceps tendon rupture

Procedure Description: The patient was brought to the operating room and after the instillation of a satisfactory spinal anesthesia, the right lower extremity was appropriately prepared and draped in the usual sterile fashion. A midline incision was made and centered over the patella and carried down to the quadriceps mechanism. Medial and lateral dissection was carried out to expose the retinaculum, which was torn approximately 2 cm laterally and medially. There was a direct avulsion of the quadriceps tendon off the patella. The quadriceps tendon and patellar surface were freshened. Three holes, center, mid lateral, and mid medial, were marked. Following this, a #5 Ethibond and #2 fiberwire were placed in the quadriceps mechanism both medially and laterally, beginning in the midportion with a Krackow suture. Following this, 3 drill holes were made longitudinally from superior to inferior through the patella and a suture passer was used to retrieve the ends of the suture. When these were secured, the quad tendon was brought down into the patellar bed. Following this, #2 Ethibond retinacular sutures were added from the superolateral and superomedial junction of the patella laterally and medially. These were then tightened. As they were tightened, the sutures in the patella were securely tightened as well. The retinacular sutures were then tightened. Supplemental 2-0 Vicryl anteriorly into the quad tendon and patellar soft tissue and retinaculum was then accomplished. This knee could be flexed to about 30 degrees before there was significant tension on this quadriceps tendon. Therefore, we will be holding him in extension. Following this, a thorough irrigation was accomplished. The subcutaneous was closed with interrupted 2-0 Vicryl and the skin closed with skin clips. A sterile dressing and a knee immobilizer were placed. The patient tolerated the procedure well and was taken to the recovery room in satisfactory condition.

Which of the following is the correct code assignment?

ICD-9-CM and CPT Code(s):

a. 844.9, 27385-RT
b. 844.9, 27430-RT
c. 844.8, 27658-RT, 27685-RT
d. 844.8, 27664-RT

ICD-10-CM Code(s): _____

8.37. The following documentation is from the health record of a 47-year-old male patient.

Hospital Outpatient Surgery Services

Operative Report

Preoperative Diagnosis: Torn medial meniscus and DJD right knee

Postoperative Diagnosis: Large flap tear, posterior horn, medial meniscus; chondral loose bodies; significant localized primary degenerative arthritis right knee

Operation: Arthroscopy of the right knee with partial medial meniscectomy; arthroscopy of the right knee, with removal of chondral loose bodies

Procedure Description: This 47-year-old male was taken to the operating room and placed in the supine position. General anesthesia was accomplished without complication. Evaluation under anesthesia of the right knee showed it was stable with a negative Lachman's test and firm end point. Negative anterior and posterior drawer, stable to varus and valgus testing. A tourniquet was placed on the midright thigh. The right leg was prepped and draped free in the usual sterile manner. Tourniquet inflated to 325 mm Hg. There were loose bodies throughout the knee, which were flushed and removed. The patient had a large flap tear of the posterior horn of the medial meniscus that was unstable. He underwent a partial medial meniscectomy with small basket forceps and small synovial resector removing the torn portion of the meniscus, leaving about a 2-mm rim posteriorly and then saucerizing this to smooth margins anteriorly. The anterior cruciate ligament and posterior cruciate ligament were normal. The lateral compartment could not be entered because of significant arthritis medially. The knee joint was thoroughly irrigated and the portals closed with interrupted 3-0 nylon mattress sutures. Sterile dressing was applied. No complications occurred. The tourniquet was deflated after 20 minutes. The patient went to the recovery room in stable condition.

Which of the following is the correct code assignment?

ICD-9-CM and CPT Code(s):

a. 717.2, 717.6, 715.16, 29881-RT
b. 717.43, 718.16, 29881-RT, 29874-RT
c. 844.8, 717.6, 29881-RT, 29877-RT
d. 717.2, 715.16, 29881-RT, 29874-RT

ICD-10-CM Code(s): _____

8.38. The following documentation is from the health record of a 68-year-old male patient.

Hospital Outpatient Surgery Services

This patient presented to the podiatrist for surgical evaluation at the request of the primary care physician. After surgery was completed, a copy of the evaluation and operative report was sent to the primary care office.

Preoperative Evaluation: This 68-year-old male of Italian descent presents with degenerative arthritis and bunion formation. On 6/30/XX, patient was sent by Dr. Brown for bunionectomy evaluation. A problem-focused history was conducted followed by an expanded problem-focused examination.

Impression: Painful left foot due to: (1) Bunion with primary localized degenerative joint disease in the toes. (2) Metatarsus primus varus. (3) Hammer toe, second digit. (4) Elongated metatarsal, second digit, left.

Plan: Surgery scheduled for 8:00 a.m. 7/12/XX, at the Hospital

Procedures: Keller bunionectomy; Austin bunionectomy; arthroplasty, second digit; and excision of the metatarsal head, second digit, left foot

Operative Report: The patient was placed in the semisupine position where Dr. Graybeard administered spinal anesthesia. After prepping and draping the patient in the usual aseptic manner and under ankle hemostasis, the left foot was approached. A dorsal linear incision was performed medial to the extensor hallucis longus tendon. Incision was carried through the skin and subcutaneous tissue and extended from midshaft metatarsal to distal proximal phalanx. The superficial fascia was separated from the deep fascia using sharp and blunt dissection techniques. An inverted L-capsulotomy was performed and sharp capsular periosteal dissection was performed with a #15 blade to expose the first metatarsal and base of the proximal phalanx. The medial eminence was resected with a micro-oscillating saw.

Next, attention was directed to the base of the proximal phalanx, where the Keller procedure was performed. One third of the proximal phalanx was resected and excised in toto.

Attention was next directed to the head of the first metatarsal where an Austin osteotomy was performed in the usual manner with screw fixation. The area was flushed with copious amounts of antibiotic flush. The capsular periosteal layer was next closed with 3-0 VICRYL. The subcutaneous tissue was reapproximated with 4-0 VICRYL.

Attention was next directed to the second digit and MPJ area, where a dorsal curvilinear incision was performed. The incision was deepened and the PIPJ was exposed. A transverse incision was performed through the capsular periosteal tissue at the PIPJ. Medial and lateral capsulotomies were performed, exposing the head of the proximal phalanx. The head of the proximal phalanx was resected and excised in toto.

Attention was next directed to the second MPJ. The incision at this area was deepened. A dorsal linear capsulotomy was performed and the head of the second metatarsal was resected and excised in toto. The surgical sites were next flushed with copious amounts of antibiotic flush. The second digit was noted to be aligned without pressure on the neurovascular structures.

Next, a .45 K-wire was placed percutaneously into the hallux distal to proximal. Capsular periosteal closure was next performed with 3-0 VICRYL. Subcutaneous closure was performed with 4-0 VICRYL. The skin was closed in 4-0 nylon. Postop anesthesia consisted of 17 cc 5.0 percent Marcaine plain and 1 cc of Decadron 4 mg/mL. Next, the sterile dressing was applied, which consisted of Betadine ointment, 4 × 4 gauze, and 4-inch Kling. The tourniquet was released, and the patient was returned to recovery in stable condition.

Which of the following is the correct code assignment for this outpatient procedure?

ICD-9-CM and CPT Code(s):

a. 727.1, 735.4, 99242-25, 28202, 28285
b. 727.1, 715.17, 754.52, 735.4, 754.59, 28299-TA, 28285-T1
c. 735.4, 754.52, 28296
d. 727.2, 715.17, 754.52, 735.4, 754.59, 28296-TA and 28292-TA-59, 28285-T1

ICD-10-CM Code(s): _____

8.39. The following documentation is from the health record of a patient who received hospital outpatient surgery services.

Preoperative Diagnosis: Deep laceration, left hand with extensive tendon disruption of the fourth and fifth digits, secondarily of the third digit, middle finger; open fracture with chip fracture from the MCP joint of the fifth digit; open fracture of the middle phalanx of the index finger

Postoperative Diagnosis: Deep laceration, left hand with extensive tendon disruption of the fourth and fifth digits, secondarily of the third digit, middle finger; open fracture with chip fracture from the MCP joint of the fifth digit; open fracture of the middle phalanx of the index finger

Operation: Extensive tendon repair, fourth and fifth digits, third digit longitudinally, index finger second digit with extensor hood, and debridement; open fracture middle phalanx; and intra-articular laceration of fourth and fifth digit

Anesthesia: Intravenous Bier block

The patient was brought to the operating theater and anesthetized with a Bier block. We explored the wound, and the joint capsule to fourth and fifth was excised into the joint. The superior pole of the articular surface of the distal metacarpal on the fifth digit was avulsed, and we excised this because it was impregnated with a lot of dirt.

The tendon of the extensor indices communis to the fifth digit was lacerated. The extensor indices proprius ulnarly was still intact. The extensor hood over the MCP joint of #4 was torn, as was the capsule. The extensor tendon along the central hood of the third digit was torn longitudinally and the point was spared. The index finger had a longitudinal tear of the extensor hood in the central portion of the midphalanx, with the lateral band on the radial side torn. The wound was copiously irrigated with bacitracin saline with a pulsatile lavage. The joint surface of the fourth and fifth were irrigated. The open fracture of the fifth digit was removed. The open fracture of the middle phalanx of the index was debrided and irrigated.

We then began the definitive repairs. We sutured the joint capsule of the fourth and fifth with a 4-0 VICRYL continuous. We sutured the extensor digitorum communis tendon to #5 with 5-0 Prolene and to #4 over the central hood, over the MCP joint with a 5-0 Prolene continuous. The extensor tendon of the third or middle finger was sutured longitudinally, and a lateral band on the radial side was repaired with a 5-0 VICRYL. The longitudinal tear, which was really a split or a double split, was sutured with over-and-over 5-0 VICRYL as well. We then increased her incision in an S-shaped fashion over the index finger to expose the central hood, which was torn, and lateral on the radial aspect, which was torn as well. This was repaired with 5-0 VICRYL, and the main extensor hood was repaired with 5-0 Prolene simple sutures. We then irrigated again with a liter of bacitracin pulsatile figure-of-8 mattress sutures, alternating with simple sutures. A bulky dressing was then applied, with a volar slab with the hand in the position of function, extension of the wrist, extension of the MCP joint, flexion of the PIP, and DIP of 30 degrees. The patient then had the tourniquet deflated fully and was sent to the recovery room in good condition.

Which of the following is the correct code assignment? Report the codes a hospital outpatient surgery department would report for this hand surgery. Do not assign E codes.

ICD-9-CM and CPT Code(s):

a. 882.1, 817.1, 26418, 26735, 26746, 11012
b. 842.12, 817.0, 26746-F4, 11010-F1, 11012-F4
c. 842.12, 817.1, 26418–F1, 26418–F2, 26418–F3, 26418–F4
d. 882.2, 816.11, 26418–F1, 26418–F2, 26418–F3, 26418–F5, 11010–F1, 11012–F4

ICD-10-CM Code(s): _____

Neoplasms

8.40.   The following documentation is from the health record of a patient who received hospital outpatient surgery services.

Operative Report

Preoperative Diagnosis:	Lesion, right forehead
Postoperative Diagnosis:	Basal cell carcinoma, right forehead
Procedure:	Excision of 1.0-centimeter lesion involving the right forehead

Technique: The skin and subcutaneous tissue around the forehead lesion were infiltrated with 0.5% Marcaine with 1:100,000 epinephrine. A total of 1.5 cc was used. The patient was then prepped and draped in the usual sterile fashion.

Microscopic excision was carried out. A 2.0-mm margin of resection was planned around the lesion. Long suture was placed on the superior margin and a short suture was placed on the inferior margin. The tissue was excised and sent for frozen section, which returned with a diagnosis of basal cell carcinoma with clear margins.

The site was closed with interrupted 5-0 plain gut. The patient was sent to the recovery area in good condition. No complications. Blood loss was 1 cc.

Which codes will be reported for this service?

ICD-9-CM and CPT Code(s):

a. 173.31, 11641
b. 173.31, 11642
c. 239.2, 11441
d. 239.2, 11442

ICD-10-CM Code(s): _____

8.41. The following documentation is from the health record of an 88-year-old female patient.

Hospital-Based Oncology Department Services

This 88-year-old white female is here to rule out the possibility of myeloma. She has been followed by Dr. Black as an outpatient and has sustained a 13-lb weight loss over a 6-week period. She seemed to stabilize at a weight of 82 lb but has recently dropped an additional 2 pounds. She is experiencing recurrent pain in the chest. Three weeks ago, she was treated by Dr. Black for a sinus infection, and sinus films showed lytic lesions of the skull, as well as the left maxillary sinus.

The patient had a left radical mastectomy 38 years ago for carcinoma of the breast without recurrence. The right breast is atrophic and without masses. Laboratory tests are attached and without noteworthy comments, except for urinalysis culture revealing over 100,000 *Escherichia coli*. A bone scan shows multiple areas of increased bony uptake and two areas of increased rib uptake and present healing osteoporotic fractures. There are multiple areas of increased uptake throughout the bony skull, suggestive of progressive metastatic disease or perhaps myeloma.

This is a delightful elderly woman who has markedly abnormal bone films and severe osteoporosis. General appearance of the bone is metastatic malignancy, supported by the weight loss history. Myeloma is consistent with her symptoms, but a normal sed rate and relatively normal globulin level are somewhat contradictory of that diagnosis. Certainly light chain myeloma is a possibility. In addition, some other metastatic disease, including the previous breast cancer, could give this appearance, but that seems unusual. I have never seen recurrent breast cancer this late (38 years).

Pertinent studies have been ordered, but I believe it would also be worthwhile to do Beta II microglobulin, which may be helpful in confirming myeloma. The UTI due to Shiga toxin-producing *E. coli* is being treated with antibiotics. Additional x-rays of the lateral skull and long bones have also been ordered. In addition, I performed a bone marrow aspiration today from the left posterior iliac crest.

At this point, my recommendation is to wait and see what the additional tests show. If we can determine that this is a myeloma, then it would be worth treating her with an alkylator-prednisone combination. In terms of any other metastatic disease, there is little we can do short of palliative radiation therapy. If this looks like recurrent breast cancer, then it may be useful to try tamoxifen. I would probably do that at any rate, if the carcinoma is further collaborated in any fashion by the bone marrow biopsy or other studies.

I cannot make any more definitive recommendations at this point. When I return next week and we see the studies ordered, we will go from there.

Procedure Note

Bone Marrow Biopsy Results: Metastatic poorly differentiated carcinoma and hyperplastic marrow with decreased iron stores

Comment from Pathologist: The features of the tumor do not suggest a definite site or origin. The most common tumors causing extensive lytic lesions of the bone are breast carcinoma, lung carcinoma, and renal cell carcinoma. With regard to the patient's previous history of breast cancer, although late recurrence has been described after more than 20 years, 38 years is an extreme interval.

Which of the following are assigned for the services performed on this date of service?

ICD-9-CM and CPT Code(s):

a. 203.01, 199.1, 38221
b. 198.5, 199.1, 733.19, 733.00, V10.3, 599.0, 041.43, 38221
c. 199.0, 27299
d. 198.5, 203.01, 174.9, 38221

ICD-10-CM Code(s): _____

8.42.   The following documentation is from the health record of a female patient who received hospital outpatient surgery services.

Operative Report

A 52-year-old female presented with abdominal pain and change in bowel habits. A barium enema suggested a diverticular stricture, so a sigmoidoscopy was performed in the clinic, finding a stricture at 25 cm. The patient was then scheduled for exploratory laparoscopy in the hospital outpatient surgical center to treat the stricture.

Preoperative Diagnosis: Stricture of the sigmoid colon, rule out carcinoma

Postoperative Diagnosis: Carcinoma of the sigmoid with invasion into adjacent tissue and suspected metastasis to the liver

The patient was brought to the surgical suite, and an NG tube was placed in the stomach and a Foley catheter in the bladder. She was placed in the lithotomy position and routine prep and draping were performed. A small incision was made in the right upper quadrant directly into the peritoneal cavity with CO_2. Once we had a good tent, we examined the peritoneal cavity and could not really see the liver because we were too close to it, but one view suggested surface lesions. After placement of the three cannulas (12 mm in the RUQ, 10 mm LLQ, and 5 mm in LUQ), we mobilized the sigmoid off the pelvic gutter and dissected down towards the bladder. She had undergone a previous hysterectomy, but there were no adhesions. We could not get the small bowel to easily come up out of the pelvis, and lesions were evident surrounding the colon, so biopsies were taken. We then used a colonoscope through the rectum and advanced to 25 cm where we saw, not a stricture, but carcinoma, and biopsies were taken for pathologic evaluation. Complete evaluation of the colon was performed with no other pathology found. The surgery was discontinued, the trocars removed, and the patient returned to recovery in stable condition. The patient will undergo evaluation and consultation with oncology before further treatment is undertaken.

Pathology report confirms invasive adenocarcinoma, moderate to poorly differentiated, of the sigmoid colon with extension to the pericolic adipose.

Which codes are assigned to this surgery?

ICD-9-CM and CPT Code(s):

a. 153.3, 197.4, 49329
b. 153.9, 49321-74, 45380-59
c. 197.4, 153.3, 197.7, 49321, 45380
d. 153.3, 198.89, 49321, 45380

ICD-10-CM Code(s): _____

8.43. The following documentation is from the health record of a female patient who received hospital outpatient surgery services.

Operative Report

Preoperative Diagnosis:	Vulvar lesion
Postoperative Diagnosis:	Carcinoma in situ of the vulva
Operative Procedure:	Vulvectomy

Indications for Procedure: This 74-year-old patient was found to have a suspicious-looking lesion on her vulva. Medically, she is diabetic, has Parkinson's disease, and is obese. On the day of surgery, her cardiac, pulmonary, and mental status were adequate.

Operative Findings: On the posterior vulva was a vulvar lesion which was superficially ulcerated and extended along the posterior vaginal introitus involving the perineum. The urethra was normal. The bladder was negative for tumor. The vaginal mucosa and remainder of the vulva appeared without any lesions.

Description of Operation: The patient received general anesthesia, was intubated and placed in the dorsal lithotomy position. A pelvic examination was performed. A vaginal prep with Betadine was done and she was draped for a vaginal procedure.

An incision was made transversely along the perineum halfway between the vaginal introitus and the rectum. The skin was dissected towards the vaginal introitus bilaterally and posteriorly. The lesion was then excised with a good margin at the posterior vagina and laterally, along the vulva. Dimensions were approximately 4 cm × 3 cm × 1 cm in a triangular shape. Bleeding points were either ligated with 3-0 Vicryl or cauterized with electrocautery. The specimen was submitted for pathology evaluation with a suture marker designating the rectal margin.

The vaginal mucosa, which was undermined for at least 2 cm, was approximated to the perineal skin by interrupted 2-0 Vicryl sutures. The entire wound was closed in this way. The patient tolerated the surgical procedure well and left the operating room in satisfactory condition.

Tissue Consultation Report

Preoperative Diagnosis: Vulvar lesion

Postoperative Diagnosis: Carcinoma in situ of the vulva

Specimen: #1. Vulvar lesion with anal margin

Gross Description: #1. Received in formalin labeled "vulvar lesion and margin tag" is a roughly triangular-shaped fragment of tissue covered on one surface with wrinkled pink-white focally hair-bearing skin and on the other surface with fibrous pink tissue. There is a suture at one apex. The specimen measures 3.5 × 2.5 cm. with a thickness that ranges from 0.3 to 0.4 cm. The surface is slightly hypopigmented and slightly rough and granular in some areas. The margins are inked. A portion of the margin containing the suture is additionally marked with yellow ink. A line diagram is drawn. The specimen is sectioned and entirely submitted in eight cassettes.

Microscopic Description: #1. The specimen consists of squamous mucosa. In the center of the specimen, there is epithelial hyperplasia with markedly abnormal maturation extending from the basal layer to the surface. The surface is composed of compact hyperkeratosis. The abnormal cells display nuclear enlargement, hyperchromasia, a disorganized growth pattern, and increased mitotic figures, many of which are abnormal. Invasive squamous cell carcinoma is not identified.

Diagnosis:

#1. Vulvar lesion, including anal margin, excision:

Carcinoma in situ (vulvar epithelial neoplasia VIN III), with clear margins

Which of the following code sets is assigned?

ICD-9-CM and CPT Code(s):

a. 239.5, 250.00, 332.0, 278.00, 57410, 56620
b. 624.02, 250.00, 332.0, 278.00, 56630
c. 233.32, 250.00, 57410, 11626, 12042
d. 233.32, 250.00, 332.0, 278.00, 56620

ICD-10-CM Code(s): _____

Disorders of the Nervous System and Sense Organs

8.44.   The following documentation is from the health record of a 22-year-old male patient who received hospital outpatient surgery services.

Operative Report

A patient injured his foot using a razor-sharp garden hoe while gardening in his yard at his home and severed the superficial branch of the external plantar nerve and the flexor digiti minimi brevis tendon in his left foot. The patient experienced loss of sensation on the outer side of the fifth toe and across the side of the foot, so a neurology consultation was requested, and the patient was taken directly to surgery. Following exploration of the wound and identification of the nerve avulsion, a repair of the nerve was undertaken using a nerve graft from the sural nerve. A lateral incision was made on the lateral malleolus of the ankle. The nerve was identified and freed for grafting, and the proximal and distal sural nerve endings were anastomosed. The wound was dissected, and the damaged area of the nerve was removed. The innervation of the external digital nerve was restored by suturing the 1.5-cm graft to the proximal and digital ends of the damaged nerve, using the operating microscope. Tenoplasty was performed on the tendon injury, and the wound closed in layers.

Which of the following would be correct? Do not assign evaluation and management service codes for the ER visit or consultation service.

ICD-9-CM and CPT Code(s):

a. 956.5, E920.4, E849.0, E016.1, E000.8, 64831, 28200
b. 892.2, 956.5, E920.4, E849.0, E016.1, E000.8, 64891, 28202
c. 892.2, 956.5, E920.4, E849.0, E016.1, E000.8, 64890-LT, 28200-LT
d. 956.5, 64890-LT, 28200-LT

ICD-10-CM Code(s): _____

8.45. The following documentation is from the health record of a patient who received hospital outpatient surgery services.

Preoperative Diagnosis:	Reflex sympathetic dystrophy
Postoperative Diagnosis:	Same
Operation:	Right stellate ganglion block #1
Location:	Outpatient Pain Clinic Surgery Center
Anesthesia:	Local with conscious sedation

Details: The patient was placed in the supine position to start the IV in his left hand for the sedation of 4 mg of Versed. Then he was positioned using a shoulder roll with the neck extended. Betadine was used for preparation. Following local anesthesia, a #22, 1.5-cm needle was introduced paratracheally at the level of the cricoid cartilage towards the stellate ganglion. Ten cc of .05 percent Marcaine with epinephrine 1:200,000 was injected, and the patient tolerated this very well. There was no paresthesia, heme, or CSF detected. The patient swallowed copiously during the procedure, but we were able to obtain an adequate block, with the patient's right hand temperature changing from 90.1 to 93 °F following the block. He was moved to the outpatient recovery area where he tolerated fluids and nutrition and was able to be discharged home to his caregiver.

Assign the correct diagnosis and procedure codes. Do not assign HCPCS Level II codes for the drug(s) injected.

ICD-9-CM Diagnosis Code(s): _____

Procedure Code(s): _____

ICD-10-CM Code(s): _____

8.46. The following documentation is from the health record of a 48-year-old female patient.

Emergency Department Services

This is a 48-year-old female presenting to the ER in the middle of the night with a complaint of unexpected right-sided weakness. It occurred during sleep, and the patient awoke and found it difficult to use her right dominant arm or leg. She denies fever, shortness of breath, cough, headache, or other symptoms, and related that she was asymptomatic until this occurred.

Medication: Glucophage for type II diabetes mellitus control. Has never used oral contraceptives.

Allergies: None.

Habits: Tobacco, one pack of cigarettes per day; social use of alcohol.

Family History: Positive for early stroke in maternal grandmother at 52; father deceased at 53 due to lung cancer.

Physical Exam: Patient is alert and oriented times three. HEENT: Pupils are round, regular, equal, and reactive to light and accommodation. Extraocular muscles are intact. Oral mucosa moist and pink. Decreased nasolabial fold on the right side and slight drooping of the angle of the mouth on the right. Neck supple, without lymphadenopathy, carotid bruit, or thyromegaly. She has impaired speech. Chest: Negative. Cardiovascular: Negative. Abdomen: Benign. Neurologic: Mild paralysis evident. Cranial nerves II through XII intact. Marked decrease in power and tone on the right side when compared to the left. Decrease in sensation on the right compared to the left. She has no visual disturbances or vertigo.

CT scan without contrast shows a small infarction in the left basal ganglia near the internal capsule. This is a small to medium-size left middle cerebral arterial embolism causing the stroke.

Plan: Will transfer for further neurologic consultation to University Medical Center for lab work per Dr. Smith on the neurology service. MRI, carotid Doppler, and two-dimensional echocardiogram were ordered to be completed there also.

Acuity Level: IV

Which of the following code set combinations will be used for reporting this ER visit for the facility?

ICD-9-CM and CPT Code(s):

a. 436, 99284-25, 70450
b. 434.11, 99283, 70470
c. 434.11, 342.90, 784.59, 305.1, 250.00, V17.1, 99284–25, 70450
d. 436, 342.90, 784.59, 305.1, 250.00, V17.1, 99284, 70470

ICD-10-CM Code(s): _____

8.47. The following documentation is from the health record of a 35-year-old female patient.

Hospital Outpatient Surgery Services

Operative Report

Preoperative Diagnosis: Right trigeminal neuralgia

Postoperative Diagnosis: Right trigeminal neuralgia

Operation: Right radiofrequency coagulation of the trigeminal nerve

Indications: This is a 35-year-old lady with intractable trigeminal neuralgia causing her considerable pain and inability to eat or speak, and who was referred for treatment of her affliction. Indications, potential complications, and risks were explained to the patient and family.

Operative Procedure: After the patient was positioned supine, intravenous sedation with propofol was administered. Lateral skull x-ray fluoroscopy was set. The right cheek was infiltrated dermally with Xylocaine, and a small nick in the skin 2.5 cm lateral to the corner of the mouth was made with an 18-gauge needle. The radiofrequency needle with 2-mm exposed tip was then introduced using the known anatomical landmarks and under lateral fluoroscopy guidance into the foramen ovale. Confirmation of the placement of the needle was done by the patient grimacing to pain and by the lateral x-ray. The first treatment, 90 seconds in length, was administered with the tip of the needle 3 mm below the clival line at a temperature of 75 °C. The needle was then advanced further to the midclival line and another treatment of similar strength and duration was also administered. Finally, the third and last treatment was administered with the tip of the needle approximately 3 cm above the line. The cerebrospinal fluid was noted. The needle was removed. The patient tolerated the procedure well and had adequate tearing and corneal sensation and had reduction, if not complete cure, of her pain by the end of the procedure.

Which of the following code sets is correct?

ICD-9-CM and CPT Code(s):

a. 350.1, 64600, 77003
b. 350.1, 64610, 77003
c. 350.1, 64610
d. 350.1, 64605

ICD-10-CM Code(s): _____

8.48. The following documentation is from the health record of a 32-year-old male patient.

Preoperative Diagnosis:	Phantom limb pain
Postoperative Diagnosis:	Phantom limb pain
Procedure:	Right lumbar sympathetic block

Findings: This patient underwent a right below-the-knee amputation approximately 7 months ago for osteosarcoma of the fibula. The patient received 3 rounds of chemotherapy following the surgery as well as rehabilitation. He presented to the office 3 months ago with some significant phantom pain which was initially managed with medication. The medications, however, are providing minimal relief and he continues to have severe pain in the foot area. Surgery was held off until the stump could achieve healing, which it has. The stump does look generally good with some small areas of irritation. Lidoderm patches are used on the stump for sensitivity issues. He is seen today for injection of Marcaine and epinephrine into the L2 space in hopes of providing more relief for the pain.

Description of Procedure: The young man was positioned prone on the operating table with a block under the abdomen. The L2 spinous process was identified. A 20-gauge spinal needle was advanced through the skin to the spinal process so that the needle is lying on the anterolateral aspect of the L2 body. The appropriate location was confirmed by US prior to the injection. Twenty mL of Marcaine and epinephrine was slowly injected into the spinal space. The patient was raised into the upright position and allowed to relax. He indicated that he felt well and that there was no pain at that time. The patient was cautioned to be careful and I discussed the possibility of continuing with oral medications although a repeat block is certainly an option if the pain returns. He was sent home in good condition.

Which of the following is the correct code assignment for this outpatient surgery?

ICD-9-CM and CPT Code(s):

a. 353.6, V10.81, 62311
b. 353.6, 729.5, V49.75, V10.81, 62311
c. 353.6, V49.75, V10.81, 0230T
d. 353.6, V49.75, 170.7, 0230T

ICD-10-CM Code(s): _____

8.49. The following documentation is from the health record of a 33-year-old female patient.

Hospital Outpatient Surgery Services

Operative Report

Preoperative Diagnosis:	Left frontal lesion
Postoperative Diagnosis:	Left frontal lesion
Operation:	Stereotactic biopsy of left frontal lesion

Indications for Procedure: The patient is a 33-year-old female transferred to the university neurosurgical service for outpatient treatment from Blank Memorial

Hospital, where she is an inpatient. She presents with neurologic deterioration, nausea, neck pain, and headache. A CT and MRI revealed a left frontal cystic mass. It was recommended that the patient undergo stereotactic biopsy and aspiration. The risks and benefits of the procedure were explained in detail to the patient and her family, who requested the procedure be performed, and the patient returned to Blank for further therapy.

Procedure: The patient was first taken to the CT suite, where a stereotactic halo was placed on the patient's head with the four-pin system using local anesthesia. The stereotactic CT was then performed, and the patient was transported to the operating room. The patient was placed on the operating room table in the supine position. General endotracheal anesthesia was smoothly induced. The left frontal area was then clipped and shaved, and the area was then prepped and draped in the usual sterile fashion. The stereotactic arm was then brought into the field and placed on the stereotactic ring. The localizing arm and the pointer were used to mark the left frontal area for skin incision. The area was then infused with 1 percent lidocaine with epinephrine, and a 2-cm skin incision was created in the left frontal region. The self-retaining retractor was placed, and hemostasis was obtained. The pointer was again used to mark the spot on the skull to make the burr hole, and a perforator was used to create a left frontal burr hole. The dura was coagulated and incised using a #15 bladed knife. The pia was then also coagulated and nicked with a #11 blade knife. The biopsy needle was then placed into the stereotactic localizing arm. The coordinates were dialed into the arm, and the biopsy needle was advanced to the appropriate depth. Upon entering the lesion, 25 cc of yellowish fluid was withdrawn from the cyst. The fluid was sent for cytology and bacteriology. The biopsy needle was then removed, and the incision was irrigated with bacitracin irrigation. The self-retaining retractor was then removed, and the incision was closed using #00 Dexon for the galea and staples for the skin. Estimated blood loss was 15 cc. No transfusion was given. The sponge, needle, and instrument counts were reported as correct at the end of the case. The patient was removed from the stereotactic halo ring. She was allowed to wake up and was extubated and taken to the recovery area. She will be transferred by ambulance back to Blank as soon as she has recovered from the anesthesia.

Assign the correct CPT codes for this procedure.

Code(s): _____

8.50. The following documentation is from the health record of a patient seen for retinal detachment.

Ophthalmologic Procedure—Nervous/Sense

Surgery Date: 04/20/XX

Preoperative Diagnoses:
1. Retinal detachment, left eye.
2. Vitreous hemorrhage, left eye.
3. Traumatic iritis, left eye.

Postoperative Diagnoses:
1. Retinal detachment, left eye.
2. Vitreous hemorrhage, left eye.
3. Traumatic iritis, left eye.

Operative Procedures:	1. Scleral buckle, left eye.
	2. Pars plana vitrectomy, left eye.
	3. Air fluid exchange, left eye.
	4. Endolaser, left eye.
	5. Injection of 16% C3F8 gas, left eye.

Anesthesia: General.

Indications: The patient presents with count-fingers vision in the left eye 4 days after blunt trauma to the left eye caused by a punch. B-scan revealed moderate vitreous hemorrhage and retinal detachment with tear at 4:30 with macula off.

Description of Procedure: After informed written consent was obtained, patient was brought to the operating room and prepped and draped in the usual sterile fashion after he was induced under general anesthesia. Speculum was placed in the left eye. A 360-degree peritomy was performed with a 0.12 forceps and Westcott scissors. Each quadrant was dissected bluntly with the curved Stevens scissors. Muscles were looped with a muscle hook and threaded with a 2-0 silk and then isolated with 2-0 silk. Quadrants were inspected and found to be pathology-free. Then a Gill knife and corneal dissector were used to perform scleral buckle procedure, 1 belt loop in each quadrant, 3 mm posterior to the muscle insertion, 3 mm long and 3 mm wide. The 41-band was threaded through each belt loop and under each muscle and tied with a Watzke sleeve superonasally. A standard 20-gauge pars plana vitrectomy was then performed with sclerotomies placed 3.5 mm posterior to the limbus with an MVR blade. The first sclerotomy placed was inferotemporal, and the trocar was used to place the cannula. Infusion line was screwed into place and turned on after it was visualized in the vitreous cavity. Other two cannulas were placed with trocars, and the BIOM viewing system was used to perform a complete vitrectomy. Tears were noted not only at 4:30, but also at the 5 o'clock that were out near the vitreous base, and there was a large tear running radially along the edge of the detachment and traction of vitreous from 6:30 all the way past the equator and about 3 disc diameters from the optic nerve head. After vitreous was removed, air fluid exchange was performed to flatten the retina and endolaser was performed 360 degrees and around the tears. Air was exchanged for 16% C3F8 gas and sclerotomies were tied with 7-0 VICRYL, as was the conjunctiva. Retrobulbar block was given, a total of 6 cc of a 50/50 mixture of 2 percent lidocaine and 0.75 percent Marcaine. Maxitrol and atropine were applied to the eye. The eye was patched with a soft pad followed by a hard pad. The patient left the room awake in a stable condition and will follow up tomorrow morning at 8 a.m.

Which of the following is the correct code assignment for this outpatient surgery?

ICD-9-CM and CPT Code(s):

a. 361.02, 379.23, 364.3, 67108
b. 361.9, 379.23, 364.3, 67108
c. 361.02, 364.3, 67108
d. 361.02, 379.23, 364.10, 67107, 67036

ICD-10-CM Code(s): _____

8.51. The following documentation is from the health record of a 17-year-old admitted for endoscopic sinus surgery.

Preoperative Diagnosis: Nasal septal deviation, hypertrophic inferior turbinates, and chronic frontal, ethmoid, and maxillary sinusitis with sinus polyposis.

Postoperative Diagnosis: Same

Procedure: Nasal/sinus endoscopy, surgical, with frontal sinus exploration, right.
Nasal/sinus endoscopy, surgical, with frontal sinus exploration, left.
Nasal/sinus endoscopy, surgical, with anterior and posterior ethmoidectomy, right.
Nasal/sinus endoscopy, surgical, with anterior and posterior ethmoidectomy, left.
Septoplasty.
Nasal/sinus endoscopy, surgical, with maxillary antrotomy and polypectomy, right.
Nasal/sinus endoscopy, surgical, with maxillary antrotomy and polypectomy, left.
Submucous resection of inferior turbinate, right.
Submucous resection of inferior turbinate, left.

History: The patient is a 17-year-old Caucasian male presenting with a history of chronic nasal obstruction and chronic sinusitis. He has been refractory to conservative therapy. Preop evaluation reveals an obvious gross nasal septal deformity, with hypertrophic inferior turbinates, causing bilateral nasal airway obstruction. His preop CT scan confirms these findings, along with evidence of polypoid degeneration involving the maxillary, ethmoid, and frontal sinuses. The recommendations for septoplasty with endoscopic sinus surgery were given to the patient and his mother. All benefits, risks, alternate therapies, and expected outcomes were discussed. Consent form signed. The patient presents at this time for this procedure.

Details of Procedure: The patient was taken to the operating suite and placed in the supine position. General anesthesia with endotracheal intubation was carried out by the Department of Anesthesia. Following adequate anesthesia, the table was turned.

Further preparation of the nasal cavity was carried out in the usual manner. Following this, the patient was properly draped and the procedure begun.

A #15 blade was used to make a Killian incision into the left aspect of the mucoperichondrium. A mucoperichondrial and mucoperiosteal flap was then developed. The cartilaginous septum was detached from the maxillary crest and from the bony septum, and a portion of reflected bony septum causing obstruction was taken down with a Gorney scissors and a biting Takahashi forceps. The large bony spur coming out the maxillary crest was then taken down with a curved chisel and mallet technique. Bone fragments were removed with a biting forceps. Following this, the cartilaginous septum was allowed to swing to the midline and attention was turned to the endoscopic portion of the procedure.

The zero-degree endoscope was inserted into the left nasal cavity and brought up to the head of the left middle turbinate. The left middle turbinate was medialized.

An infundibulotomy incision was made, followed by uncinectomy. The maxillary antrum was then entered. The antrotomy opening was widened with the Xomed straight shot microdebrider. Polypoid tissue encountered in the left maxillary sinus was then visualized and evacuated with a series of biting forceps. Following this, the debrider was used to gain access to the anterior, then the posterior, ethmoid air cells, removing diseased mucoperiosteal tissue along the way. The nasal frontal recess was then identified. Polypoid tissue in this region was evacuated. The nasofrontal duct was then cannulated. Further disease around the duct was removed with the debrider. Following these maneuvers, submucous resection of the left inferior turbinate was then carried out. Next, attention was turned to the opposite maxillary, ethmoid, and frontal sinuses. Identical procedures and findings were noted here. Submucous resection of the right inferior turbinate was then carried out.

The middle turbinates were then sutured in the midline, utilizing 4-0 VICRYL on a PS2 cutting needle. Silastic splints, Merocel sinus and nasal packs were then placed. The oral cavity was then suctioned of all blood and debris. The patient tolerated these procedures well. He was turned back over to the Department of Anesthesia, and was taken to the recovery room in satisfactory condition.

Report of Surgical Pathology

Final Diagnosis: Nasal sinus mucosa with septal bone and cartilage
Mild chronic allergic sinusitis; nasal bone and cartilage showing no specific gross abnormality specimen(s)
Nasal septum—with sinus products
Clinical diagnosis: recurrent sinusitis

Gross Examination: Received are multiple portions of somewhat mucinous mucosa accompanying bits of platelike, wedge-shaped, and sail-shaped bone and cartilage. The latter present no specific gross abnormalities. The mucosa has an estimated aggregate volume of 2 cc and is submitted for histologic processing (1 block).

Microscopic Examination: Sections disclose edematous sinonasal mucosa with mild chronic inflammation, basement membrane thickening, and a somewhat mucinous epithelium. The inflammatory infiltrate is dominantly lymphoplasmacytic with foci of eosinophilic admixture. There is no evidence of squamous metaplasia or dysplasia.

Select the correct code set to report for this patient.

ICD-9-CM and CPT Code(s):

a. 470, 478.0, 473.0, 473.2, 473.1, 471.8, 31276-50, 31255-50, 30140-50-59, 30520, 31256-50
b. 470, 478.0, 473.0, 473.2, 473.1, 471.8, 31276, 31255, 30140, 30520, 31256
c. 470, 478.0, 461.0, 461.1, 461.2, 471.8, 31276-50, 31255-50, 30520, 31256-50
d. 470, 478.0, 461.0, 461.1, 461.2, 471.8, 31276-50, 31255-50, 30140-50-59, 30520, 31256-50

ICD-10-CM Code(s): _____

Newborn/Congenital Disorders

8.52. The following documentation is from the health record of a 3-year-old child.

Hospital-Based Clinic Outpatient Services

Parents bring their 3-year-old boy, who was born with hydrocephalus, to the pediatric neurology clinic at University Hospital to have the child evaluated by the pediatric neurologist and have his VP shunt lengthened to accommodate a growth spurt. Their pediatrician requested a consultation to evaluate the shunt and replace the peritoneal catheter if needed. Outpatient surgery had been previously scheduled tentatively pending this evaluation for the afternoon.

The catheter used in the shunt was removed and replaced in the outpatient surgery suite following a follow-up consultation, which included a detailed interim history, a detailed examination, and medical decision making of moderate complexity. Findings documented in the consultation include "Assessment: Shunt valve malfunction requiring replacement." The VP shunt valve was replaced, along with a new peritoneal catheter in a longer length.

Which of the following code sets will be reported for this service?

ICD-9-CM and CPT Code(s):

a. V53.01, 62230
b. 996.2, 742.3, 62230
c. 742.3, V53.01, 62225
d. 742.3, 62230

ICD-10-CM Code(s): _____

8.53. The following documentation is from the health record of a 4-week-old baby.

Emergency Department Services

A 4-week-old baby is rushed to the hospital after the parents found her cyanotic. While in the ER, she suffered respiratory arrest followed by cardiac arrest and was given cardiopulmonary resuscitation. The baby was born at 36 weeks, with a birth weight of 2400 g. Her current weight is 2700 g. An emergency intubation was performed, and then she was placed on a ventilator and transferred to the neonatal intensive care unit at the university hospital across town for monitoring and further workup. The ER physician provided 1 hour and 20 minutes of critical care, not including the cardiopulmonary resuscitation. His final diagnosis for the ER service is "Hypoxia with respiratory failure in a preterm infant—etiology unknown."

Which of the following code sets (diagnoses and CPT codes) will be reported for the hospital emergency room encounter?

ICD-9-CM and CPT Code(s):

a. 770.84, 765.19; 765.28, 99285
b. 770.84, 779.85, 765.18, 765.28; 99291, 92950, 31500
c. 770.84, 779.85, 765.18, 765.28; 99468, 92950
d. 770.84, 779.85, 765.18, 765.28; 99291

ICD-10-CM Code(s): _____

Pediatric Conditions

8.54. The following documentation is from the health record of a female patient who received clinic services.

Chief Complaint: Spina bifida clinic follow-up visit

History: The patient is a 12-year-old girl with T11-12 spina bifida and shunted hydrocephalus. She also has neurogenic bladder and neurogenic bowel and is status post congenital scoliosis, repaired with rodding. When I saw her last, she also complained of some right-sided lower abdominal pain but that resolved shortly after her last visit. Today, she denies headache, nausea, vomiting, diarrhea, any change in bowel or bladder function, upper extremity weakness, cognitive changes, or difficulties swallowing or chewing. Mother has requested a modular wheelchair with hand rails, platforms, and switchback, which I ordered today.

Examination: Normocephalic. Shunt catheter is taut over the right clavicle. Heart regular rate and rhythm. Lungs clear to auscultation. Abdomen has positive bowel sounds. She has some tenderness in the right lateral latissimus area around the inferior border of her scapula. It does not appear to be point tender. It appears to be either musculoskeletal or tendon tenderness. Upper body strength is 5/5. Grip is excellent. There is no weakness noted at all. Lower extremity, she is 0/5. Her skin is clean and dry. She has multiple healed scars on her back from various surgeries. Her toes are clean and dry with no breakdown. Perineal area is clean and dry.

Diagnoses:
1. 12-year-old girl with T11-12 spina bifida and shunted hydrocephalus
2. Neurogenic bladder and bowel
3. Status post scoliosis repair with rodding

Disposition: Continue current catheterization. Keep next week's appointment with Neurology to assess VP shunt.

Which is the correct diagnosis code set for this clinic service?

ICD-9-CM Code(s):

a. 741.02, 596.54, 564.81, 737.30, 996.2
b. 741.02, 596.54, 564.81, V45.2, V13.68
c. 741.90, 596.54, 331.4, 737.30
d. 741.92, 596.54, 564.81, V45.2, V13.68

ICD-10-CM Code(s): _____

Conditions of Pregnancy, Childbirth, and the Puerperium

8.55. The patient is seen in the Women's Clinic in this Ambulatory Surgery center:

Admission Diagnosis: First trimester intrauterine pregnancy in a patient desiring suction evacuation followed by laparoscopic tubal ligation.

Procedures Performed: Suction evaluation of products of conception; bilateral tubal fimbriectomy.

Indications for Procedure: This is a 37-year-old gravida 5, para 3, ab 1 who desires termination of her current pregnancy followed by a tubal ligation. Two of her children were born with significant congenital deformities and she is concerned about the possibility that this will occur with the current pregnancy. She has discussed this at length with her husband and wishes to proceed with the surgeries.

Past history includes three vaginal deliveries and one spontaneous abortion. No other significant past medical or surgical history to date. There are no mitigating factors in her family history. Patient has a history of tobacco use but quit smoking 4 years ago. She does not drink alcohol or use illegal drugs.

Review of Systems: HEENT: negative; cardiorespiratory: negative; GI: negative; GU: deferred

Physical Examination revealed a well-nourished, well-developed female of 37 years. She is presenting today for abortion and tubal ligation. Vital signs include temperature of 98.5 and blood pressure of 110/75 in her left arm. HEENT: normal. Breasts: Normal with no masses or lumps palpable. Heart and lungs are normal to percussion and auscultation and no rales or rhonchi are heard. Her abdomen is soft without tenderness or masses. Her pelvic examination confirms a first trimester (9 weeks) pregnancy.

Consent for the procedures was obtained after a thorough discussion of the risks of each of the surgeries and the combination of surgeries. The possibility of occurrence of complications including death were explained and all questions answered.

Description of Procedure: The patient was anesthetized, prepped, and draped in a normal sterile fashion for a vaginal procedure. The cervix was stabilized with a Lahey clamp and the uterus sounded to 10 cm. The internal os accommodated a #8 Hegar dilator and the uterine contents were vacuumed out until no more evidence of products of conception was noted. A light curettage of the uterine wall revealed no additional fetal remnants. The dilator was removed and attention turned to the tubal ligation. Through four strategically placed trocars, the contents of the abdominal/pelvic cavities were examined and no abnormalities noted. Sufficient insufflation had been achieved. Attention was turned to the right fallopian tube which was cut with a curved Kelly and clamped and fulgurated then tied with #1 chromic. The left fallopian tube was dissected in a similar manner. The trocars were removed and the patient tolerated the procedure well. There was blood loss of approximately 100 ml. The patient was sent to PACU in excellent condition.

Pathological Findings: Tissue submitted consisted of products of conception and portions of the right and left fallopian tubes.

Gross examination revealed pieces of irregularly shaped placenta and fetal tissue. Two grossly identifiable pieces of fallopian tubes each about 18 mm in length and 6 mm in diameter were examined.

Final Diagnoses based on Pathological Findings: Products of conception; fallopian tubes.

The patient was allowed to go home after being given her discharge instructions including a return visit to the physician's office in 2 weeks.

What is the correct code assignment for this outpatient surgery?

ICD-9-CM and CPT Code(s): _____

ICD-10-CM Code(s): _____

8.56.   The following documentation is from the health record of a 33-year-old woman who received hospital observation services.

Observation Patient

Admit Note: 2/28/XX, 07:30

This is a 33-year-old G2, P0, estimated delivery date of 2/28 and estimated gestational age of 40 weeks. She presents for induction secondary to gestational DM. She has required insulin since 28 weeks with adequate control. PNL: O positive, rubella immune. PE: AVSS, abdomen FH 40 cm, EFW 3800–4000 g. Cervix is closed/50 percent/-3/post/ceph. Plan is for Prostin EZ induction and insulin infusion when in active labor.

Progress Note: 2/28/XX, 09:15

Patient is having uterine contractions every 3 to 8 minutes. Cervix is 1 cm/100 percent/floating. Patient does not want to start Pitocin yet. Feels that she is in labor. FHR reactive, baseline 120s with accelerations.

Progress Note: 2/28/XX, 19:25

Patient's uterine contractions have resolved. Cervix unchanged. Discussed options, would like to go home to sleep and return in a.m. for Pitocin induction. Discharged home for tonight to sleep. Admit in a.m., start IV Pitocin as per protocol, start insulin drip, clear liquid diet.

Which of the following is the correct code set for this outpatient encounter?

ICD-9-CM and CPT Code(s):

a. 648.81, 250.01, V58.67, 99235
b. 648.83, 250.81, 99235
c. 648.83, V58.67, 99235
d. 648.83, 790.29, V58.67, 99235

ICD-10-CM Code(s): _____

8.57.   The following documentation is from the health record of a female patient who was seen in the Emergency Department.

Emergency Department Record

This is a 30-year-old G2 P1 female who is 13 weeks pregnant who came in following a motor vehicle crash today. The patient was a passenger in the vehicle and appeared unhurt at the scene. She accompanied her daughter, who had obvious injuries, to the ED in the ambulance. During the initial exam of the child, this patient became lightheaded and had mild abdominal cramping. She was triaged and care began for her. She has had passage of 2 clots since the initial cramping episode. Pregnancy was confirmed as intrauterine on ultrasound at 7 weeks. There has been no dizziness, no syncope, and no other complaints on review of systems. She has a history of a left-sided conductive hearing loss following several childhood illnesses. The patient has a poor obstetrical history with pre-term labor during her first pregnancy.

Vital Signs: 37.0. 78, 18, 132/73, 98%. Alert and oriented × 3. HEENT is generally normal with significant hearing loss demonstrated on the left. Chest is clear to auscultation bilaterally. Heart shows RRR. Back is normal. Normal bowel sounds, nontender and nondistended. + VB from cervical OS. No POC seen. Musculoskeletal does show tenderness over the right olecranon and proximal ulna on palpation. Motion is slightly painful but full. Neuro, Nodes and Skin are all normal. Fetal heart tones are appropriate for gestational age. On reexam after two hours of bedrest, VB appears to have stopped. Fetal heart tones continue to be strong. Patient's VS are stable.

Thirty-year-old female with threatened AB and contusion to right elbow, status post MVA, restrained passenger. Doubt ectopic given positive IUP on ultrasound. She is anxious to join her daughter at her bedside and agrees that she will be re-seen here if she has any further symptoms. Agrees that nurses on pediatric floor will monitor her closely, and they are alerted to the situation. She will be seen by her OB tomorrow AM if she is not seen here in the ED later today.

Assign the correct codes for this encounter.

ICD-9-CM Code(s): _____

ICD-10-CM Code(s): _____

8.58. The following documentation is from the health record of a 36-year-old female patient.

Hospital Outpatient Surgery Services

Preoperative Diagnosis: Left ectopic pregnancy

Postoperative Diagnosis: Same

Anesthesia: General

Operation: Diagnostic laparoscopy
Left salpingostomy with removal of ectopic pregnancy

Rationale for Surgery: This patient is a 36-year-old gravida III, para I, AB I, at 9 weeks gestation, who has a positive pregnancy test with left adnexal mass that is a gestational sac with FHTs, and left ectopic pregnancy diagnosis was made. She was admitted at this time for laparoscopy with removal of this left ectopic pregnancy. We did talk about possibly sacrificing the tube on that side if we did get into problems with bleeding. This patient has a history of pelvic adhesions with blocked right tube. She is aware that we may have to sacrifice the left tube and that essentially she would be unable to become pregnant in all probability if we're not able to save the tube. She is also aware of the risks and benefits of surgery, including hemorrhage, bowel and bladder injury, and infection.

Procedure: With the patient in the lithotomy position and under satisfactory general anesthesia, the abdomen and perineum were prepped and draped in the usual manner. A weighted speculum was placed in the vaginal vault. The anterior lip of the cervix was grasped with a single-toothed tenaculum. The uterus was sounded to about 9 cm, and it was retroverted. The endocervical canal was dilated with Pratt dilators, and the Zumi uterine manipulator was placed and the bulb insufflated with approximately 8 cc of air. A red rubber catheter was placed to gravity and attached to the Zumi uterine manipulator. Attention was then turned to the abdominal area, where a small skin incision was made with a scalpel. A large trocar was placed in the direct insertion technique, and pneumoperitoneum was established without difficulty. It is noted she did have some blood in the cul-de-sac. The right tube and ovary looked grossly within normal limits except the fimbriated end on the right was somewhat blunted. The ectopic pregnancy was really at the fimbriated end and had a small clot that was extruded from the fimbriated end. She also had the ovarian cyst on that side, which was not complicating this pregnancy. It was opened and drained. She also had a peritubular cyst, which I left intact. I isolated the ectopic pregnancy and then made a small cut using the needle coagulator over the ectopic pregnancy and extruded this with the needle nose forceps. Had some oozing along the fimbriated end. I did put Avitene in this area and then topped it with some Surgicel. We watched it for several minutes, and it seemed to control the small amount of oozing. We irrigated the pelvic region with copious amounts of irrigation and then aspirated it. We again checked the operative field, and it seemed to be dry. We watched it as we deflated the abdominal pressure. I then removed all the instruments, used .25 mg of Marcaine injection at the injection sites, and closed the incisions with staples. Vaginal instruments were removed. She was taken to the recovery room in good condition. Estimated blood loss approximately 50 cc. Sponge and needle count was correct × 2. Patient did tolerate the procedure well and left the operating room in good condition.

Which of the following is the correct code set for this outpatient surgery?

ICD-9-CM and CPT Code(s):

a. 633.20, 620.2, 59121, 49320
b. 633.10, 620.2, 620.8, 59150, 58662
c. 633.10, 620.2, 58673, 49320
d. 633.20, 654.43, 58673, 58662

ICD-10-CM Code(s): _____

Disorders of the Respiratory System

8.59.   A patient is respirator-dependent and has a tracheostomy in need of revision due to redundant scar tissue formation surrounding the site. Under general anesthesia and establishing the airway to maintain ventilation, the scar tissue is resected, and then repair is accomplished using skin flap rotation from the adjacent tissue of the neck. What codes will be used to report this procedure, which was performed in the hospital outpatient surgical department?

ICD-9-CM Diagnosis Code(s): _____

CPT Code(s): _____

ICD-10-CM Code(s): _____

8.60. The following documentation is from the health record of a 72-year-old female patient.

Hospital-Based Clinic Services

This 72-year-old female presented to the hospital-based urgent care clinic with a chief complaint of recurrent epistaxis for 3 days prior to admission. The bleeding occurred in the right nostril. She also complained of weakness and dizziness when standing. At the last clinic visit, hematocrit was 35, and this morning it is 27. Her past medical history is positive for COPD, with a negative surgical history.

A right anterior limited nasal pack was placed in the clinic treatment room. Because of the weakness and dizziness, we decided to admit the patient to an observation bed. In the evening, the anterior pack required replacement with extensive cauterization in the right nares because of refractory bleeding. Due to falling hematocrit, two units of packed red cells were transfused for the blood-loss anemia resulting. The next morning, the patient was still experiencing some bleeding around the anterior nasal pack. For this reason, she was taken back to the treatment room, and a posterior nasopharyngeal pack in the right nares was placed by another physician. No further bleeding occurred throughout the day, and the patient was discharged to home healthcare follow-up following pack removal.

Which of the following should appear on the UB-04 claim for the outpatient services rendered to this Medicare patient?

Note: The facility purchases its blood from the blood bank.

ICD-9-CM and CPT Code(s):

a. 784.7, 30901-RT, 30903-RT, 30905-RT, 36430-RT
b. 784.7, 280.0, 496, 30901-RT, 30901-RT-76, 30905-RT-77, P9021
c. 784.7, 285.9, 30901-RT, 30903-RT-59, 30905-RT-77, 36430-RT, P9021 (two units)
d. 784.7, 280.0, 496, 30901-RT, 30903RT-59, 30905-RT-59, 36430-RT, P9021 (two units)

ICD-10-CM Code(s): _____

8.61. The following documentation is from the health record of a 66-year-old male patient.

Emergency Department Services

The patient is a 66-year-old male who presented to the Emergency Department with a 2-day history of severe shortness of breath, nonproductive cough, and slight fever. His medical history includes non-small cell lung cancer in the right middle lobe, 2 months post completion of radiation therapy. Surgery was contraindicated because of atrial fibrillation and long-term use of Coumadin. The Oncologist documented that chemotherapy was not indicated in this case and felt that the tumor was eradicated. The patient also has been plagued with chronic dermatitis over the radiation port area on the right lateral chest wall following the 2nd radiation treatment. The skin continues to show the infection on exam. A 2-view chest x-ray showed consolidation in the right lower lobe of the lung.

The physician diagnosed pneumonitis as an aftereffect of radiation therapy and prescribed both the inhaled corticosteroid, Beclomethasone Dipropionate, and long-term oral corticosteroids on a tapering dose.

Which of the following represents correct coding for this service, including the chargemaster-assigned codes?

ICD-9-CM and CPT Code(s):

a. 486, 692.3, V10.11, E879.2, 71010
b. 508.0, 692.82, 427.31, V58.61, V10.11, E879.2, 71020
c. 508.0, 990, E926.5, 162.4, 427.31, V58.69, 71030
d. 508.1, 692.82, 162.4, 427.31, V58.69, E926.5, 71020

ICD-10-CM Code(s): _____

8.62.   The following documentation is from the health record of a patient who received hospital outpatient surgery services.

Operative Report

Preoperative Diagnosis: Chronic sinusitis

Postoperative Diagnosis: Sinusitis of the maxillary, ethmoid, and sphenoid sinuses

Procedure: Bilateral endoscopic sinusotomies, anterior and posterior ethmoidectomies, and sphenoidotomy, with debris removal in all sites

EBL: <100 cc

Description of Operation: The patient was placed in the supine position after appropriate preparation, draping, and induction of endotracheal anesthesia. The nose was cocainized and injected with Xylocaine 2 percent with 1:100,000 epinephrine.

The endoscope was then used to examine the maxillary sinus structures on the left side. There were several polyps present, and these were carefully injected with Xylocaine 0.5 percent with 1:200,000 epinephrine and removed. The maxillary sinus opening was identified by blunt dissection and was then opened, and with various rongeurs, the tissue was debrided. We then started through the posterior of the middle meatus region involving the ethmoid floors. Care was taken to preserve the parietal mucosa while performing the ethmoidectomies; then we proceeded posteriorly and entered into the sphenoid posteriorly and inferiorly. Gelfilm was folded and placed in the areas involved.

Attention was then directed to the right side in similar fashion. Again, polyps were removed from the maxillary sinus. The uncinate was prominent and was resected, and more polyps were debrided. We then identified the maxillary sinus opening on the right and opened it in a satisfactory manner. We then proceeded anterior through posterior ethmoidal cells into the sphenoid cavity posteriorly, opening and removing large amounts of polypoid mucosa, polyps, and some mild purulence. When this was completed to our satisfaction, Gelfilm was folded and placed. The posterior throat was suctioned clear, and the patient was awakened and taken to recovery in good condition.

Which codes will be reported for this ambulatory surgery service?

ICD-9-CM and CPT Code(s):

a. 473.9, 31256-50, 31287
b. 473.0, 473.2, 473.3, 471.8, 31256-50, 31287–50
c. 473.0, 473.2, 473.3, 471.8, 31255-50, 31267–50, 31288–50
d. 473.0, 473.2, 473.3, 471.8, 31255, 31267

ICD-10-CM Code(s): _____

Trauma and Poisoning

8.63.   The following documentation is from the health record of a 25-year-old female patient.

Emergency Department Services

A 25-year-old female fell off of her horse in the morning, sustaining an injury and fracture of the spinal cord and vertebra at the C4 level. The patient was leisurely riding her horse at the stables at her home. The patient was brought to the nearest ED by ambulance in a full-body air splint. CT scan revealed the injury to be a complete injury to the spinal cord (tetraplegia). The patient was having some difficulty breathing, and after endotracheal intubation, ventilator support was initiated. Vital signs were unstable in the ED. The patient had no feeling below the level of the injury. The patient was closely monitored throughout her stay in the ED. Later that day, when it was thought that she was stable enough for transport, she was transferred to the neurosurgical intensive care unit at the teaching hospital downtown for definitive treatment at the fracture site.

Critical care services were provided according to the acuity system. The ED physician who managed this patient recorded extensive progress notes, which included the specific time he spent with the patient on and off throughout the day. Times noted included the following: 0800–0900, 1000–1030, 1100–1115, 1300–1315, 1500–1600.

Which of the following sets of codes would be appropriate for facility reporting of this ED service in addition to the CT scan, 72125, assigned via the chargemaster?

ICD-9-CM and CPT Code(s):

a. 805.04, 344.01, E828.2, E849.0, E006.1, E000.8, 99291, 31500
b. 805.04, 344.01, E828.2, E849.0, E006.1, E000.8, 99291, 31500
c. 806.01, E828.2, E849.0, E006.1, E000.8, 99291, 31500
d. 806.01, E828.2, E849.0, E006.1, E000.8, 99291, 31500, 22305

ICD-10-CM Code(s): _____

8.64.   The following documentation is from the health record of a male patient with a hand injury.

Hospital Outpatient Surgery Services

Preoperative Diagnosis: Open fracture, shaft of the middle phalanx of the left small finger, on the oblique

Postoperative Diagnosis: Open fracture, shaft of the middle phalanx of the left small finger, on the oblique with disruption of collateral ligament and extensor tendon

Procedure: Irrigation and debridement, open reduction of fracture, repair of extensor tendon and lateral collateral ligament, left small finger

Indications: This 42-year-old man sustained this injury at his single-family home while using a powered hedge trimmer which slipped. The medial ligament, soft tissue, and skin are intact. Because of this wound, the patient was brought to the operating room today.

Description: Two grams of Ancef were administered prior to the start of the case. The patient was identified by site of surgery, by direct communication with the patient, and by consent form. Following induction of general anesthesia, the left upper extremity was prepped and draped in the usual manner. A tourniquet was placed. Attention was first directed to the wound, and the margins of the wound were trimmed of devascularized tissue. There was a significant amount of debris in the wound. It was debrided of bone chips using the operating microscope and lavaged with 4 liters of Kantrex saline solution. Following this, the oblique fracture of the middle phalanx was approximated over a metal pin using fluoroscopic guidance. This provided excellent alignment of the fracture and appropriate positioning of the finger. The extensor tendon was repaired with acceptable extension being achieved. The lateral collateral ligament was repaired and the PIP joint was again stable. The wound was closed using 4-0 nylon suture, apposing his soft tissues. The tourniquet was released. Tourniquet time was 40 minutes. Vascularization appeared adequate. Sterile bandage of bacitracin, Adaptic, 2 × 2s, and a tube gauze bandage were applied. Estimated blood loss was minimal during the procedure.

Which of the following code sets is appropriate for this service?

ICD-9-CM and CPT Code(s):

a. 816.00, 26756-F4, 13131-F4
b. 816.01, E920.1, 11012, 26735-F4
c. 816.11, E920.1, E849.0, E016.1, E000.8, 26735-F4
d. 816.11, E920.1, E849.0, E016.1, E000.8, 26756-F4, 26418-F4, 26540-F4, 11012, 13131

ICD-10-CM Code(s): _____

8.65. Emergency Department Visit

HPI: This white female, aged 28 years old, was brought to the emergency room by her friends after she took approximately 60, 15 mg Dalmane, approximately 100, 7.5 mg Tranxene and several glasses of wine. This was done out of sight of the friends. They noticed that the patient became very drowsy and unable to ambulate. She got up from the sofa to go to the kitchen when she fell and hit her forehead on the corner of the table. There is a 2.2-cm laceration on the forehead which is bleeding profusely. The patient admitted to the friends what she had done and they brought her to the hospital immediately. She actually appears to be alert but somewhat combative. Her speech is slurred but she is oriented as to time, date, and place. There is a question of exactly how many pills she took.

Past Medical/Surgical History: Patient is gravida 3, para 1, AB 2. Her most recent spontaneous abortion occurred a little more than a month ago and she has been very depressed since the miscarriage.

Social History: Patient is married with one small child. She married quite young at age 16. The patient has never smoked and usually drinks very little alcohol. She works as a teacher's aide.

Family History: Her mother is deceased from complications of diabetes. Her father died of colon cancer complicated by cirrhosis of the liver. The father was an alcoholic. No family history of mental illness.

Review of Systems: A very brief ROS was taken. Cardiovascular: patient has no trouble with SOB, dyspnea or exertion, palpitations, or chest pain.

Neuropsychiatric: Patient did have postpartum depression following the birth of her child. This was mild to severe and she continues to seek outpatient treatment for it. The Tranxene was prescribed by her psychiatrist. The depression was exacerbated by her recent miscarriage.

Vital Signs: BP 130/50 and P 95.

Services Provided: 1. Patient underwent gastric lavage to remove all pills that she ingested. Following this the patient's forehead wound was sutured with single layer closure. The wound was debrided prior to suturing.

The patient's husband arrived at the hospital and the patient was released to his care to be admitted to the local mental health hospital for suicide prevention.

What codes are reported for this emergency department service?

ICD-9-CM and CPT Code(s): _____

ICD-10-CM Code(s): _____

8.66. Emergency Department Services

This 17-year-old girl was a passenger on a motorcycle and was thrown from the back of the motorcycle. She sustained multiple contusions and reported pain in her left forearm and ribs. Patient was taken to x-ray to have the hand and ribs examined. While waiting for the results, the nurse cleaned an abrasion on her left knee, on her left cheek, and on the scalp. She had a 1.1-cm. laceration on her right palm which the physician examined. It was debrided to remove a significant amount of dirt, gravel, and even wood chips. It was then copiously washed with sterile water. The physician examined the palm and was able to suture it using single layer 3.0 chromic sutures.

X-ray results showed a non-displaced fracture of the distal one-third of the left ulna. The radius was not involved. A long-arm plaster cast was applied to the arm. There were no injuries sustained to the ribs. There appears a large ecchymosis to the right upper quadrant but there is no flank tenderness or swelling of the organs.

The patient is given a prescription for Lortab l q. 6 hrs. p.r.n. and told to see her family physician in the morning.

What codes are reported for this emergency department visit?

ICD-9-CM and CPT Code(s): _____

ICD-10-CM Code(s): _____

Chapter 9

Case Studies from Physician-Based Health Records

Note: Although the specific cases are divided by setting, much of the information pertaining to the diagnosis is applicable in most settings. Even the CPT codes in the ambulatory and physician sections may be reported in the same manner. The differences in coding in these two settings may involve modifier reporting, evaluation and management CPT code reporting, and other health plan reporting guidelines unique to settings. If you practice or apply codes in a particular type of setting, you may find additional information in other sections of this publication that may be pertinent to you.

Every effort has been made to follow current recognized coding guidelines and principles, as well as nationally recognized reporting guidelines. The material presented may differ from some health plan requirements for reporting. The ICD-9-CM codes used are effective October 1, 2012, through September 30, 2013, and the HCPCS (CPT and HCPCS Level II) codes are in effect January 1, 2013, through December 31, 2013. The current standard transactions and code sets named in HIPAA have been utilized. The 2013 draft edition of ICD-10-CM was utilized.

Instructions: Assign all applicable ICD-9-CM diagnosis codes including V codes and E codes. Assign all CPT Level I procedure codes and HCPCS Level II codes. Assign Level I (CPT) and Level II (HCPCS) modifiers as appropriate. Final codes for billing occur after codes are passed through payer edits. Medicare utilizes the National Correct Coding Initiative (NCCI) edits. CMS developed the NCCI edit list to promote national correct coding methodologies and to control improper coding leading to improper payments for Medicare Part B. The purpose of the NCCI edits is to ensure the most comprehensive code is assigned and billed rather than the component codes. In addition, NCCI edits check for mutually exclusive pairs.

Cases in this workbook are presented as either multiple choice or fill in the blank.

- For multiple-choice cases:
  - Select the letter of the appropriate code set.
- For fill-in-the-blank cases:
  - Sequence the primary diagnosis first followed by the secondary diagnoses including appropriate V codes and E codes (both cause of injury and place of occurrence).
  - Sequence the primary CPT procedure code first followed by additional procedure codes including modifiers as appropriate (both CPT Level I and HCPCS Level II modifiers).

> ○ Assign HCPCS Level II codes **only if instructed** (case specific).
>
> ○ Assign evaluation and management (E/M) codes **only if instructed** (case specific).
>
> The scenarios are based on selected excerpts from health records. In practice, the coding professional should have access to and refer to the entire health record. Health records are analyzed and codes assigned based on physician documentation. In physician practice, valuable information for coding purposes is available on the superbill; however, documentation for coding purposes must be assigned based on medical record documentation. A physician may be queried when documentation is ambiguous, incomplete, or conflicting. The queried documentation must be a permanent part of the medical record.
>
> The objective of the cases and scenarios reproduced in this publication is to provide practice in assigning correct codes, not necessarily to emulate complete coding, which can only be achieved with the complete medical record. For example, the reader may be asked to assign codes based on only an operative report; in real practice, a coder has access to documentation in the entire medical record.
>
> The *ICD-9-CM Official Guidelines for Coding and Reporting of Outpatient Services*, published by the National Center for Health Statistics (NCHS), supplements the official conventions and instructions provided within ICD-9-CM. Adherence to these guidelines when assigning ICD-9-CM diagnosis codes is required under the Health Insurance Portability and Accountability Act (HIPAA) of 1996. Additional official coding guidance can be found in the American Hospital Association (AHA)'s *Coding Clinic* publication.

Anesthesia Services

9.1.   A neonatal patient is brought to the operating room for repair of complete transposition of the great arteries under cardiopulmonary bypass. The infant is in critical condition and may not survive. Assign the correct diagnosis codes and CPT codes to report the administration of anesthesia, including physical status, Level I and II modifiers, and qualifying conditions for this procedure.

ICD-9-CM and CPT Code(s):

a.   745.10, 00562–AA–23, 99100
b.   745.11, 00561–AD–P5, 99140
c.   745.10, 00561–AA–P5
d.   745.19, 00563–AA–P5, 99100, 99140

ICD-10-CM Code(s): _____

9.2.   A patient came into the pain clinic for management of chronic neck and shoulder pain after a car accident one year ago. The vehicle she was driving struck a bus on a country road. The pain extended down into her left hand, and the patient had difficulty lifting or moving anything with that hand. She also reported inability to sleep well due to pain. Her attending physician requested that Dr. Jones, a pain specialist, take over the care for her pain. Dr. Jones performed an expanded problem-focused history and expanded problem-focused physical exam with medical decision making of low complexity. He and the patient discussed the injection of Marcaine and steroids into the cervical plexus for relief. The patient agreed to this plan, and after consents were signed, the injection was performed. The patient noted approximately 40 percent relief in pain almost immediately. Dr. Jones requested that the patient come back in one week and again in two weeks for another injection.

Diagnosis: Cervicobrachial syndrome, due to auto accident one year ago.

Assign the correct diagnosis and CPT codes (including E/M) for this scenario.

ICD-9-CM and CPT Code(s):

a. 723.3, 907.3, E929.0, 99202, 64413
b. 907.3, 723.3, E929.0, 99242, 64413
c. 723.3, 907.3, E929.0, 99212, 64415
d. 907.3, E929.0, 99203, 64490

ICD-10-CM Code(s): _____

9.3.   A 55-year-old patient is brought into the operating room for elective decompression of the median nerve for carpal tunnel syndrome. She is in excellent health otherwise. The surgeon places an Esmarch bandage on the arm, and the arm is exsanguinated. A tourniquet is then placed and the surgeon administers Bier block anesthesia.

Tourniquet time was approximately 50 minutes. Assign the ICD-9-CM diagnosis code and CPT surgical and anesthesia codes with any applicable modifiers.

ICD-9-CM and CPT Code(s):

a. 354.0, 64719
b. 354.0, 64722–47
c. 354.0, 64721–47
d. 354.1, 64721, 01810

ICD-10-CM Code(s): _____

Disorders of the Blood and Blood-Forming Organs

9.4.   A 32-year-old female has recently had surgery for melanoma of the right lower leg, Clark level IV. She had no other signs of metastasis or adenopathy. Under general anesthesia, a sentinel node biopsy of the deep axillary nodes was performed with a gamma counter probe. An injection of isosulfan blue dye was performed and the nodes followed carefully to the single -bright-blue node. This node was excised and sent for frozen section, which proved to be negative for melanoma. Before the procedure, the radiologist performed a lymphoscintigraphy. Which of the following code sets would the surgeon report? (Do not report supplies.)

ICD-9-CM and CPT Code(s):

a. 173.69, 38525
b. 172.7, 38525, 38792
c. 172.7, 38525, 38792–51, 78195
d. 172.9, 38525, 38790–51

ICD-10-CM Code(s): _____

9.5.   The following documentation is from the health record of a male patient.

History: This is a 66-year-old male who had a coronary artery bypass graft in February. He did well. He was discharged home. Some time after that when he was home, he had two days of black stools. He mentioned it to the nurse, but I'm not sure anything was done about it. He has not had any other evidence of hematemesis, melena, or hematochezia but was feeling rather weak and fatigued. He had blood work done, which showed a hemoglobin of 5.7, hematocrit of 20.9, MCV of 80. Serum iron of 8, 2 percent saturation. No indigestion or heartburn. No abdominal pain of any kind. No past history of anemia or GI bleed.

Past Medical History: General health has been good.

Allergies: None known

Previous Surgeries: Coronary artery bypass graft

Medications: At the time of admission include Glucotrol, Lasix, potassium, and aspirin

Review of Systems: Endocrine: He does have diabetes, controlled with medication. Cardiovascular: History of coronary artery disease with coronary artery bypass graft. No recent symptoms of chest pain or shortness of breath. Respiratory: No chronic cough or sputum production. GU: No dysuria, hematuria, history of stones, or infections. Musculoskeletal: No arthritic complaints or muscle weakness. Neuropsychiatric: No syncope, seizures, weakness, paralysis, or depression.

Family History: His mother had cardiovascular disease and diabetes. No history of cancer.

Social History: The patient is married. Never smoked. Doesn't drink any alcohol. Works in a factory.

On physical examination, a well-developed, well-nourished, alert male in no acute distress. Blood pressure 146/82. Respirations 18. Heart rate 78. Skin: Good turgor and texture. Eyes: No scleral icterus. Pupils are round, regular, equal, and react to light. Neck: No jugular venous distention. No carotid bruits. Thyroid is not enlarged. Trachea in the midline. Lungs are clear. No heart murmur noted. Abdomen is soft. Bowel sounds present. No masses, no tenderness. Liver and spleen are not palpably enlarged. Extremities: Good pulses. Trace edema of the feet.

Laboratory values show severe anemia with a hemoglobin of 5.7. Hemoccult is also positive. His iron studies showed low iron and low ferritin, consistent with chronic blood loss anemia. His B_{12} and folate levels were normal. His SMA-12 was essentially unremarkable.

Impression: 1.   Anemia. Probably he is anemic post bypass and then had stress gastritis with a little bit of bleeding and has never recovered from that. No evidence of acute or active bleeding at this time. The patient is stable. Possibility of occult malignancy or active peptic ulcer disease does exist.

2.   Arteriosclerotic heart disease of native vessel, stable

Recommendations: Admit patient as an outpatient for blood transfusion. Patient is being transfused. He should have an esophagogastroduodenoscopy and colonoscopy, possible biopsy or polypectomy, which has been explained to the patient along with potential risks and complications, including bleeding, transfusion, perforation, and surgery. These tests will be scheduled for a later date.

Discharge Note

Final Diagnosis: Severe blood loss anemia, weakness, diabetes mellitus, history of coronary artery disease status post coronary artery bypass graft.

The patient received three units of packed red blood cells; he felt better with subsidence of his shortness of breath and his weakness improved. His last hemoglobin was 8.4, with a hematocrit of 27.7.

The patient was scheduled for EGD to rule out peptic ulcer disease and colonoscopy to rule out occult malignancy in one week. The patient will be discharged home, and he will have a clear liquid diet. He is to call for any problems. He will continue with his home medications, and he was placed on ferrous sulfate one tablet twice a day.

What diagnosis codes are reported for this hospital outpatient encounter reported by the physician?

ICD-9-CM Code(s):

a. 280.0, 792.1, 414.01, 250.00, V45.81
b. 285.9, 780.79
c. 280.0, 578.1, 414.01, 250.00, V45.81
d. 998.11, 285.1, 792.1, 414.01, 250.00, V45.81

ICD-10-CM Code(s): _____

Disorders of the Cardiovascular System

9.6. A patient who is six weeks post anterior MI with congestive heart failure has been taking Lanoxin and is experiencing nausea and profound fatigue. The evaluation and treatment were focused on adjustment of medication only. Blood levels show 4 ng/mL. Which of the following diagnosis codes will be reported?

ICD-9-CM Code(s):

a. 972.1, E858.3, 787.01
b. 410.12, 428.0
c. 787.02, 780.79, E858.3
d. 787.02, 780.79, E942.1, 410.12, 428.0

ICD-10-CM Code(s): _____

9.7. The following documentation is from the health record of a female patient.

History: This is a 70-year-old female who had noted exertional tachyarrhythmia described as palpitations, diaphoresis, and presyncope. She had noted no frank syncopal episodes. Prior to this admission, she had been on Lopressor, Norpace, and Lanoxin in combination but was still experiencing breakthrough atrial flutter.

Hospital Course: Upon admission, the patient underwent echocardiography. This revealed moderate left ventricular dysfunction, mild to moderate aortic regurgitation, mild mitral regurgitation, and the left atrium proved to be within the upper limits of normal. At that time, it was recommended that the patient begin on amiodarone therapy due to drug refractory atrial flutter. Pulmonary function test and thyroid function test were also performed. Thyroid function test results proved within normal limits. Pulmonary function test results revealed normal lung volumes with mild loss of alveolar capacity. Amiodarone loading continued. The patient was taken to the electrophysiology lab, and overdrive pacing was attempted. This was unsuccessful. The patient therefore underwent direct-current external atrial cardioversion and at that time converted to normal sinus rhythm. The patient was discharged with a scheduled follow-up in 1 month.

Final Diagnoses: 1. Drug refractory atrial flutter
2. Successful cardioversion to normal sinus rhythm

Which of the following is the correct code assignment?

ICD-9-CM and CPT Code(s):

a. 429.9, 424.0, 92961
b. 429.9, 394.1, 33240
c. · 427.32, 394.1, 429.9, 33211
d. 427.32, 396.3, 429.9, 92960

ICD-10-CM Code(s): _____

9.8. The following documentation is from the health record of a 66-year-old male patient.

Discharge Summary

Admission Date: 6/19/XX

Discharge Date: 6/28/XX

History of Present Illness: This patient is a 66-year-old male admitted on 6/19 because of unstable postinfarct angina. He underwent cardiac bypass surgery here 15 years ago. He did well until 1989, when he developed angina and underwent angioplasty here. On 6/9, he was awakened by severe chest pain and was taken to a nearby community hospital where he was found to have a small anterior wall myocardial infarction with the CPK only slightly elevated. He had cardiac catheterization performed at that time. Because of this small infarction, he was referred here for consideration for further surgical intervention. He was discharged from the hospital on 6/16. On 6/19, as the patient was walking from the car to the office, he developed significant chest pain and was therefore admitted to rule out further infarction.

Documentation of recent cardiac catheterization showed that complete left heart catheterization, left ventricular cineangiography, coronary arteriography, and bypass visualization were performed. The left ventricle showed severe anterior hypokinesis, although it did still move. The left main coronary artery was narrowed by about 70 percent. The bypass to the circumflex looked good, but the bypass to the left anterior descending had a very severe stenosis in the body of the graft. There was a very large, marginal circumflex artery that had an orificial, 80 percent stenosis. He was thought not to be a candidate for angioplasty but bypass surgery instead.

Surgical Procedure: Using extracorporeal circulation, the left internal mammary artery was anastomosed to the left anterior descending coronary artery, and a venous graft was placed from the aorta to the marginal circumflex. It was found that the old venous graft to the main circumflex was in excellent condition with very soft, pliable walls so that the vessel was left intact. There were no complications of this surgery. His postoperative course was singularly uncomplicated. He never had any arrhythmia problems; his wounds healed nicely. He had a tiny left pleural effusion that never needed to be tapped. He was walking about the ward participating in the cardiac rehab program at the time of discharge.

Discharge Instructions: Discharge medications will simply be aspirin grains 5 q.d., Tylenol with Codeine 1 or 2 p.r.n. for pain, Lopressor 50 mg a day, and Colace, as necessary. He was instructed to contact his private physician upon return home for resumption of his medical care. He is to call me here at the medical center if there are any questions or problems that he wishes to discuss.

Discharge Diagnoses:
1. Unstable angina (intermediate coronary syndrome)
2. Recent incomplete, anterior wall myocardial infarction
3. Coronary atherosclerosis, three vessel
4. Successful double-bypass surgery

What are the correct codes for this admission?

ICD-9-CM and CPT Code(s):

a. 414.01, 414.05, 410.12, 411.1, 33517, 33533, 33530
b. 414.01, 414.05, 410.12, 411.1, 33510, 33533
c. 414.00, 414.05, 410.11, 411.1, 33530
d. 414.01, 414.05, 410.12, 412, 33518, 33530

ICD-10-CM Code(s): _____

9.9. The following documentation is from the health record of an 85-year-old female patient.

Admission Date: 12/10/XX

Discharge Date: 12/22/XX

Discharge Diagnoses:
1. Acute pulmonary edema with acute systolic congestive heart failure
2. Myocardial infarction ruled out
3. Chronic obstructive pulmonary disease
4. Pneumonia
5. Senile dementia

History of Present Illness: This 85-year-old female was admitted via the emergency room from the nursing home with shortness of breath, confusion, and congestion. There was no history of fever or cough noted. Patient has a history of senile dementia and COPD. Prior to admission, the patient was on the following medications: Prednisone, Lasix, Haldol, and Colace.

Physical Examination: Blood pressure 140/70, heart rate of 125 beats per minute, respirations were 30, temperature of 101.4°F. The eyes showed postsurgical eyes, nonreactive to light. The lungs showed bilaterally bibasilar crackles. The heart showed S1 and S2, with no S3. The abdomen was soft and nontender. The extremities showed leg edema. The neurological exam revealed no deficits, and she was alert × 3.

Laboratory Data: ABGs were 7.4, PO_2 of 63, CO_2 of 43, bicarbonate 26, saturation of 89. Hemoglobin 11.7, hematocrit was 31.5, platelets of 207,000. Sodium 139, chloride 107, potassium 4.4, BUN 42, creatinine 1.2. The EKG was unremarkable.

Hospital Course: Basically, this patient was admitted to the coronary care unit with acute pulmonary edema, rule out myocardial infarction. Serial cardiac enzymes were done, which were within normal limits, therefore ruling out myocardial infarction. A chest x-ray performed on the day of admission confirmed acute systolic congestive heart failure and pneumonia. The patient was started on Unasyn and tobramycin for the pneumonia, which improved. The congestive heart failure, however, was not improving with administration of Lasix. The patient was not taking foods and liquids well and, at the family's request, she was labeled DNR. On hospital day 12, she was found without respirations, with no heart sounds, and pupils were fixed. She was pronounced dead by the physician, and the family was notified.

Which of the following answers demonstrates the correct ICD-9-CM code assignment?

ICD-9-CM Code(s):

a. 428.21, 486, 496, 290.0, V49.86
b. 428.21, 518.4, 486, 496, 290.0
c. 428.0, 410.91, 486, 496, 290.0, V49.86
d. 518.4, 428.21, 486, 496, 290.0, V49.86

ICD-10-CM Code(s): _____

9.10. Dr. Hiram performs an endovascular repair of a very long aneurysm of the descending thoracic aorta, with placement of two distal extension components due to the extensive length of the aneurysm. The left subclavian artery was not covered during this procedure. Assign the appropriate CPT code(s) to report this procedure.

a. 33880
b. 33779
c. 33881
d. 33881, 33883, 33884

9.11. Ms. Jones has a pseudoaneurysm of her left iliac artery that has developed proximal to an area of occlusion. She is admitted to Community Hospital for iliac artery endovascular revascularization and repair. She undergoes a percutaneous transluminal balloon angioplasty of the area of occlusion, with placement of a drug-eluting stent, and an endovascular repair of the pseudoaneurysm using ilio-iliac tube endoprothesis. An endovascular ultrasound is performed after the procedure to assure patency of the vessel. Assign the appropriate CPT code(s). You do not need to assign modifiers for this exercise.

    a. 34900, 37221, 37250
    b. 34900, 37221
    c. 37221
    d. 34825, 37221, 37250

9.12. In the cardiac catheterization laboratory of Big City Hospital, Dr. Hart performed a PTCA on a patient's right coronary artery, with placement of a drug-eluting stent. He also performed a PTCA of the left circumflex coronary artery and placement of two stents. The patient had undergone a complete diagnostic cardiac catheterization at an outlying hospital the previous day, so complete cardiac catheterization was not performed. Dr. Hart performed the procedure via femoral artery cutdown without left heart catheterization. Assign the appropriate CPT codes and HCPCS Level II modifiers that Dr. Hart would use to report these procedures.

CPT and HCPCS Level II Code(s):

    a. 92928-RC, 92929-LC
    b. 92928-RC, 92929-LC, 92920-RC, 92921-LC
    c. 93455, 92928-RC, 92929-LC
    d. 93455, 92928-RC, 92929-LC, 92920-RC, 92921-LC

9.13. This is a progress note from the office records of a physician's office:

Chief Complaint: Chest pains in a 44-year-old man

HPI: Patient indicates that he woke up this morning with what he thought was indigestion but as the morning progressed he began to have some intermittent chest pains. He comes to the office for check-up.

Past Medical History: Patient has mild open angle glaucoma, mild hypertension, and DJD. He does smoke a pack of cigarettes per day. In light of his family history, I have repeatedly suggested that the patient attempt a smoking cessation regime. I have offered prescription meds but patient refuses.

Family History: Patient's father died at age 43 of myocardial infarction. His older brother has had one minor MI at age 51.

Vital Signs: BP 163/78; pulse 89; respirations 17.

Physical Examination:

HEENT: Glaucoma, diagnosed 8 months ago, is in control. He last saw his ophthalmologist just about 3 weeks ago. I will continue to monitor in between visits with the specialist.

Pulmonary: Chest is clear to percussion and auscultation. No rales or rhonchi heard. Hiatal hernia noted.

Abdomen: Obese. No gross hepatosplenomegaly. Bowel sounds are normal.

Extremities: Pedal edema in the lower extremities. There did not appear to be any lesions or open wounds on the lower extremities. Patient complained of some pain in the right knee. He has a history of a right knee replacement some 10 years ago. I see no obvious abnormalities with the knee but if it continues to cause him discomfort he should see an orthopedist.

Cardiovascular: Heart sounds were regular. No murmurs or ectopic beats heard.

Plan: Because of the patient's hypertension and family history of myocardial infarctions, the chest pains are extremely worrisome. I have arranged for the patient to have a cardiac catheterization today. He was instructed to report to the hospital immediately.

What codes would be recorded for this office visit?

ICD-9-CM Code(s): _____

ICD-10-CM Code(s): _____

9.14.   Operative Report

Preoperative Diagnoses: Atrial fibrillation with sick sinus syndrome.

Postoperative Diagnoses: Atrial fibrillation with sick sinus syndrome.

Procedure: Insertion of Medtronics N rhythm dual chamber pulse generator pacemaker, model number P1501DR with atrial and ventricular leads under fluoroscopic guidance.

Anesthesia: 1% Xylocaine local with sedation.

Estimated Blood Loss: Minimal.

Comment: This is an elderly gentleman with atrial fibrillation and sick sinus syndrome who had a dual chamber pacemaker placed with a screw-in atrial lead in the operating room. During the time of implantation, the permanent lead parameters were recorded in the patient's permanent medical record and the entire procedure was performed under fluoroscopy. The patient has been on Coumadin for several years but blood loss was minimal. The patient tolerated the procedure well.

Procedure: The patient was taken to the operating room and placed on the table in supine position. After adequate intravenous sedation was given, the left chest wall was prepped with DuraPrep and draped with sterile drapes in the usual fashion. After infiltration with 1% Xylocaine, an oblique incision was fashioned inferomedial to the deltopectoral groove. The incision was deepened to the skin and subcutaneous tissue to the pectoralis fascia where a pocket was fashioned inferiorly for the pulse generator. Through the wound, two Seldinger wires were placed uneventfully into the left subclavian vein with the patient in Trendelenburg and these were then exchanged for dilator and breakaway sheaths through which were introduced a tinned-tipped ventricular lead advanced to the central circulation under fluoroscopic guidance with the tip brought to rest in the apex of the right ventricle until satisfactory parameters were obtained in this location and the lead was then secured to the chest wall with three interrupted #2-0 Ethibond sutures. More medially, the dilator and breakaway sheath in this position was then replaced with a screw-in type pre-formed, J-shaped atrial lead advanced in the septal circulation under fluoroscopic guidance with the tip implanted in the right atrium with the screw-in device until satisfactory parameters were obtained in this location. This lead was secured to the chest wall in a similar fashion. The two leads then firmly connected to the pre-programmed Medtronics pulse generator model as noted above, which was placed into the previously fashioned subcutaneous pocket with the leads coiled beneath it. The subcutaneous tissues were irrigated with Ancef saline and the superficial subcutaneous tissues were closed over the top of the pacemaker leads with interrupted #3-0 Polysorb suture and the skin closed with running inverted, interrupted subcuticular #4-0 Biosyn followed by application of a Bioclusive dressing. Sponge, needle, and instrument counts were reported to be correct × 2 at the termination of the procedure. The patient tolerated the procedure well and left the Operating Room in satisfactory condition.

What are the correct codes for this outpatient surgery?

ICD-9-CM and CPT Code(s):

a. 427.41, 427.81, 33202, 33213
b. 427.41, 427.81, 33212, 33217
c. 427.31, V58.61, 33201
d. 427.31, 427.81, V58.61, 33208

ICD-10-CM Code(s): _____

Disorders of the Digestive System

9.15.   This is the documentation from the record of a patient seen in the outpatient surgery suite.

Procedure: Upper GI endoscopy

Indications: Heartburn

Complications: No immediate complications

Procedure: After obtaining informed consent, the endoscope was passed under direct vision. Throughout the procedure, the patient's blood pressure, pulse, and oxygen saturations were monitored continuously. The Olympus GIF-Q160 gastroscope (Serial No. 2306352) was introduced through the mouth, and advanced to the third part of the duodenum. The upper GI endoscopy was accomplished without difficulty. The patient tolerated the procedure well.

Findings: Biopsy of esophageal mucosa with a cold forceps was performed for histology, evaluation for microscopic esophagitis, and evaluation to rule out Barrett's Esophagus.

Diffuse mildly erythematous mucosa with no bleeding was found in the gastric antrum. Biopsies were taken with a cold forceps for histology. Biopsies were taken with a cold forceps for Helicobacter pylori testing.

The examined duodenum was normal. Biopsy with a cold forceps was performed for histology, evaluation of celiac sprue, evaluation of celiac disease, and evaluation of chronic inflammation.

Impression: GERD.

Mild antral gastritis/gastric mucosal abnormality characterized by erythema. Normal examined duodenum. This was biopsied.

Recommendations:
- Continue present medications.
- Use sucralfate tablets at 1 gram PO QID.
- Telephone endoscopist for pathology results.
- Await pathology results.

Which codes would the physician use to report these services?

ICD-9-CM and CPT Code(s):

a. 530.81, 535.40, 43239
b. 530.81, 535.50, 43239
c. 530.81, 535.40, 43202, 43605, 44010
d. 530.81, 535.40, 43239

ICD-10-CM Code(s): _____

9.16. A 48-year-old man came in to the emergency department complaining of vomiting material resembling coffee grounds several times within the past hour. He has abdominal pain and has been unable to eat for the past 24 hours. He is dizzy and lightheaded. Two stools today have been black and tarry. While in the emergency department, he vomited bright-red blood and some material resembling coffee grounds. A nasogastric tube was inserted by the ED physician and attached to suction. An abdominal exam showed a fluid wave consistent with ascites. CBC and clotting studies were drawn. A detailed history and physical exam with high-complexity medical decision making were documented. A GI consultant was called and the patient was taken to Endoscopy for further evaluation of upper GI bleeding. Diagnosis: Hematemesis, rule out esophageal varices; blood loss anemia, acute; ascites.

Which of the following is the correct diagnosis and CPT procedure code assignment for the independent ED physician?

ICD-9-CM and CPT Code(s):

a. 578.0, 285.1, 789.59, 99285, 43752
b. 578.0, 789.00, 780.4, 99284-25, 91105
c. 789.51, 578.0, 280.0, 99284, 43752
d. 578.0, 285.1, 789.59, 99284-25, 43752

ICD-10-CM Code(s): _____

9.17. This 35-year-old man has had a history of diverticulosis with frequent bleeding in the past. He came in to have a colonoscopy and rule out any other pathology, such as carcinoma. During the colonoscopy, severe diverticulosis was noted. This is definitely the cause of the bleeding. Also noted were a polyp at the splenic flexure and a polyp in the transverse colon. The polyp at the splenic flexure was removed by hot biopsy, and the second polypectomy was done by snare technique. The polyps were both classified as adenomatous with no signs of malignancy. What are the correct codes for this case?

ICD-9-CM and CPT Code(s):

a. 562.12, 211.3, 45385, 45384-51 or 45384-59
b. 211.3, 562.10, 578.1, 45384
c. 562.12, 211.3, 578.9, 45385
d. 562.12, 211.3, 45384

ICD-10-CM Code(s): _____

9.18. The patient had a laparoscopic Nissen fundoplasty performed for gastroesophageal reflux with esophagitis. He also has Barrett's esophagus. These conditions have not been responding to conservative treatment, and the patient wishes to undergo surgery at this time. The patient has also had many instances of treatment for chronic cholecystitis. It has been decided to pursue a laparoscopic cholecystectomy at the same time that the fundoplasty is done. Which of the following is the correct code assignment?

ICD-9-CM and CPT Code(s):

a. 530.81, 530.85, 47562, 43289-51
b. 530.11, 530.85, 574.10, 43327, 47600-52
c. 530.11, 530.89, 575.11, 43326
d. 530.11, 530.85, 575.11, 43280, 47562-51

ICD-10-CM Code(s): _____

9.19. The following documentation is from the health record of a 58-year-old male patient:

Preoperative Diagnosis:	Diverticular disease of left colon Non-continuity of bowel
Postoperative Diagnosis:	Diverticular disease of left colon
Operation:	Laparoscopic left colon resection with coloproctal anastomosis Laparoscopic splenic flexure mobilization
Anesthesia:	General endotracheal, Marcaine 0.5% local
Estimated Blood Loss:	20 cc.

Indications: This 58-year-old male presents back to the operating room four months after his sigmoid colon perforation due to diverticular disease. A temporary ostomy was performed, along with sigmoidectomy at that time. In the interim, the patient has undergone a colonoscopy identifying additional diverticular disease in the left colon. Upon discussion with him, we plan today for reanastomosis of the bowel but also additional colon resection on his left colon in light of this additional disease. The risks, benefits, and alternatives of the procedure are explained, and he is agreeable.

Gross Findings: Appropriate splenic flexure mobilization was completed to allow for advancement of the colon down to the rectal stump providing a tension-free anastomosis.

Description of Procedure: The patient was placed in a supine position after sterile prep and drape was complete. Marcaine was infiltrated in the area of about 1.0 centimeters around the midline incision site and blunt dissection was then done, including sharp dissection to the fascia. This was then opened and entrance was gained into the abdomen. #11 port was placed and CO2 insufflation was then obtained. Additional ports were placed for laparoscopic approach to the procedure. With the aid of a ligature, the splenic flexure was completely mobilized. After completion of this, additional mobilization was done for the colon. The rectal stump was identified easily with the Prolene sutures that were utilized for its location, placed on the last procedure. After adhesions were taken out of this area, the ostomy on the left side of the abdomen was then excised with sterile technique and dissection was done about the subcutaneous tissues to the fascia freely mobilizing the colon. Advancement of the left colon was then done outside of the abdomen and a pursestring device was then used to fire across the proximal portion of the left colon; this bowel was then sent to Pathology. A 25 mm EEA device was then utilized and its anvil was placed at the end of the colon. This was then placed back into the abdomen and towel clips were used to temporarily approximate the skin allowing pneumoperitoneum to exist.

Next, re-evaluation of the rectal site was done with the assistance of the surgical assist. Advancement of the EEA device was then done in the rectum, and this trocar was advanced through the anterior portion of the rectum. The phenol end of the device was then attached to the trochar and approximation of the tissues was then done. Minimal tension and no twist were appreciated on the anastomosis. Once it was fired, two donuts were appreciated. Irrigation and aspiration was done revealing minimal blood loss with the procedure.

C02 pneumoperitoneum was then released into the air and additional irrigation was done at the old ostomy incision site. This fascia was re-approximated with one Vicryl suture and the other port sites 10 mm or larger were re-approximated with 0-Vicryl suture. All incisions were closed with Vicryl and the ostomy site was also closed with skin clips in light of the higher chance of infection. The patient tolerated the procedure well and went to the recovery room in stable condition.

Which of the following is the correct CPT code assignment?

a. 44207, 44213
b. 44207, 44213, 44620
c. 44227
d. 44626

9.20. The following documentation is from the health record of a 33-year-old female patient.

History and Physical

The patient is scheduled for surgery today.

Chief Complaint: Anal pain with bleeding

History of Present Illness: This is a 33-year-old woman with a 2-year history of anal pain and bleeding, which has been markedly worse lately. Has been on stool softener and sitz baths; symptoms have not improved. She presents for ligation of internal hemorrhoids.

Past History: General health is good. There are no major medical illnesses. She has had a tubal ligation in the past.

Family History and Review of Systems: Otherwise noncontributory

Physical Examination: HEENT: Grossly intact. Neck: Supple. Chest: Clear. Heart: Regular rate and rhythm. Abdomen: Soft, without mass, tenderness, or organomegaly. Anal exam: There is marked posterior tenderness and pain.

Impression: Bleeding, prolapsed internal hemorrhoids, not responding to conservative therapy

Recommendations: Internal rubber band ligation. The procedure has been explained in detail to the patient, and she understands and accepts.

Operative Report

Preoperative Diagnosis:	Internal prolapsing hemorrhoids
Postoperative Diagnosis:	Same
Surgery Performed:	Proctosigmoidoscopy, rubber band ligation of the internal hemorrhoids, done with an anoscope

Procedure: The patient was placed on the operating table in a sitting position. The patient was placed in prone jackknife position and the buttocks were retracted. Proctosigmoidoscopy was then carried out to 20 cm and was normal except for the anal findings mentioned above. The proctoscope was withdrawn, and the anus was prepped and draped in antiseptic fashion. A field block with Marcaine 0.25 percent was then placed. The anoscope was inserted. There was a prolapsing hemorrhoid in the anterior midline. This was rubber-band ligated above the dentate line by applying two bands. In the posterior midline, there was another hemorrhoid, which was banded in the same manner. Bleeding was checked, and none was noted.

The patient was taken to the recovery room in stable condition. Blood loss was negligible. Counts correct; no drains.

Which of the following is the correct code assignment?

ICD-9-CM and CPT Code(s):

a. 455.2, 46221, 45300-51, 46600-51
b. 455.2, 46221, 46221-59, 45300
c. 455.0, 46945, 45300
d. 455.8, 46083, 45300-51, 46600-51

ICD-10-CM Code(s): _____

Evaluation and Management (E/M) Services

9.21. **Physician Encounter:** A primary care physician in the patient's very small hometown sees the patient and recommends a partial lumpectomy for a 0.9-cm lesion in the right breast. The general surgeon completes a very thorough preoperative evaluation and refers the patient to a general surgeon in a neighboring, much larger community, for the actual removal of the lump. The PCP asks that the general surgeon perform the lumpectomy only. The patient has the lumpectomy and returns back home to the care of the primary care physician. How would the surgeon's service be coded? The primary care practitioner's (PCP)?

a. Surgeon: 19120-52; PCP: 19120
b. Surgeon: 19120-54; PCP: 19120-55-56
c. Surgeon: 19101-54; PCP: 19120-55-56
d. Surgeon: 19101-54; PCP: 19120, 99213

9.22. Dr. Bill admitted a patient to observation care services after seeing him in the emergency department with severe nausea, vomiting, and dizziness from dehydration. The initial observation services documentation supported a comprehensive history, comprehensive exam, and moderate complexity medical decision making. IVs were started, and the plan was to hydrate the patient and discharge him to home the next morning. The patient, however, had not improved enough the next day (day two) and was observed an additional 24 hours. The subsequent care documentation supported a problem focused examination and low complexity medical decision making. On day three, the physician's documentation supported an observation care discharge service and the patient was discharged home.

Choose the correct sequence of CPT procedure E/M codes for Dr. Bill's observation service coding.

a. 99219, 99231, 99217
b. 99219, 99224, 99217
c. 99283, 99219, 99217
d. 99283, 99231, 99217

9.23.   Dr. Smith sent a patient to observation care at the local hospital following his visit to the nursing facility. The patient was admitted for observation to rule out stroke due to a change in mental status. The next morning, Dr. Smith left town, and his partner, Dr. Johnson, admitted the patient to inpatient care because of sudden worsening symptoms. The patient expired later the same day. Assuming documentation guidelines were met, how would E/M services for these two physicians be coded?

   a. Dr. Smith: 99315, 99219; Dr. Johnson: 99236
   b. Dr. Smith: 99219; Dr. Johnson: 99217, 99236
   c. Dr. Smith: 99219; Dr. Johnson: 99236
   d. Dr. Smith: 99315, 99222; Dr. Johnson: 99238

9.24.   An 85-year-old patient of Dr. Smith's was brought to the clinic from her home after her family failed to get her to respond to their phone calls. She was poorly nourished, dehydrated, and confused. Dr. Smith admitted her to the hospital to stabilize her, then discharged her to a nursing facility the next day. Assuming that all documentation guidelines for each level of service have been met, assign the correct CPT codes for Dr. Smith's services to the hospital and nursing home.

   a. 99214, 99222, 99239, 99305
   b. 99222, 99239, 99305
   c. 99214, 99235, 99305
   d. 99222, 99305

9.25.   Dr. Donahue had an elderly Hispanic male come to his office for an initial visit. The patient had multiple medical problems and had not had any care for at least 10 years. The patient brought his 12-year-old granddaughter to interpret; however, she was of minimal assistance due to her unfamiliarity with medical terms and problems. Dr. Donahue's nurse called the local hospital and requested the services of their Spanish-speaking interpreter. By putting the interpreter on speakerphone, Dr. Donahue was able to finish his examination of the patient, prescribe medications, and give instructions for follow-up care. He documented a comprehensive history, a physical examination, and medical decision making that was moderate. He spent an additional 50 minutes counseling and coordinating the care of this patient, for a total of 95 minutes of care.

   Assign the correct CPT code for Dr. Donahue's services.

   a. 99204, 99354
   b. 99205, 99354, 99355
   c. 99205, 99354
   d. 99204

9.26.   The following documentation is from the health record of a 56-year-old female.

Preventive Medicine Visit

This patient is a 56-year-old female who comes in today for a complete physical, which is covered by her insurance company. Patient is known to me, although has not been in to see me since last year.

Past Medical History:
1. History of proctosigmoiditis, probably ischemic, treated 1/93
2. History of TAH-BSO for endometriosis
3. History of NSVD × 2
4. History of correction of bunion and hammer toe, 1996

The only concern that she has is some problems with headaches in the frontal area in the morning. The headaches seem to be worse fairly consistently in the morning. She has also had some problems with hips aching, and her eyes occasionally have been a little blurry. Other than that, she has no other concerns on ROS. She has no jaw claudication, joint pains, etc.

Family History: Her mother died of CVA and colon cancer at age 76. Her father died of heart disease at age 80.

Social History: She has been married for 25 years. She has two children and is a homemaker. She does not smoke or drink. Her husband is a farmer.

Allergies: No known allergies

Medications: ASA, Premarin, Caltrate

ROS is otherwise entirely unremarkable.

Physical Exam: She appears to be in no acute distress.

HEENT:	Head is normocephalic. PERRLA: Fundi benign. TMs are clear. Pharynx is negative. There is no temporal artery tenderness.
Neck:	Without adenopathy or thyromegaly
Lungs:	Clear
Heart:	Showed a normal S1, S2, with regular rate and rhythm and no murmur
Breasts:	Without masses. Self breast examination was taught and encouraged on a monthly basis. Axillary is unremarkable.
Abdomen:	Soft and nontender with no hepatosplenomegaly present
Genitalia:	External genitalia normal. Cervix was absent. Vaginal Pap smear was done. Bimanual exam revealed an absent uterus and nonpalpable ovaries. Rectal exam was normal.
Neurological:	Exam intact

Assessment:
1. Headaches, exact etiology not clear. I am going to check her sed rate. If that is normal, then will proceed with CT scan of the head.
2. Routine physical

I will write to her with the test results. If she does not hear from me in two weeks, she will give me a call. Otherwise, I will see her right after her head CT.

Assign the correct codes for this visit:

ICD-9-CM and CPT Code(s):

a. V72.31, V76.47, V45.77, 99396, 784.0, 99213-25
b. V70.9, 99396, 784.0, 99213
c. V76.2, V76.47, V45.77, G0101, Q0091, 784.0, 99213-25
d. 784.0, V72.31, V76.47, V45.77, 99214

ICD-10-CM Code(s): _____

9.27. The following scenario involves a female patient in the intensive care unit.

Hospital Emergency Visit

Subjective: I was called regarding endotracheal tube cuff leak and copious secretions suctioned through ETT. N/G sounds not heard in stomach per nurse, though no evidence by exam that N/G was withdrawn partially. Anesthesia called in. Patient is very afraid of losing airway.

Objective: Vital signs stabilized. Endotracheal tube replaced by anesthesia and verified with good bilateral breath sounds. There are a few mild right expiratory rhonchi. Cor 50s to 60s. O_2 saturation remained in the 90s.

Assessment:
1. Respiratory failure: Holding own; chest x-ray ordered
2. Congestive heart failure: Retaining fluid despite increased diuretics
3. Nutrition: Improved
4. Heart: Remains in normal sinus rhythm
5. Atelectasis and pneumonia: Now afebrile, still needs frequent pulmonary toilet
6. INR 1.9

Critical Care Time: 2 a.m. to 3 a.m.—Emergent

Plan:
1. Transfer to ICU
2. Increase Coumadin
3. Continue respiratory care and IV antibiotics
4. Increase diuresis: She is above her dry weight

Determine the correct E/M code(s) for the ER physician for this scenario.

a. 99233
b. 99291, 99292
c. 99233, 99354
d. 99291

9.28. The following documentation is from the health record of a male patient.

Well Child Check—Newborn

This 4-day-old male patient is seen in clinic today for his routine well check following release from the newborn nursery with his first-time mom. He is spitting up much of his feedings and also is not latching on as well as he had been for the first 2 days. His weight is down 6 ounces to 6 pounds, 2 ounces and he is again below his birth weight. Remainder of the exam is normal.

The mom is advised to reinstitute supplemental bottle feedings with pumped breast milk. She will see the lactation nurse this afternoon in the Woman's Care Center for additional counseling on feeding problems. The patient will be seen again tomorrow in follow-up. If spitting up continues after appropriate latch response is achieved and it's not related to excess air intake, will discuss switching to formula feeds.

Diagnosis: Normal newborn with feeding problems

Determine the correct code assignment for this physician's services.

ICD-9-CM Code(s):

a. V20.2, 779.31
b. V20.2, 783.21
c. V20.31
d. V20.31, 779.31

ICD-10-CM Code(s): _____

9.29.   Office Visit

Chief Complaint: Patient claims he has no problem swallowing, no shortness of breath, or chest pains.

Past Medical History: Patient has hypertension and hyperlipidemia. Patient is taking atenolol, lovastatin, and cimetidine.

Social History: Patient is married and was in the military for 25 years until his health problems necessitated an honorable discharge.

The patient is a 51-year-old African-American male who has long-standing hyperlipidemia and hypertension. He has a history of esophageal dilatation for swallowing difficulties. Today he denies any SOB or chest pains. He mentions that his reflux is much improved on the cimetidine. I will schedule a follow-up EGD for three months. The patient is severely overweight but he is not motivated to lose weight. He does not restrict his diet in any way and refuses to engage in any sort of physical activity. His morbid obesity is of no concern to the patient. Nor is the possibility of stroke or MI.

Vital signs today show a slightly elevated blood pressure of 145/89, heart rate of 100 beats per minutes, and a weight of 267. Patient has gained 3 pounds since his last appointment 2 months ago.

However his physical examination today is relatively normal. His GERD is much improved on the cimetidine so we will continue that and do a repeat EGD in 3 months. Patient is moderately depressed although can't really find a cause. He did suffer a setback at work 6 months ago and this seems to be contributing to his depression. I will put him on a trial of Celexa until his next visit to see if this will help with the depression.

History is of detailed level; examination is comprehensive; MDM moderate complexity.

Which of the following answers best reflects the code assignment for this encounter?

ICD-9-CM and CPT Code(s):

a. 272.4, 278.00, 530.81, 311, 401.9, 99204
b. 272.4, 278.00, 530.81, 311, 401.9, 99214
c. 272.4, 278.01, 530.81, 311, 401.9, 99214
d. 272.4, 278.00, 530.81, 311, 401.9, 99213

ICD-10-CM Code(s): _____

Endocrine, Nutritional, and Metabolic Diseases and Immunity Disorders

9.30. A 13-year-old male patient is being evaluated in the children's clinic for delayed puberty. He is 4'1" and does not exhibit any signs of puberty or secondary sexual characteristics. His parents wonder if the necrotizing enterocolitis that he had at birth is the cause of his short stature. Other than his short stature, the patient seems in normal health. Blood tests indicated a deficiency of growth hormone. The patient returned to the clinic for follow-up of test results and parents were given the option of starting him on growth hormone treatments. Diagnosis on the second visit is HGH deficiency. Give the codes for both the first and second visits.

ICD-9-CM Code(s):

a. First visit: 259.4, 259.0; second visit: 253.3
b. First visit: 259.0; second visit: 253.3
c. First visit: 259.0; second visit: 253.4
d. First visit: 259.4; second visit: 253.4

ICD-10-CM Code(s): _____

9.31. An 18-year-old female was referred to an endocrinologist by her family doctor with symptoms of a right-sided neck mass that is increasing in size. A thyroid ultrasound completed today shows a complex cystic structure in the right lobe of the thyroid with recent hemorrhage of the thyroid. There was also a small thyroid nodule located in the left lobe.

The endocrinologist requests a surgical consultation for treatment options because of the likelihood of a re-bleed if the thyroid is drained and a potential for malignancy, given the two areas of concern in the thyroid.

Which of the following is the correct diagnostic code set for this visit to the endocrinologist?

ICD-9-CM Code(s):

a. 240.9
b. 241.0, 246.2
c. 241.0, 246.3
d. 241.0, 246.2, 246.3

ICD-10-CM Code(s): _____

9.32. The following documentation is from the health record of a 69-year-old female.

HPI: The patient is a 69-year-old female with a large pituitary tumor found after lymph node biopsy that demonstrated lung cancer. The lung cancer is apparently non–small cell adenocarcinoma. This is being followed by Dr. Smith who is planning chemotherapy, I believe, for the future. The pituitary gland appears to be nonfunctioning. She underwent transphenoidal surgery 3 days ago and is doing well without complaints.

Physical Exam: Vital signs normal. General: Elderly white female in no acute distress. HEENT: Normocephalic and atraumatic. Pupils are equal, round, and reactive to light. Lids and conjunctivae are normal. Throat unremarkable. No blurred vision. Lungs: Clear, but with decreased basilar breath sounds. Cardiac: Regular rate and rhythm without any murmurs. Abdomen: Positive bowel sounds. Soft and nontender, without hepatosplenomegaly. Extremities: Negative; no edema. Neuro: Oriented × 3. Cranial nerves II–XII intact.

Lab Data: WBC 6.9, hemoglobin 12.1, hematocrit 36.2, platelets 314,000

Glucose 116, BUN 9, creatinine 0.7, sodium 134, potassium 3.9, Chloride 85, CO_2 26, calcium 8.2

Assessment and Plan: Pituitary tumor, status post resection. Currently on steroids, 50 mg q. 8 hours. Wean to 20 mg in the morning and 10 mg in the evening starting tomorrow. Recommend follow-up in 2 weeks with Dr. Smith; he will further evaluate that. We will watch urine output and look for any evidence of diabetes insipidus.

Which of the following is the correct code set for this physician?

ICD-9-CM Code(s):

a. 227.3, 162.9, V77.1
b. 194.3, 162.9
c. 239.7, 162.9, 253.5
d. 239.7, 162.9

ICD-10-CM Code(s): _____

Disorders of the Genitourinary System

9.33.   This is the documentation from the record of a patient admitted to the hospital.

Chief Complaint: Gross hematuria, headache, dizziness, feeling lousy.

HPI: Patient is a 39-year-old white male with C5-6 quadriplegia managed with a suprapubic tube for urinary diversion. He was in the hospital about three weeks ago and at that time had a cystoscopic examination, biopsy of polypoid cystitis, bled for a day or two but that seemed to clear up. He awoke this morning, had some mild gross hematuria which progressed throughout the day, started passing clots and then developed headache, feeling lousy. He was seen in the ER and found to have a blood pressure of 168 systolic and bradycardia and was felt to be having autonomic dysreflexia as a manifestation of his bladder distension. His bladder was irrigated; blood pressure promptly fell back into the 98 range. He is admitted at this time for control of his gross hematuria.

Past Medical History: He has had a penile implant for condom catheter drainage. He has also had tracheostomy in the past, chest tubes on the left side, and a suprapubic tube. Current medication includes Ditropan, Vitamin C, and Metamucil.

Allergies: Penicillin caused a rash.

Social History: Does not smoke, drinks occasionally. He is disabled but currently attending school.

Family History: Both parents are living and well.

Review of Systems: Negative except for HPI

Physical Examination:

General:	Shows a cooperative male in no acute distress.
Skin:	Warm and dry.
HEENT:	Pupils are equal, round, reactive to light and accommodation. Pharynx is clean.
Lungs:	Clear
Heart:	Regular without murmur or gallops.
Abdomen:	Soft. There is a suprapubic tube present.
Genitalia:	Penis has a small implant in it. Testes are down bilaterally without induration.
Rectal:	Shows a normal size prostate. No rectal masses are appreciated.
Neurological:	Shows C5-6 quadriplegia, limited use of arms and hands, decreased triceps musculature.
Neck:	Regular

Impression: Gross hematuria secondary to cystitis, probable urinary tract infection, autonomic dysreflexia, C5-6 quadriplegia, and catheter dependence.

Discharge Summary

Admission Diagnoses: Gross hematuria, suprapubic catheter dependent, quadriplegia, autonomic dysreflexia, anemia secondary to hematuria.

Discharge Diagnoses: Same

Transfusion: Two units packed cells

Laboratory values on admission: His admitting HGB was 13.2; later that evening it had fallen to 9.8 and the patient received two units. The next morning his HGB was 11.3 but again the following morning it had fallen to 9.3. His BUN was 18, creatinine 0.6.

Hospital Course: Patient was admitted, started initially on intermittent catheter irrigations. He had persistent problems with clotting and then a Foley catheter was inserted per urethra and the patient was placed on a continuous irrigation with prompt clearing of his urine. He was also treated with oral Amicar. At the time of discharge, even though the patient's HGB was 9.3, the patient declined further transfusion and wished to be discharged.

Which of the following code sets (excluding E&M) would be reported for this hospital admission?

ICD-9-CM and CPT Code(s):

a. 599.71, 280.0, 344.04, 337.3, 596.54, 599.0, 51700, 36430
b. 599.71, 280.0, 344.03, 337.3, 596.54, 599.0, 51700, 36430
c. 599.71, 280.0, 344.04, 337.3, 596.54, 51700, 51702, 36430
d. 599.71, 280.0, 344.04, 337.3, 51700, 51702, 36430

ICD-10-CM Code(s): _____

9.34. A patient has a transrectal ultrasound-guided placement of prostatic radiation palladium seeds with a cystoscopy for localized adenocarcinoma of the prostate.

Procedure Description: The patient was given general anesthesia, placed in the lithotomy position, and prepped and draped in sterile fashion. The bladder was drained, and 100 cc of half contrast and half saline were placed into the bladder. The scrotum was then draped up out of the way. The BUK 7.5 MHz transrectal ultrasound probe was then introduced into the rectum, and the prostate was imaged. The probe was placed into the stabilization bar mechanism. We then centered the prostate image on the template screen and established our base image. Stabilization needles were then put into position. We then passed the needles using a perineal approach at the corresponding positions to the corresponding depth, using ultrasound and fluoroscopy for guidance. After satisfactory placement of all the needles, the ultrasound probe and needles were removed. A total of 60 palladium seeds were put in place. We had good distribution of the seeds and good images on the ultrasound. Using the #22 French cystoscope, a cystoscopy was performed, and the bladder was fully inspected with the 30- and 70-degree lenses without notable findings. The bladder demonstrated no tumors, lesions, or other abnormalities, there were no seeds present, and there was very minimal bleeding. The bladder was drained and the patient was taken to the recovery room in stable condition.

Which of the following code sets would be reported for this service in addition to the HCPCS Level II supply codes for the implants and contrast used? The procedure was performed in the cancer center.

ICD-9-CM and CPT Code(s):

a. 233.4, 55875, 52000, 77763, 76965, 76000-59
b. 185, 55875, 77778, 76965, 76000-59
c. 185, 55875, 77787, 76872, 77790
d. 185, 52000, 77762

ICD-10-CM Code(s): _____

9.35. A female Medicare patient is scheduled for breast biopsy of a palpable lump in the right breast. In the left breast is a much smaller lesion as shown on mammography and identified by a radiological marker. An excisional biopsy is performed on both sides. The specimen on the right is diagnostic for breast malignancy with clear margins, while the small lesion in the left breast is found to be only fibrocystic disease without evidence of malignancy.

Which of the following is reported for the physician services? The procedure is completed at the hospital surgery center.

ICD-9-CM and CPT Code(s):

a. 611.72, 610.1, 19120-50
b. 174.9, 610.1, 19125-50, 19290-50, 19120-50
c. 174.9, 610.1, 19120-RT, 19125-LT-51, 19290-LT-51
d. 174.9, 610.2, 19120, 19125-59, 19290-59

ICD-10-CM Code(s): _____

9.36. The following documentation is from the health record of a 48-year-old female patient.

Surgical Procedure

The patient is here for office hysteroscopy. She has a long history of dysfunctional bleeding. She is known to have multiple fibroids. Recent ultrasound did demonstrate normal appearing ovaries but several large fibroids, the largest of which is 5 cm in diameter.

After informed consent and taking the preop medication, the patient was sterilely prepped. We then injected her with a total of 12 cc of 2% Lidocaine without Epinephrine. We then performed an office hysteroscopy using a uterine sound. The uterus sounded to 8 cm. We then dilated the cervical OS with Pratt dilators. The hysteroscope was placed with good visualization of all portions of the endometrium. We were able to identify both tubal ostium. There was a very large fibroid posterior that does press in on the endometrium and occupies much of it. This is not a pedunculated endometrium and is intramural. There are other fibroids that also affect the cavity size and shape, but again these are intramural fibroids and not accessible through the hysteroscope. D&C was performed without difficulty and the patient tolerated the procedure well. Instrument, needle, and sponge count were correct.

I advised the patient to see how her symptoms proceed in the next few months. Her last FSH level was 30, suggesting a perimenopausal state. She does understand that the fibroids should shrink in size or at least remain the same once she is menopausal. However, if she feels her bleeding problems are persistent, we may have to consider hysterectomy. The patient will follow up in three or four months and will document her bleeding.

Which diagnosis and CPT procedure codes does the surgeon assign?

ICD-9-CM and CPT Code(s):

a. 626.8, 218.1, 58558
b. 626.8, 218.9, 57800, 58558
c. 627.0, 218.9, 58558, 58120
d. 627.0, 218.1, 58558

ICD-10-CM Code(s): _____

9.37. The following documentation is from the health record of a female patient.

Operative Report

Preoperative Diagnosis: Cystocele, urinary stress incontinence

Postoperative Diagnosis: Incomplete cystocele, urinary stress incontinence

Operation: Monarch trans obturator tension free suburethral sling and anterior repair of cystocele

Indication: The patient is an 80-year-old G4, P4, status post hysterectomy done for benign reasons, now with a cystocele and urinary stress incontinence. I presented her with options and she wished to proceed with the surgical correction.

Description of Procedure: The patient was taken to the operating room suite and anesthesia was administered. The patient was placed into the dorsal lithotomy position and her vagina, perineum, and inner thighs were prepped and draped in the usual fashion for a sling procedure. A Foley catheter was placed into the urinary bladder and then a weighted speculum was placed into the vagina.

A small mid-urethral vaginal incision was then made to a distance of approximately 2.0 cm. Dissection was carried out beneath the vaginal mucosa up toward the inferior edge of the pubic bone. The notch along the internal edge of the ischiopubic ramus was palpated on the patient's left side and then a small stab wound incision was made. This was repeated in the same fashion on the patient's right. The Monarch helicopasser was now placed into the incision on the patient's left and then a guiding finger placed through the vaginal incision until the tip of the Monarch passer was palpated. The Monarch passer was now guided around the ischiopubic ramus and through the vagina incision keeping direct contact with the surgeon's finger. The Monarch sling was attached to the passer and the passer rotated out and through, bringing the Monarch sling through the incision. Using the opposite Monarch passer on the patient's right side, this was repeated in a similar fashion, again guiding the passer with the surgeon's finger in direct contact throughout. The other end of the Monarch sling was then attached and the Monarch helicopasser brought back out through the obturator foramen. Now with the two ends of the sling still attached to the Monarch passers on each side, the sling was positioned using the alignment marks on the sling. It was placed and then the helicopassers cut from the sling. Now the plastic sheaths were withdrawn and the sling placed without tension. The mesh was then cut at subcutaneous level adjacent to the lateral skin incisions.

Once that was done, attention was turned to the cystocele. A longitudinal injection with 1% Lidocaine was made. Vaginal mucosa was dissected away from the cystocele. Anterior repair was performed by placing purse string sutures of 2-0 Vicryl to correct for the cystocele, and the excess vaginal tissue was trimmed away. The vaginal mucosa was repaired with a locking stitch of 0-Vicryl. The lateral skin incisions were reapproximated using DermaBone tissue adhesive. The patient was returned to the supine position. She was then awakened and transferred to the recovery room in stable condition.

Which of the following code sets is reported for the surgeon for this hospital-based ambulatory surgical service?

ICD-9-CM and CPT Code(s):

a. 618.2, 57288
b. 618.2, 625.6, 57240, 53440
c. 618.2, 625.6, 57240, 57288
d. 625.6, 57288

ICD-10-CM Code(s): _____

9.38.   The following documentation is from the health record of a male patient.

Operative Report

A patient with an elevated prostate-specific antigen (PSA) of 35.7 comes to the surgery center for a transrectal, ultrasonic-guided (TRUS) prostate biopsy.

Technique: The patient is placed in the Sims position with the left side down. The anus was generously lubricated with 2 percent Xylocaine jelly. The ultrasound probe was then introduced and scanning initiated. A great deal of calcification was noted in the outer margin of the central zone. The area proximal and anterior to the calcifications was hypoechoic but may have been influenced by the stones. There was very thin peripheral zone tissue available. Three needle biopsies were taken from each side, starting in the periphery and working toward the midline and trying to biopsy anterior to the stones on the more medial biopsies from each side.

The pathology report confirmed carcinoma in situ of the prostate.

Which codes will be reported for this service? The facility bills for the technical and professional components and also reports procedure codes for radiologic procedures for reimbursement. Do not include surgical supplies in this example.

ICD-9-CM and CPT Code(s):

a. 185, 55700
b. 233.4, 790.93, 55705, 76872
c. 185, 790.93, 602.0, 55700, 76872, 76942
d. 233.4, 602.0, 55700, 76872, 76942

ICD-10-CM Code(s): _____

Infectious Diseases/Disorders of the Skin and Subcutaneous Tissue

9.39.   A 53-year-old male is seen in the office for a skin problem on the left shin. It started two days ago as mild redness and has developed into an area of severe itching, is swollen with dark red blotches, and has an area of open weeping. The patient has Type II diabetes mellitus, diabetic peripheral vascular disease, and a previous MRSA infection. A detailed history and a comprehensive examination are documented.

The physician diagnoses cellulitis of the left leg and obtains cultures from the open area. To speed the start of treatment, the physician administers one dose of 300 mg Clindamycin IV push at the office before sending the patient to the observation unit at the hospital for continued doses of antibiotic every 6 hours for the next 48 hours. The patient's primary insurance is Blue Cross.

Which of the following code sets is appropriate for physician reporting of these services? Do not code laboratory services.

ICD-9-CM and CPT Code(s):

a. 686.9, V12.04, 250.00, 443.81, 99214, 96372
b. 682.6, V02.54, 250.70, 443.81, 99214, 96374, S0077
c. 682.6, V12.04, 250.70, 443.81, 99215, 96374, S0077
d. 891.1, V02.54, 250.70, 443.81, 99215, 96372, J3490

ICD-10-CM Code(s): _____

9.40. The following documentation is from the health record of a 73-year-old male patient.

Physician Office Record

This 73-year-old male slipped and fell while carrying a pane of glass. He was changing an outside window at his single-family home. He sustained three lacerations—one on his left ankle, one on his right ankle, and one on his left hand.

Left ankle: 3.5-cm laceration, involving deep subcutaneous tissue and fascia, was repaired with layered closure using 1 percent lidocaine local anesthetic.

Right ankle: 4.2-cm laceration was repaired under local anesthetic with a single-layer closure.

Left hand: 2.5-cm laceration of the dermis was repaired with simple closure using DERMABOND tissue adhesive.

Assessment: Wounds of both ankles and left hand requiring repair.

Plan: Follow-up in 10 days for suture removal. Call office if there are any problems or complications.

What are the correct diagnosis and CPT procedure codes?

ICD-9-CM and CPT Code(s):

a. 891.0, 882.0, E920.8, E849.0, E013.9, 12004
b. 891.1, 882.0, 12002, 12032-51
c. 894.0, 12032, 12002, supply code for the DERMABOND adhesive
d. 891.0, 882.0, E920.8, E849.0, E000.8, E013.9, 12032, 12002-51, G0168

ICD-10-CM Code(s): _____

9.41. An operative report provides the following information.

Preoperative Diagnosis:	Ductal carcinoma in situ of the right breast
Postoperative Diagnosis:	Ductal carcinoma in situ of the right breast
Procedure:	Right needle-localized lumpectomy

Indications: The patient is a 68-year-old woman who was noted to have abnormal calcifications at roughly the 6 o'clock position of the areola. These were biopsied and found to be ductal carcinoma in situ. She was inclined to proceed with needle-localized lumpectomy. The risks of bleeding, infection, poor wound healing, and unappealing cosmetics were discussed. The possibility we could find invasive carcinoma was also discussed. The need for postoperative radiation therapy was also discussed. She was well aware of the possibility of positive margins which would lead to further surgery or a mastectomy.

Procedure Description: The patient was initially taken to the Center for Breast Diagnostics where the radiologist placed a needle at the inferior aspect of the breast. The patient was then taken to the Operating Room. General anesthesia was administered. SCDs were placed. A curvilinear incision was made on the inferior aspect of the areola. This was taken down to the subcutaneous tissue. Flaps were raised in each direction for approximately 2 cm and taken down to the chest wall. A long stitch was placed medially, a short stitch superiorly.

The specimen was removed. The cavity was then thoroughly irrigated. 0.25% Marcaine was used for local anesthesia. The subcutaneous tissue was then approximated using 3-0 Monocryl. The skin was approximated using 4-0 Monocryl in a running subcuticular fashion. A sterile dressing was applied. The patient tolerated the procedure well and was taken to the Recovery Room.

What is the correct code set for the services of the surgeon?

ICD-9-CM and CPT Code(s):

a. 174.0, 19290, 19301
b. 174.9, 19290, 19125
c. 233.0, 19125
d. 233.0, 19301

ICD-10-CM Code(s): _____

9.42. The following documentation is from the health record of a patient who received outpatient surgical services.

Operative Report

Preoperative Diagnosis:	Full-thickness burn wound to anterior left lower leg
Postoperative Diagnosis:	Same
Operation:	Split-thickness skin graft, approximately 35 cm; preparation of the wound
Anesthesia:	General

Procedure: The left lower leg was prepped and draped in the usual sterile fashion. The ulcer, which measured approximately 8 × 4 to 4.5 cm, was debrided sharply with Goulian knife until healthy bleeding was seen. The bleeding was controlled with epinephrine-soaked lap pads. Split-thickness skin graft was harvested from the left lateral buttock area approximately 4.5 to 5 cm × 8 cm at the depth of 14/1000 of an inch. The graft was meshed to 1 to 1.5 and placed over the prepared wound. This was stabilized with staples, and then Xeroform dressings and dry dressings, wrapped with gauze and finally immobilized in a posterior splint. The donor site was covered with Xeroform and dry dressings.

What is/are the correct procedure code(s) reported by the physician for this procedure performed in the hospital outpatient surgical suite?

a. 15220, 15221-51, 15002-51
b. 15100
c. 14021, 15002-51
d. 15100, 15002-51

9.43. The following documentation is from the health record of a patient who received outpatient surgical services.

Operative Report

Preoperative Diagnosis: Basal cell carcinoma of the forehead

Postoperative Diagnosis: Same

Procedure: Excision of basal cell carcinoma with split-thickness skin graft

The patient was given a local IV sedation and taken to the operating room suite. The face and left thigh were prepped with pHisoHex soap. The cancer was outlined for excision. The cancer measured approximately 2.5 cm in diameter. The forehead was infiltrated with 1 percent Xylocaine with 1:1,000,000 epinephrine.

The cancer was excised and carried down to the frontalis muscle. The area of the excision measured 5 × 4 cm in total. A suture was placed at the 12 o'clock position. The specimen was sent to pathology for frozen section.

Attention was then turned to the skin graft. A pattern of the defect was transferred to the left anterior thigh using a new needle. A local infiltration was performed on the thigh. Using a free-hand knife, a split-thickness skin graft was harvested. The thigh was treated with Tegaderm and a wraparound Kerlix and ACE wrap. The skin graft was applied and sutured to the forehead defect with running 5-0 plain catgut.

Xeroform with cotton soaked in glycerin was sutured with 4-0 silk. A sterile dressing was applied. The patient tolerated the procedure well with no complications or blood loss.

What are the correct codes reported by the physician for this procedure performed in the hospital outpatient surgical suite?

ICD-9-CM and CPT Code(s):

a. 195.0, 15120
b. 173.31, 15120, 11646
c. 173.31, 15100, 11646
d. 195.0, 15004, 15120

ICD-10-CM Code(s): _____

9.44. The physician sees an established patient in the office. She is a 2-year-old girl with a two-day history of fever to 100.5 degrees, fuzziness, fatigue, and headache. She also has been complaining for five days of pain in the left buttock with an area that is swollen and red as of today, with no known injury. She is a known asthmatic. A detailed history is obtained. Physical exam reveals a 4 cm × 4 cm abscess over the left upper buttock that is fluctuant and red, as the only finding on a comprehensive exam. Laboratory done in the office today reveals: Elevated WBC on the automated complete CBC with differential and an abnormal automated urinalysis with microscopy. A moderate level of medical decision making is used.

After obtaining consent, the physician and the staff observer prepare the patient for conscious sedation in the procedure room. The physician injects 5 cc of 2% Lidocaine as anesthetic and incises the abscess with a #11 blade straight scalpel. 10 cc of pus is drained and the area is packed with Iodoform gauze. Culture and sensitivity of the drainage is sent to an outside laboratory for evaluation. Total intra-service time was 30 minutes. The patient was given Ceftin 300 mg b.i.d. for 10 days to treat both the UTI and the abscess and will return to clinic in two days for a wound check.

What are the correct diagnosis and CPT procedure codes for the services provided?

a. 599.0, 682.5, 780.60, 493.90, 99214-25, 99143, 10061, 99000
b. 599.0, 682.5, 780.61, 99215, 99143, 10061, 36415, 85025, 85009, 81001
c. 599.0, 682.2, 99214, 99144, 10060, 99000, 36415, 85025, 81003
d. 599.0, 682.5, 493.90, 99214-25, 99143, 10060, 99000, 36415, 85025, 81001

ICD-10-CM Code(s): _____

9.45. Office Progress Note

Chief Complaint: The patient presents today for removal of a scalp cyst.

HPI: This patient has had a cyst present in the scalp for the last several months. She has been monitoring it as instructed but feels that it has grown significantly in the months since her last appointment.

Physical Exam: The original lesion was approximately 1.5 cm but today seems to have grown to approximately 2.0 cm. The cyst rests in the frontal lobe close to the hairline—patient is beginning to feel very awkward in public.

Procedure: After obtaining informed consent from the patient, I injected the periphery of the cyst will 2% buffered lidocaine. The hair around the scalp was carefully shaved leaving a clear field. A linear incision was made through the scalp and the cyst was removed followed by lavage to the wound. The contents of the cyst appeared to be clear with no pus or infection. 2-0 nylon was used to approximate the edges and to maintain hemostasis. The area was treated with an antibiotic ointment and a bandage was carefully placed on the wound site.

Patient is instructed to not shower or wash her hair for 2 days and to put ice on the wound 20 minutes at a time throughout the next 24 hours. She will be seen in 1 week for removal of sutures.

Assign the correct codes for this office visit:

ICD-9-CM and CPT Code(s): _____

ICD-10-CM Code(s): _____

9.46.   This is the documentation from the record of a patient presenting with a mass in the right breast.

Chief Complaint: Mass in the right breast

Past Medical History: No serious illnesses. She has had a tubal ligation. She has had an appendectomy. She has had an exploratory laparotomy.

Systemic Review: She does have headaches. She has had abdominal pain and has to get up at night to urinate. Her menses are usually every 28 days and last 7 days. She has four children who are living and well. She has had three miscarriages.

Family History: There is cancer, epilepsy, diabetes, and heart attacks in the family.

Social History: She does not smoke and takes a rare social drink. She is a housewife, married and lives with her family.

History of Present Illness: This 31-year-old white female is admitted with the chief complaint of a nodule in her right breast and a lump in her left axilla. She has had this lump for several months but it is getting larger, was tender for a while, but is no longer tender. She had a mammogram which suggests a benign process in the right breast but there are concerns about the lesion in the axilla.

Physical Examination:

Blood Pressure 108/78; Pulse 68; Respirations 16

HEENT:	Head and neck are normal. Eyes—pupils are round, regular and equal. Reactive to light and accommodation. EOM are normal. Sclera—white. Conjunctiva—pink. Oral cavity is within normal limits. Tympanic membranes are clear bilaterally.
Neck:	No venous distention; no palpable thyroid.
Chest:	Clear to A&P. Breath sounds are normal and no rales are heard.
Cardiac:	The apex beat is in the fifth interspace, midclavicular line. Normal sinus rhythm is present and no murmurs are heard.
Abdomen:	Soft. No masses, tenderness, or palpable organs. Peristalsis is present and normal.
Breasts:	There is a nodule about 1.5 to 2 cm at the lower border of the areola in the right breast. There is a fairly large lymph node in the left axilla.
Extremities:	No edema. No deformity.
Pelvic:	Not done as she had one last week with a PAP and these were all ok.
Diagnosis:	Lesion of the right breast; nodule in the left axilla.

Laboratory: The urine was negative; HGB was 13.8; HCT 39.8; WBC was 4,900 and 46 polys.

Operative Record

Preoperative Diagnosis:	Nodule of the right breast; lymphadenitis left axilla.
Postoperative Diagnosis:	Same
Operation Performed:	Excision of nodule of the right breast and excision of 3 or 4 lymph nodes in the left axilla.

Findings: The patient was found to have at least 1 large lymph node and 2 or 3 small lymph nodes deep in the left axilla and these were all excised. She had a nodule, sort of like an oval nodule, at the areolar skin junction of the right breast. This was about 2 cm × 1 cm.

Operative Note

Under satisfactory general anesthesia, the patient is in the supine position and both breasts and left axilla were prepared with Hibiclens and draped with sterile drapes. A semi-lunar incision was made at the skin, areolar junction of the right breast. Subcutaneous tissue was divided, bleeding points were picked up with hemostats and ligated with 4-0 sutures. The nodule was excised by sharp dissection and bleeding points were again ligated with 4-0 Vicryl. The breast tissue was closed with interrupted 2-0 Vicryl sutures in a figure-of-eight manner. The skin and subcutaneous tissue were closed with continuous 4-0 sutures. The wound was cleansed with Hibiclens and a sterile Opsite dressing and sterile pressure dressings were applied. Incision was made at just about the apex of the axilla on the left side and the subcutaneous tissues were divided; bleeding points were picked up with hemostats and ligated with 4-0 sutures. Superficial lymph nodes were picked up with Allis forceps and dissected free and after we got these all dissected and free and the bleeding controlled we found another larger lymph node, much deeper, and this we excised by sharp dissection and bleeding points carefully ligated. Following this the deep tissues were closed with interrupted 2-0 Vicryl sutures. Subcutaneous tissues were closed with continuous 4-0 sutures. Sterile dressings were applied. The patient withstood the procedures well and returned to PACU in good condition.

Pathological Findings: Sections labeled as specimen "A" consist of portions of fibrofatty breast tissue containing duct ectasia, small cyst formation, and aprocrine metaplasia. Sections labeled as "B" reveal the large ovoid structure and the small fragment of homogenous gray-tan tissue to consist of lymph nodes. The large lymph node shows some evidence of follicular hyperplasia with abundant mitotic and phagocytic activity. Lymphocytes are also noted in the surrounding fibrous capsule. The small lymph nodes contain general lymphoid-like tissue.

Pathological Diagnoses: 1. RT Breast Nodule: Mild fibrocystic disease

2. LT Axillary Nodule: Lymph nodes containing hyperplasia. The large lymph node has signs of toxoplasmosis but this can not be determined without further testing.

What codes are reported for this physician service?

ICD-9-CM and CPT Code(s):

a. 610.1, 289.3, 19120-RT, 38525-LT, 38500-LT
b. 610.2, 130.9, 19120-RT, 38525-LT, 38500-LT
c. 610.2, 289.3, 19100-RT, 38525-LT
d. 610.1, 289.3, 19101-RT, 38525-LT, 38500-LT

ICD-10-CM Code(s): _____

Behavioral Health Conditions

9.47. A patient was brought to the emergency department by her mother after she was found to be groggy after an intentional overdose of a "handful" of aspirin approximately one-half hour before. The mother thought the bottle was almost empty. The patient was beginning to experience dizziness and loud ringing of the ears. The physician inserted a gastric tube and lavage was performed. The patient was stabilized in the ED, during which time bleeding studies and urinalysis were completed. A detailed history and physical examination were performed, and medical decision making was of moderate complexity. The diagnosis was suicide attempt with unknown quantity of aspirin, dizziness, and tinnitus. A psychiatric consult was arranged, and the patient was transferred to the psychiatric hospital by ambulance.

What are the correct diagnosis and CPT codes for this visit?

ICD-9-CM and CPT Code(s):

a. 965.1, 780.4, 388.30, E950.0, 99284-25, 43753
b. 965.1, 780.4, E980.0, 99284
c. 780.4, 388.30, E935.3, 99284-25, 43752
d. 780.4, 388.30, 965.1, E935.3, 99284, 43752

ICD-10-CM Code(s): _____

9.48. A 20-year-old patient was brought into the emergency department in nearly comatose condition following an evening of drinking beer and vodka with friends. Vital signs were depressed. A blood-alcohol level was measured, which was reported as 0.38. The patient had vomited several times before passing out. There was a 1-cm laceration on the patient's eyebrow. This was treated with a Steri-Strip. The patient was stabilized in the ED for one and a half hours and admitted to intensive care by the Internal Medicine physician on call. Documentation in the ED record supports a level 5 ED visit. Diagnosis was alcohol poisoning, acute alcohol intoxication, and 1-cm laceration, right eyebrow.

What is the correct ICD-9-CM and CPT code assignment?

a. 303.00, 980.9, 99291, 99292
b. 980.9, 305.00, 99285-25, 12011
c. 980.0, 305.00, 873.42, E860.0, 99285
d. 980.0, 303.00, 99291, 12011

ICD-10-CM Code(s): _____

9.49. The following psychiatric biopsychological assessment documentation is from the health record of a 22-year-old female patient.

Date of Admission: 02/10/XX

Date of Evaluation: 02/12/XX

Amount of Time of Evaluation: The patient participated in a direct interview for 40 minutes.

Sources of Information: The patient participated in a 40-minute direct interview. Patient's commitment documents from ABC facility were also reviewed. Patient's records from Dr. S. were also reviewed.

Chief Complaint: "I came here because someone was hurting me, and they thought that I wasn't eating enough and that I was throwing up too much."

History of Present Illness: The patient is a 22-year-old female with a past history of anorexia nervosa and attention deficit disorder. She was committed after a six-week stay at ABC. Her parents brought her to this facility after her mother noticed that she was fasting and vomiting and was not sleeping. Her mother also noted that she was more weak than usual and was only able to work her job for one or two hours rather than a full day. It was also noticed that she was losing track of time, appearing confused, fearful, and angry. Patient notes that, prior to admission, she was actually sleeping fairly normally for her, about five hours of sleep per night, though she does agree that she was eating rather little and vomiting because of some abuse that was troubling her. On admission, she was noted to be withdrawn and refused to talk to staff and was very tearful. Later that day, however, she did not remember this incident of being tearful. On admission she was noted to be 84 pounds at a height of 5 feet. She at that time admitted to vomiting as much as three times a day and that she had to have her teeth resurfaced due to purging. At ABC facility, staff noted she was hoarding condiments in her room and was also noted to purge in front of staff during her stay there. The patient, however, does not think that her purging was due to an eating disorder; rather, she thinks that it was due to stress and anxiety over a previous abuse. Previous records reveal potassium levels as low as 2.0. She states that the low potassium is due to a kidney disorder; however, a nephrologist thought that the low potassium was most likely due to her purging behavior. Her weight at discharge from ABC was 85.5 pounds. Patient notes that her sleep has not been disrupted prior to her hospital stay. She states that she usually gets about five hours of sleep per night, which is normal for her. She notes that her appetite has been decreased for the past several months because of stress regarding prior abuse. She denies any thought racing or excessive energy for the past several months. She also denies any suicidal thoughts or behaviors. She also denies any obsessive-compulsive actions. She denies feeling hopeless or depressed.

Chemical Dependency History: Patient denies any current or previous use of alcohol or drugs.

Current Prescribed Medications: Claritin 10 mg p.o. q. d.; potassium chloride 20 mEq t.i.d. to q. i.d. p.r.n. hypokalemia; Dexedrine SR 40 mg t.i.d.

Past Psychiatric History: Patient has a history of problems with eating disorders that goes back to the age of 14. Over the past eight years she has been involved in a variety of treatment programs. She was first treated in an inpatient setting at the age of 14. She was subsequently hospitalized at the age of 15, age 16 × 2, and age 17. From the age of 17 to 18 she was placed in foster care. She has attempted suicide three times in her life. Each time the attempt was made by trying to overdose on her asthma medication, theophylline. She has been hospitalized five times for hypokalemia. She notes that she currently sees a psychiatrist and a psychologist as an outpatient. In the past, she has exhibited some features of self-injurious behavior. She burned a cross into her arm at age 13. She also has a past history of scratching her arm.

Family Psychiatric History: She notes that her younger sister attempted to overdose one time in the past and that her father has been treated for depression with ECT, which was successful.

Mental Status Examination: The patient is a petite, too-thin young female who appears younger than her stated age of 22. She is clean, well groomed, and dressed in jeans and a large hooded sweatshirt. Her general behavior is noted to be normal and appropriate throughout the interview. She is cooperative throughout our question-and-answer session. Her mood is somewhat subdued, and she seems slightly anxious. Her affect is rather flat throughout the interview. No abnormal movements are noted during the interview. Her speech is fairly soft and rather monotone in nature. Speech is noted to be of normal speed. Stream of mental activity is normal and appropriate. The form of thought processes appears to be normal without any tangential thinking. Thought content appears to be normal as well. She denies delusions, hallucinations, and suicidal or homicidal ideation at present. She does not seem to be impulsive in her speech or thought processes throughout the interview. She does seem to have some insight into her illness in that she is able to name her illness as anorexia. She states that her weight now is OK. Her judgment, concentration, and orientation all appear to be within normal limits. Recent and remote memory appears intact. Her general fund of knowledge is above average. Her calculations, abstractions, proverbs, and similarities are all within normal limits. Estimated IQ would be 120 based on educational background and verbal skills. The patient does not appear to be dangerous or suicidal at present.

Biopsychosocial Discussion and Discussion of Differential Diagnosis: The patient is a 22-year-old female with a past history of anorexia and subsequent hypokalemia. She notes that recent exacerbation in her anorexia and vomiting seems to be due to stress over abuse in the past by a physician with whom she had previous professional contact and subsequently became friends. She has limited insight into her eating disorder in that she is able to name it as anorexia now. In the past, however, she has denied the existence of an eating disorder. In the past, she has had suicidal attempts. However, at this time she does not appear to be depressed and does not indicate any suicidal thoughts or plans. At this time, she does not indicate feeling particularly anxious but, rather, regards her main symptom as stress. She states that her only fear right now is that of being in the hospital for her first commitment. She appears to have a long history of hospitalizations for her eating disorder and subsequent hypokalemia. Her family history does appear to have a history of mental illness, with depression in her father and a suicide attempt by her younger sister. She also was noted to have burned a cross into her arm as a young child, as well as a history of scratching her arm. There is a possibility that she has a personality disorder with borderline features. Though she does not seem to be in danger of suicide right now or hurting others, it is felt that because of her history of severe hypokalemia and history of anorexia, as well as purging behavior, she will require a long-term inpatient hospitalization for her safety.

Admitting Diagnosis

Axis I:	1. Anorexia nervosa, purging type
	2. Attention deficit hyperactive disorder
Axis II:	Personality disorder with predominant borderline features
Axis III:	1. Asthma
	2. Hypokalemic periodic paralysis (per patient report)
Axis IV:	Severe with stresses incurred due to previous abuse

Axis V: Current GAF—50 to 60

Prognosis: Guarded due to her history of multiple hospitalizations for her eating disorder

Strengths:
1. Patient is very intelligent.
2. Patient is enrolled in school and has had a high level of education.
3. Patient has a therapeutic relationship with her therapist and psychiatrist as an outpatient.
4. Patient's weight is near her target weight already.
5. The patient has some insight into her eating disorder.

Problems:
1. Patient lacks a deep insight into her eating disorder.
2. Patient clings to a diagnosis of hypokalemia periodic paralysis, which she claims is a kidney disorder that she has. Nephrologist cannot corroborate this theory.
3. Patient has a high rate of recidivism in the hospital system for treatment of her eating disorder.

Short-Term Goals:
1. Patient will identify and discuss high-risk situations.
2. She will listen.
3. She will demonstrate four alternative coping skills to purging.
4. She will seek out assistance from staff before acting on urges to purge.
5. Patient will identify triggers.
6. Patient will be able to discuss short- and long-term consequences of her eating disorder.
7. Patient will complete a crisis plan to control purging urges.
8. Patient will maintain personal safety by not engaging in purging.
9. Patient will maintain her current weight or increase that weight to 90 lb.

Long-Term Goals:
1. Patient will reduce the frequency of purging.
2. Patient will complete community passes without reports of purging in preparation for transition to home.
3. Patient will develop the ability to control impulses and demonstrate strategies to deal with dysphoric moods.
4. Patient will maintain her current weight or increase that weight.
5. Patient will maintain normal potassium levels and will not require supplemental potassium treatment.

Biopsychosocial Treatment Plan:
1. Because of her anorexia nervosa and possible personality disorder, she would likely benefit from a referral to dialectical behavior therapy.
2. She would also benefit from a referral to the eating disorders group.

3. We will weigh her three times a week in order to monitor her progress here. We will expect that she maintain her current weight or increase it.

4. She will be allowed initially to go to the cafeteria on her own and choose what she eats, assuming that her weight stays at her current level or increases.

5. She will be started at level B privileges.

Discharge Criteria: 1. She will maintain or increase her weight during her stay here.

2. She will participate in dialectical behavior therapy as well as the eating disorders group.

3. She will reduce the frequency of her purging behaviors while here.

4. She will complete community passes without reports of purging in preparation for transition to home.

Estimated Length of Stay as Per UM Norms: 45 days

Which of the following is the correct code set for reporting this physician's service?

ICD-9-CM and CPT Code(s):

a. 307.1, 314.01, 301.83, 493.90, V17.0, 90791
b. 301.1, 314.01, 301.83, 276.8, 493.90, 359.3, 90791
c. 307.1, 314.01, 301.83, 493.90, V17.0, 99223
d. 301.1, 314.01, 301.83, 276.8, 493.90, 359.3, 99223

ICD-10-CM Code(s): _____

Disorders of the Musculoskeletal System and Connective Tissue

9.50. The following documentation is from the health record of a patient having surgery on facial trauma.

Preoperative Diagnosis: Complicated left facial fracture

Postoperative Diagnosis: Complicated left facial fracture

Operation: 1. Open reduction internal fixation of comminuted left tripod fracture

2. Open reduction internal fixation of left lateral orbital wall telescoped fracture

3. Endoscopic exam of left orbital floor

Findings: A comminuted fracture involving the left tripod and mid face. There were two fractures in the left lateral orbital rim with a central fragment telescoped in the lateral orbital wall. The Zygoma was depressed and rotated. There was a comminuted fracture of the distal zygomatic arch. The orbital floor showed a nondisplaced fracture. There is no evidence of orbital herniation into the antrum. Several mucosal lacerations of the lateral antral wall.

Description of Procedure: After an adequate induction, the oral cavity was examined. The occlusion was deemed class I, thus an oral intubation was performed. The patient's face was prepped with Betadine paint, ophthalmologic. The patient was draped in the usual manner. The original laceration over the left zygoma was opened. There was some serosanguineous fluid expressed. The wound extended to the large zygomal fragment.

A sublabial incision was made from the right piriform aperture to the left zygomaticomaxillary buttress. This incision had previously been injected with 1% Lidocaine with 1:100,000 Epinephrine. The incision was taken to the face of the maxilla and then all soft tissue was elevated off the piriform aperture, the anterior maxilla, zygomaticomaxillary buttress, and zygoma. The left lateral orbital wall was also skeletonized through the previous laceration, which was extended superiorly into the left brow. At this point, a Carol Gerard screw was placed in the left zygoma, and the zygoma was reduced into its native position. The telescoped fragment in the left lateral orbital wall was also reduced. The zygomaticomaxillary buttress fracture was identified and found to be reduced in its native position.

The following plates were placed: On the left lateral orbital rim, a 2 mm orbital rim plate was placed with six 6 mm $\times$ 2 mm diameter screws. On the left zygomaticomaxillary buttress, an L-shaped plate was placed using four 6 mm screws $\times$ 1.5 mm in diameter.

The nasal cavity was examined and a simple reduction was performed. There appeared to be slight medial displacement of the nasal bones. The orbital floor was examined endoscopically. All the antral contents of devitalized mucosa and old blood was debrided. There was no evidence of fat herniation into the antrum, but there appeared to be a few small nondisplaced fractures with gentle palpation of the globe.

All the areas were then copiously irrigated. The left lateral orbital incision was then closed in layers with 4-0 Vicryl and 5-0 plain gut. Sublabial incision was closed with interrupted 3-0 Chromics.

Total blood loss 10–20 cc. No complications. The patient emerged and was sent to recovery in stable condition.

Which CPT code(s) is/are assigned to the surgical services?

a. 21365-LT
b. 21315-LT, 21365-LT
c. 21365-LT, 31292-LT
d. 21315-LT, 21365-LT, 21406-LT, 31237-LT

9.51. The following documentation is from the health record of a patient having orthopedic surgery on the leg.

Operative Report

Preoperative Diagnosis: Left distal femur osteosarcoma

Postoperative Diagnosis: Left distal femur osteosarcoma

Operation:
1. Resection of left distal femur
2. Prosthetic reconstruction of the left knee
3. Osteotomy of the left femur
4. Femoral artery exploration

Anesthesia: General

Estimated Blood Loss: 500 ml. The patient received 4 units of packed RBCs.

Complications: None

Indications for Procedure: The patient is a 23-year-old female who was diagnosed with a left distal femur osteosarcoma on biopsy and has undergone preoperative chemotherapy. Risks, benefits, complications, and alternatives of resection and reconstruction were discussed with her, and consent was obtained.

Description of Procedure: The patient was seen in the preoperative area and a history and physical examination were performed. Consents were reviewed. She was taken to the operating room and given general anesthesia. She received preoperative antibiotics, and a Foley catheter was placed. Both legs were prepped and draped out. An external incision was made on the anteromedial aspect of the left thigh, extending towards the anterior aspect of the proximal tibia, including excision of the previous biopsy tract.

Dissection was carried down to the subcutaneous tissue leaving a cuff of healthy tissue on the biopsy tract, and also a cuff of muscle was left. Dissection was carried subvastus, elevating the muscle but leaving the fat and other loose tissue including fascia on the tumor. Medially the vastus medialis was elevated off the medial septum. Dissection was carried further subvastus as well as laterally. The patella was preserved. Distally the subpatellar tendon fat pad was left with the knee to be resected. Following dissection, an Osteotomy site was located further laterally and proximally at 16 cm from the articular surface of the femoral condyle. This was based on the recent MRI. An osteotomy was performed, parts of the posterior cortex were curetted, and marrow was removed and passed off to the pathologist for evaluation. Both of these were read on frozen sections as being normal and not containing any malignant tissue.

With these findings known, the remaining posterior attachments to the femur were dissected/transected. The femoral artery extending towards the popliteal space was carefully explored and retracted, and any branches of the tumor were either clipped or suture ligated. The tumor was dissected and the resection was carried out under tourniquet at 270 mmHg.

The tourniquet was let down and hemostasis was achieved with Bovie cautery, vascular clips, or suture ligations. The wound was slightly irrigated. The specimen was sent off to the pathologist for evaluation. The tibial surface was reamed and trial implants were placed. The femoral canal was reamed to 15 mm, which gave satisfactory chatter suggestive of a good fit. A 15-mm-diameter, 150-mm-long stem was placed into the femur with various length trials. A regular femoral condyle was chosen along with a regular tibial component. Following adequate leg length, which gave us satisfactory soft tissue tensioning and rotation as well as the ability to close the wound and patella tracking, but also about 1 extra cm length on the left side, the appropriate components were chosen. The tibial plastic component was cemented into place. An uncemented 150-mm-long, 15-mm-diameter stem with the components in place was gently impacted into the femur and was checked under fluoroscopy. It was noted to be satisfactorily placed. After placement of the bushings, the hinge, and the bumper, the components were reduced. The soft tissue tension was adequate and the vessels seemed to be without any undue stress, and adequate pulsation of the femoral artery was present extending down to the popliteal space. With these findings, patella tracking was again checked and noted to be satisfactory. The wound was thoroughly irrigated, 2 drains were placed, and the various layers were reapproximated with either #1 Ethibond, #1, 0, or 2-0 Vicryl sutures, and then the skin was closed with 4-0 Monocryl. Steri-strips were applied, and the dressings were applied as well as the knee immobilizer with a slight flexion of the knee.

Postoperatively, the foot showed adequate blood flow with a palpable dorsalis pedis pulse. The patient was extubated. She will be admitted for postoperative pain control as well as rehabilitation and discharged when stable.

Which of the following is the correct code assignment for the services of the surgeon?

ICD-9-CM and CPT Code(s):

a. 170.7, 27360, 27447, 35741, 27448, 76000
b. 170.7, 27365, 27445, 35721, 27448-59, 76000-26
c. 238.0, 27329, 27445, 27448-59, 76000-26
d. 239.2, 27360, 27447, 27448, 76000

ICD-10-CM Code(s): _____

9.52. The following documentation is from the health record of a 42-year-old male patient.

Physician Office Record Entries

Hospital Copy: History and Physical

Admitting Diagnosis: Herniation of intervertebral disc, L5–S1 right side

Present Medical History: Patient is a 42-year-old Native American male who initially developed problems with his back in July of this year. He was treated with anti-inflammatory agents and started on an exercise program; his condition improved enough to return to work. About 1 month ago, he had recurrence of pain, which has become steadily worse in the past week. He noticed some numbness of his right foot, primarily the toes and right heel. The patient was initially evaluated by his family physician and is now admitted to the orthopedic service for microdiskectomy after MRI revealed herniation and protrusion of the disc encroaching on the nerve root.

Past Medical History: Patient denied any known allergies or drug sensitivities. He has been taking Advil on a p.r.n. basis. Also takes Lotensin 10 mg daily for hypertension and has a history of incomplete bundle branch block, hyperlipidemia (no meds), hiatus hernia with gastroesophageal reflux.

Previous Surgeries: Tonsillectomy as a child and also tendon repair to the right hand in 1989. Does state that he injured his kidney in a motorcycle accident at age 21 years and was hospitalized with viral pneumonia in 1983.

Family History: Father is 62 years with heart disease and hypertension problems. Mother is 64 years and in good health, without significant illness. Three siblings, all in good health.

Social History: Patient is employed full-time at the Harley-Davidson dealership. At the present time, he is divorced and has one child who lives with her mother. He does not smoke, is sexually active, and admits to sporadic alcohol use.

Review of Systems

HEENT: Patient denies any unusual problems with headaches and dizziness, or visual or hearing difficulty. Cardiorespiratory: Denies chest pain; does have occasional asthma symptoms with some wheezing but does not use medications. Hypertension for 2 years, well controlled on medication. Gastrointestinal: Denies distention, diarrhea, and constipation. Genitourinary: Negative. Musculoskeletal: See present complaint.

Physical Examination: Reveals a well-developed, well-nourished male in no acute distress. Does have a hard time sitting due to pain on the right side. Height 6910, weight 210 lb, blood pressure 122/90, pulse 72, respiration 20. Skin is clear, normal temperature and texture. HEENT: Head normal cephalic. Pupils are round, equal, and reactive to light accommodation. Canals are clear. Tympanic membranes, nose, and throat are clear of infection. Neck: Supple, thyroid negative. No adenopathy, no distomegaly or carotid bruits. Chest: Symmetrical, lungs clear to P & A. Heart: Normal sinus rhythm, no thrills or murmurs. Abdomen: Soft, no tenderness or masses. No organomegaly. Normal male genitalia. Extremities: Normal development. Patient does have tenderness in the area of the right sciatic knot and in the lower lumbar area on the right side. Has positive leg raising and some decrease in the deep tendon reflexes on the side.

Impression: Herniation of intervertebral disc at L5–S1 right side

Plan: Microdiskectomy tomorrow morning

Operative Report

Preoperative Diagnosis: Herniated nucleus pulposus, right

Postoperative Diagnosis: Same

Operation: Right L5–S1 diskectomy with minifacetectomy foraminotomy

Complications: None

Indications: The patient is an otherwise healthy 42-year-old Native American male who has had 6 months of disabling right leg pain. He has tried extensive physical therapy, nonsteroidal -anti-inflammatory drugs, and an epidural injection, without relief. He has a positive straight -leg-raising test on the right side and an absent ankle jerk. MRI scan confirms the disk herniation at L5–S1 on the right side.

Description of Procedure: The patient was brought to the operating room, and general anesthesia was administered in the usual fashion. He was positioned in the prone position onto a -well-padded Andrews frame. All pressure points were well padded. The back was prepped and draped in a sterile fashion. He received 1 g of Ancef prior to the beginning of the case, along with 30 mg of IV Toradol.

Initially, an x-ray was checked that showed we were at the L4–5 interspace, so we went down one level. A 3/4 skin incision was made in the midline of the lumbar sacral spine, and this was carried down to the subcutaneous tissue. The fascia over the L5–S1 lamina was then dissected away. The paraspinal muscles were then elevated above the lamina, and a laminotomy was performed in between L5 and S1. The superior facet of S1 was undercut using a Kerrison rongeur. The S1 nerve root was well visualized and this area was protected throughout the procedure. Following this, a foraminotomy was performed over the top of the S1 nerve root. The S1 nerve root was then gently retracted medially, and a very large extrusive disk fragment was pulled out from underneath the S1 nerve root. The annulotomy that had been made from the disc herniation was then explored, and no further fragments could be found. The wound was thoroughly irrigated with a bacitracin solution. Gelfoam and thrombin were placed over the top of the dura, and the deep fascia was closed with interrupted 0 VICRYL sutures. The subcutaneous tissue was closed with 2-0 VICRYL suture, and the skin was closed with 4-0 VICRYL suture. Benzoin and Steri-Strips were applied to the wound. The patient was returned to recovery in stable condition. EBL 10 cc.

Pathologic Diagnosis: Intervertebral disc L5–S1 resection, herniated nucleus pulposus

Which of the following is the correct code assignment for physician service? Code for surgical services only.

ICD-9-CM and CPT Code(s):

a. 722.52, 401.9, 63047
b. 722.73, 401.9, 63030
c. 722.10, 63047
d. 722.10, 401.9, 63030

ICD-10-CM Code(s): ────────────────────────

9.53.   The following documentation is from the health record of a male patient.

Operative Report

Preoperative Diagnosis: 1. ACL deficient, right knee
2. Medial and lateral meniscal tear, right knee

Operation: 1. Examination under anesthesia, right knee
2. Arthroscopic-assisted anterior cruciate ligament reconstruction, right knee
3. Partial medial and partial lateral meniscectomy

Anesthesia: General

Complications: None

The patient was identified and taken to the operating room and general anesthesia administered. The patient's lower extremity was examined under anesthesia. The patient had evidence of +2 Lachman and +2 pivot shift. After examination under anesthesia, the right lower extremity was prepped and draped in the usual sterile fashion. Routine arthroscopic portals were placed. Examination of the patellofemoral joint was fairly unremarkable. Coming down the medial gutter and the medial compartment, there was a complex tear of the posterior horn of the medial meniscus. Using a combination of basket and 4.2 shaver, partial medial meniscectomy was carried out. This resected about 50 percent of the posterior horn of the medial meniscus. There was a horizontal cleavage component remaining that was stable to probing; it was left alone. Intercondylar notch revealed a complete tear of the anterior cruciate ligament. Going to the lateral compartment, there was a flap tear of the posterior horn of the lateral meniscus, and, again utilizing the lateral meniscus, partial lateral meniscectomy was carried out. This resected about 30 percent of the posterior horn. At this point, the scope was removed from the knee. We did make a longitudinal incision based upon the tibial tubercle medially. This was carried down through the skin and down the subcutaneous tissue. We readily identified the hamstring tendon and harvested the gracilis and semitendinosus. These were taken to the back table and a #2 ETHIBOND leader was placed on the leading edge, and the graft was doubled over for quadruple graft. The scope was placed back into the knee. Notchplasty was performed. Subsequently, we made a tibial tunnel utilizing the Arthrex tibial guide referenced off the posterior cruciate ligament. We then made a femoral tunnel, again utilizing the Arthrex femoral guide referenced off the posterior cortex. Both of these were 8-mm tunnels. We subsequently placed the graft on the knee, and we fixed it on the femoral side with 8 × 23 Arthrex bioabsorbable screw. Visualization of the graft revealed no evidence of impingement, no roughing on the medial aspect of the lateral wall. We subsequently held the knee in just short of full extension with appropriate amount of tension and fixed it on the tibial side with an 8 × 28 Arthrex bioabsorbable screw. Examination after placement of the graft revealed a negative Lachman and negative pivot shift. Multiple intraoperative photos were obtained. At the end of the procedure, subcutaneous tissue was closed with 2-0 VICRYL, the skin with running 2-0 nylon, and portals with 3-0 nylon. Sterile dressing was placed followed by ACE wrap and total thigh and knee immobilizer. The patient tolerated the procedure well, and there were no complications.

Assign the correct codes for this case.

ICD-9-CM Primary (First-Listed) Diagnosis: ————————————————

ICD-9-CM Additional Diagnoses: ————————————————

CPT Procedure Code(s): ————————————————

ICD-10-CM Code(s): ————————————————

9.54. The following documentation is from the health record of a patient admitted for a right total hip.

Preoperative Diagnosis:	Right hip osteonecrosis, Ficat stage IV
Postoperative Diagnosis:	Right hip osteonecrosis, Ficat stage IV
Procedure Performed:	Right total hip arthroplasty
Blood Loss:	350 cc
Complications:	None

Implants Used:

1. DePuy Articul/EZE femoral head 28 mm + 1.5, lot #1169939
2. DePuy large AML femoral component, 150 mm long, 45-mm offset, lot #YDZCV1000
3. DePuy hole eliminator, lot #YH9DH1000
4. DePuy pinnacle acetabular liner 28 mm, lot #X69AR1000
5. DePuy cancellous bone screw 25 mm long, lot #X2BEN1000
6. DePuy acetabular cup 36 mm, lot #X60CK1000

Indications for Operation: The patient is a 54-year-old man who is presented with long-standing right hip pain secondary to osteonecrosis. Nonsurgical treatment was unsuccessful. After risks, benefits, and alternatives of the surgery were explained to the patient, informed consent was obtained for this procedure.

Details of Procedure: Patient was taken back to the operating room and placed on the operating table in a supine position. After induction of general anesthesia, the patient was placed in the left lateral decubitus position and the left lower extremity was prepped and draped in usual sterile manner. Lateral incision was made over the greater trochanter. This incision was approximately 15 cm long. It was carried down through subcutaneous tissue to the iliotibial band, which was incised longitudinally. The gluteus medius was identified and split in line with its fibers down to the level of the greater trochanter. The gluteus medius was then split. This ran along with greater trochanter and was lifted anteriorly off the greater trochanter in line with vastus lateralis as well. These structures were dissected off of the greater trochanter. The gluteus minimus was exposed and its tendon was transected longitudinally as well. Capsule was delineated just lying underneath the gluteus adducted and placed in a sterile bag as it was dislocated. The neck was cut with an oscillating saw. Retractors were placed inferiorly, posteriorly along the acetabulum, as well as superiorly. The acetabulum was then debrided off the remaining capsular and labral tissue as well as ligamentaries. The acetabulum was then reamed starting with a 49-mm reamer and reamed sequentially in 1-mm increments to 55; 56 was trailed and it was deemed to be appropriate. Version was checked at each sequential reaming. The 56-mm acetabular component was then inserted and hammered into place. Trial liner was placed. The limb was then placed in the bag and the medial aspect of the greater trochanter was cut with the use of a box cutter. The femoral canal was then reamed sequentially and increments to a 13.5. The lateral side cutter was then used to cut out the cancellous bone from the calcar. A small broach was replaced with 13.5 large broach. The head component was placed and was trailed. The hip was deemed to be too tight. Intraoperative x-ray was obtained and demonstrated the femoral neck cut to be insufficient. The hip was dislocated. The trial head and neck were removed and the femur was then reamed further distally. The calcar planar was used to take down the femoral neck cut. The broach was placed prior to calcar planning often reaming the femoral canal sufficiently, the 13.5 large broach did in fact sink further end of the canal and after the hip was reduced it was deemed to be both stable and not in too much tension. The hip was then dislocated. The broach was removed as well as the trial liner. The true liner was then placed as well as the femoral stem component. Femoral head was placed and the hip was located. Tension was deemed to be adequate. The hip was tested and position of instability was deemed to be stable. The wound was copiously irrigated to sterile saline. The minimus was repaired with interrupted #0 VICRYL sutures. The medius was reapproximated with running #0 VICRYL sutures as well as drill holes placed into greater troch and #5 Tycron sutures. The IT band was repaired with interrupted #0 VICRYL sutures and subcutaneous tissue was repaired with interrupted #2-0 VICRYL sutures. The skin was closed with staples. Sterile dressings were applied. The patient was extubated and recovered in a holding area uneventfully.

Code the orthopedic surgeon's code sets.

ICD-9-CM and CPT Code(s): _____

ICD-10-CM Code(s): _____

Neoplasms

9.55.   The patient is a four-year-old male with acute lymphocytic leukemia who has had a fever for the last 24 hours. It has been nine days since his last chemotherapy, which was his first. A comprehensive history is documented. On examination, the skin over his Hickman site is extremely red and starting to break down. No other abnormal findings are noted in the comprehensive exam. Labs show that the patient is not neutropenic. The physician lists the diagnoses as: ALL not in remission, infected Hickman. The patient is given 770 mg of Ceptaz over 10 minutes through a new peripheral IV site and admitted for continued treatment. Medical decision making is moderate.

What code set is reported for the services of the emergency physician?

ICD-9-CM and CPT Code(s):

a. 204.00, 996.62, 780.60, 99284-25, 96374
b. 204.00, 999.31, E878.8, 99284
c. 208.00, 996.69, 780.61, 99285
d. 208.00, 999.31, 99285-25, 96374

ICD-10-CM Code(s): _____

9.56. A patient with a chronic cough and shortness of breath is scheduled for a pleural biopsy following a chest x-ray that revealed a significant mass in the left lower lobe of the lung. Due to the position of the mass, a pleural biopsy is planned rather than a bronchoscopic biopsy.

Following the administration of local anesthetic in the interventional radiology suite of the hospital, a pleural biopsy needle is passed over the left side of the ribs. Fluoroscopic guidance is used to guide needle placement into the mass, so that tissue is obtained for pathologic evaluation.

Which of the following code sets would the physician assign for this procedure if carcinoma of the lung is diagnosed?

ICD-9-CM and CPT Code(s):

a. 162.9, 32400, 77002
b. 786.09, 786.2, 32405
c. 162.5, 32405, 77002-26
d. 162.5, 786.09, 786.2, 32405, 77002-26

ICD-10-CM Code(s): _____

9.57. A patient with hemoptysis, hoarseness, and chronic cough was scheduled for an outpatient flexible fiberoptic laryngoscopy including a biopsy of the cricoid. Procedure: Patient was taken to operating outpatient suite #2. IV sedation was administered at 1300 and topical anesthetic spray was applied. Next, a flexible fiberoptic laryngoscope was introduced. Biopsies were taken from multiple sites of the affected areas. The pathology report states "metastatic carcinoma of the arytenoid cartilage and the posterior commissure and -well-differentiated carcinoma of the cricoid and extrinsic larynx." The operative note states suspected involvement of the thyroid cartilage with primary malignancy believed to be from the esophagus. The patient experienced an increase in blood pressure after the biopsies were obtained, and the procedure was discontinued at 1316. An esophagoscopy will be scheduled after the patient's blood pressure is stabilized.

Which of the following code sets would the physician report?

ICD-9-CM and CPT Code(s):

a. 197.3, 199.1, 796.2, 31576, 99144
b. 161.8, 198.89, 401.9, 31510
c. 150.9, 197.3, 197.3, 197.3, 197.3, 997.1, 31576-53
d. 150.9, 161.8, 796.2, 31576, 99144, 99145

ICD-10-CM Code(s): _____

9.58. A Medicare patient with a personal history of colon cancer, considered to be at high risk for recurrent disease, presents to the office for a screening colonoscopy. The gastroenterologist also examines the anastomosis sites following a previous hemicolectomy.

Procedure: The patient was prepped in the usual fashion, followed by placement in the left lateral decubitus position. I administered 3 mg of Versed. Monitoring of sedation was assisted by a trained RN.

A colonoscopy to the terminal ileum was performed with lesions found just beyond the splenic flexure, which were biopsied. In the sigmoid colon, two polyps were found and excised by hot biopsy forceps.

The pathology report showed the descending colon lesions to be a recurrence of the malignancy and the polyps to be adenomatous.

Which of the following code sets would be reported for the procedure performed in the office?

ICD-9-CM and CPT Code(s):

a. 153.2, 45384
b. 153.2, 211.3, 45384, 45380-59
c. V67.09, V10.05, 153.2, G0105, 45384-59
d. 153.9, V10.05, V45.89, 45384, 45380

ICD-10-CM Code(s): _____

9.59. The following documentation is from the health record of a 23-year-old female patient.

Preoperative Diagnosis:	Osteochondroma of the right scapula
Postoperative Diagnosis:	Same
Procedure:	Excision of osteochondroma of right scapula

Indication: This 23-year-old female has noticed a growing lump coming out of the back of her right scapula over the past year. It has become unsightly and recently has become tender, especially when it's bumped. CT scan has shown a pedunculated osteochondroma coming off the scapula, right at the base of the spine on the medial border. There is no thickened cartilage cap, and simple excision should be adequate.

Findings: Classic osteochondroma of right scapula

Specimen Sent: Osteochondroma

Description of Procedure: After induction of adequate general anesthesia and appropriate timeout, the patient was positioned on her left side with the right side uppermost. The right upper extremity was prepped and draped in the standard fashion with the arm free in the field. We marked out a 4-cm incision over the medial border of her right scapular spine and made this incision through the skin and subcutaneous tissues down to the fascia. I could palpate the osteochondroma easily. We worked our way down through the fascia and separated a 3-cm-wide section of trapezius over the bump, which let us see the pseudocapsule over the bump. We then dissected bluntly down around the osteochondroma to its base, where we could feel that it was right at the takeoff of the scapular spine. The osteochondroma had a well-defined pedunculated stem as we had seen from the CT scan, and with the 3/4-inch osteotome, we went around part of it and were able to come from the other side and separate it from the scapula. There were a couple of rough edges, which were rongeured and smoothed, and then we bone waxed the stalk of the osteochondroma. We removed the excess bone wax. The osteochondroma was inspected and the cartilage cap was seen to be intact. We then infiltrated the bone in the local area with 0.5% Marcaine with epinephrine, of which about 6 mL stayed in the wound. We also infiltrated the skin edges. We then closed the trapezius muscle with three 2-0 mattress sutures after a copious round of irrigation and cauterizing a few little bleeders. The subcutaneous tissue was then approximated with 2-0 inverted mattress Vicryl sutures, and the skin was closed with 3-0 running subcuticular Prolene. The wound was then dressed in two layers with a 4 × 4 and Tegaderm on the first layer and a bulky dressing on the top, which can be taken off in a couple of days. The patient was then awakened and taken to the recovery room in satisfactory condition.

Which of the following will be reported for the surgical service?

ICD-9-CM and CPT Code(s):

a. 170.4, 23182
b. 170.4, 23190
c. 213.4, 23140
d. 213.4, 23190

ICD-10-CM Code(s): _____

9.60. The following documentation is from the health record of a 78-year-old male patient.

Preoperative Diagnosis: Need for permanent venous access

Postoperative Diagnosis: Same

Description of Procedure: Placement of Infuse-A-Port, right subclavian vein

The patient is a 78-year-old Hispanic male with widely disseminated metastatic colon carcinoma under chemotherapy management. His oncologist has requested placement of a permanent venous access catheter.

The patient was brought to the operating room and placed in the supine position. The initial request was for placement in the left subclavian vein. However, after cannulation of the vein and injection of contrast, there was not adequate flow to allow passage of the guidewire through the vein into the superior vena cava. Therefore, the left-sided procedure was aborted.

The right subclavian vein was cannulated without difficulty, and the guidewire was passed centrally down into the superior vena cava. The location was confirmed with fluoroscopy. A subcutaneous pocket and tunnel were then created for the port. The port was placed just above the pectoral fascia. The dilator and peel-away catheter and sheath were passed off the guidewire into the subclavian vein. The sheath was peeled away, and the catheter that had been previously trimmed to the appropriate length and flushed with heparinized saline was passed through the sheath into the subclavian vein. The sheath was peeled away, and hemostasis was achieved. The port was sutured into the pocket with 3-0 Dexon. The 2.5-cm wound was irrigated with saline and closed in layers with 3-0 Dexon subcutaneously followed with 4-0 Dexon subcuticular for the skin. Steri-Strips were applied with sterile dressing and tape. Following the procedure, a chest x-ray in the holding area revealed no pneumothorax and the catheter in excellent position.

Which of the following code sets would the surgeon report for this ambulatory surgical service performed at the hospital?

ICD-9-CM and CPT Code(s):

a. 199.0, 153.9, 36561, 36556-59
b. 153.9, 36563, 36410-53
c. 199.0, 153.9, 36561, 36410-59
d. V58.81, 199.0, 153.9, 36561, 12031

ICD-10-CM Code(s): _____

9.61.   The following documentation is from the health record of a patient with a lesion on the left calf.

COMPREHENSIVE VISIT

History

Referring Doctor:	Primary care physician
Chief Complaint:	Lesion lt. calf
History of Present Illness:	4 to 5 yr. HX pigmented lesion posterior lt. calf. Lesion changed (divided into 2, became rough). Pt. saw primary care physician and lesion was biopsied. Path positive for malignant melanoma in situ. Pt. referred for wide re-excision.
Medications:	Indural 40 mg 2 qd, Norvasc 5 mg 1 qd, Lasix 80 mg 2 qd, Potassium 20 meq 2 qd
Allergies:	Septra
Medical History:	Wears glasses, high BP
Surgery:	Tonsillectomy 1945, partial hysterectomy 1963, lumpectomy rt. breast 1965, lumpectomy rt. breast 1967

Physical

HT:	5'1"
WT:	147

TEMP:	
BP:	160/72
P:	64
R:	
General:	NDWF
HEENT:	No bruits or JVD
Heart:	RSR without murmur
Extremities:	Lt. posterior calf recent biopsy site—greater than 1-cm-diameter defect—dermal based
Diagnosis:	Melanoma in situ, lt. posterior calf
Plan:	Will need wide local excision with STSG to excision site. Donor site—thigh or hip.

Select the correct codes for this physician.

ICD-9-CM Code(s):

a. 172.7
b. 232.7
c. 232.7, 172.7
d. 172.7, 709.9

ICD-10-CM Code(s): _____

Disorders of the Nervous System and Sense Organs

9.62. A patient presents to the neurology clinic for assessment of apraxia at the request of her primary care physician. The patient has a history of CVA and has expressive aphasia. She is unable to carry out purposeful movements, even though she has normal muscle tone and coordination. A full assessment is performed using the Boston Diagnostic Aphasia Examination including interpretation and report (one hour). The consulting neurologist conducts a detailed history and examination, performs medical decision making of low complexity, and dictates a complete report to the requesting physician, along with the finding of the aphasia assessment.

Which of the following code sets is reported for this service?

ICD-9-CM and CPT Code(s):

a. 438.11, 438.81, 99203, 96105
b. 784.3, 784.69, 99244
c. 438.81, 99243
d. 438.11, 438.81, 99243-25, 96105

ICD-10-CM Code(s): _____

9.63. This 35-year-old female patient was admitted with the diagnosis of cerebral aneurysm. The following procedure was performed: intracranial aneurysm repair by intracranial approach with microdissection, carotid circulation. The patient continued to improve with no residual defects. During the hospital stay, she did experience postoperative pneumonia due to *Pseudomonas*.

In addition to the E/M codes submitted by the office, what other codes are assigned?

ICD-9-CM and CPT Code(s):

a. 437.3, 61700
b. 430, 482.1, 61700, 69990-51
c. 437.3, 997.3, 482.1, 61700, 69990
d. 747.81, 997.3, 61703, 69990

ICD-10-CM Code(s): _____

9.64. A patient presents to the neurology clinic for a consultation with a neurologist for intention tremors with periodic muscle weakness in the upper body.

Short-latency somatosensory-evoked potential studies were conducted immediately following a comprehensive history, comprehensive neurologic examination, and decision making of moderate complexity. Both arms and the head and trunk were tested. The results of the interpretation of the tests state "Rule out MS," and a report was sent to the requesting physician stating that a diagnosis of multiple sclerosis could not be ruled out at this time and further testing would be undertaken at a later date. Which of the following is correct?

ICD-9-CM and CPT Code(s):

a. 333.1, 728.9, 99244-25, 95925, 95927-51
b. 340, 99245-25, 95927
c. 333.1, 728.9, 99204, 95925, 95927-51
d. 728.9, 781.0, 99244-25, 95927

ICD-10-CM Code(s): _____

9.65. A Medicare patient has a persistent pain syndrome of the low back and leg subsequent to an automobile accident five years ago in which he sustained back injuries. The patient is brought to the outpatient surgery center nerve block area and is premedicated so he is relaxed enough to be positioned appropriately. The sacral area is prepped with Betadine and a 25-gauge needle, followed by a 22-gauge needle, and is placed under lidocaine anesthesia in the caudal space. The area is injected with 29 cc of solution containing 150 cc of Xylocaine and 16 mg of Decadron LA. The patient remained in good condition in the block room and the recovery area.

Which of the following procedure code sets is reported?

a. 64449
b. 62319
c. 62311
d. 62311, 77003

9.66. This 45-year-old patient has been followed for left ear conductive hearing loss. It was decided to proceed with surgery to correct the condition. The postoperative diagnosis is left ear otosclerosis. During the procedure, a markedly thickened stapes footplate was observed; however, the eustachian tube was intact, and there was normal mobility of the malleus and incus. The left ear stapedectomy with drillout of the footplate proceeded uneventfully. During recovery, the patient experienced atrial fibrillation. This was felt to be due to the surgery because the EKG was normal during the preoperative evaluation. The patient was admitted to the hospital from the outpatient surgical area, and a consultation was requested from the cardiologist.

With the exception of E/M codes, what are the correct diagnosis and procedure codes for physician reporting?

ICD-9-CM and CPT Code(s):

a. 387.9, 997.1, 427.31, 69661-LT
b. 387.9, 69661-LT
c. 387.9, 427.31, 69661-LT
d. 387.9, 69660-LT

ICD-10-CM Code(s): _____

9.67. The following documentation is from the health record of a patient seen in the ambulatory surgery center.

Chief Complaint: Bilateral decrease in vision especially in the right eye.

History of Present Illness: The patient is a 62-year-old woman who has had very poor vision in her right eye for some time which was the result of a cataract and is finding increasing difficulty with reading and watching television because of a cataract developing in the other eye at this time.

Allergies: Sulfa

Family History: She has a brother who had a retinal detachment.

Social History: She denies smoking or drinking alcohol.

Review of Systems: Neuro: Negative. Eye, ear, nose and throat: Bilateral decrease in vision as well as occasional sinus problems. Cardiovascular: Negative except for a very long history of hypertension. HTN is well controlled when the patient takes her meds. She tends to be somewhat noncompliant with taking her medication for high blood pressure. Patient states "I really don't need the little pills for my blood pressure." Pulmonary: She does have COPD which is well controlled on her medications. GI: History of liver biopsy in the past—reason unknown. GU: Occasional frequent urination and she does have a history of kidney stones in the past. Gynecologic: Negative. Endocrine: Negative. Hematologic: Patient has a history of a platelet disorder for which she had a splenectomy several years ago. Skin: Negative.

Physical Examination:

Vital Signs:	BP 145/76; Pulse 72; Respirations 16
Neck:	Negative
Cardiovascular:	S-1, S-2 without murmur, gallop, or rub
Chest:	Clear to A&P. Characteristic for patient with history of COPD
Abdomen:	Negative
Extremities:	Shows 1+ pedal edema
HEENT:	Bilateral cataracts
Impression:	Bilateral cataracts, right eye greater than left. Plan: Cataract extraction with implant in the right eye.

Operative Report

Preoperative Diagnosis: Cataract right eye

Postoperative Diagnosis: Same

Procedure: Extracapsular cataract extraction with implantation of a 16 Diopter posterior chamber lens (a Sinskey style posterior chamber lens) in the ciliary sulcus.

Operative Note: A honan balloon was placed in the right eye for 30 minutes at 35 mm of Mercury pressure. The patient was then prepped and draped in the usual fashion and an O'Brien block and a retrobulbar injection of Marcaine and Lidocaine and Wydase were performed on the right. The lid speculum was inserted, superior rectus suture was placed. A fornix-based flap was made, limbal hemostasis was obtained with bipolar cautery. A corneal groove was made with a 64 Beaver blade and a microsharp entered the anterior chamber. Healon was injected into the anterior chamber and an anterior capsulotomy was performed. The wound was enlarged with corneal scleral scissor to the right and to the left and 8-0 silk 10 o'clock and 2 o'clock sutures were placed. Nucleus expression was performed without difficulty and temporary sutures were tied. Site irrigation aspiration was performed and Kratz scratcher was used to polish the posterior capsule. The 16 Diopter implant was inspected, irrigated and Healon placed on the implant and in the anterior chamber. The implant was then inserted beneath the iris at 6 o'clock into the sucus avoiding the capsule. The superior Haptic was then placed beneath the iris at 12 o'clock. The lens was rotated to approximately 9 and 3 o'clock positions with excellent centration. The peripheral iridectomy was performed. The wound was closed and the superior rectus suture was removed. Ointment was placed on the eye followed by a patch and shield.

How would the physician report his services for this outpatient surgery?

ICD-9-CM and CPT Code(s):

a. 366.1, 401.9, 496, V15.81, 66984-RT
b. 366.9, 401.9, 496, V15.81, 66984-RT
c. 366.9, 401.9, 496, V15.81, 66985-RT
d. 366.9, 401.9, 496, 66984-50

ICD-10-CM Code(s): _____

Newborn/Congenital Disorders

9.68. The following documentation is from the health record of a newborn infant.

Newborn Care

Delivery Note: 11/20/XX, 2300. Called to provide pediatric standby during delivery for suspected nuchal cord. Mother G2, P1. Onset of labor 0730 with normal progression. Entered stage 2 labor at 2100. Fetal monitor showed occasional decelerations. Spontaneous rupture of membranes at 2110, fluid was clear. Noted to have nuchal cord at time of delivery. Otherwise uneventful course.

O: Initial Apgar score 8/9. Weight 3,340 g. Approximate gestational age 38 weeks.

General: Pink with lusty cry. HEENT: Normal, moderate molding, minimal caput. Spine intact. Lungs: Clear bilaterally. Cardiovascular: No murmur noted, capillary refill less than 2 seconds.

Assessment: Normal full-term newborn, noted to have nuchal cord with occasional decels, otherwise uneventful delivery.

Plan: No further intervention at this time. Transferred to newborn nursery for routine newborn care and monitoring.

Progress Note: 11/21/XX, 0630

Subjective: Female newborn, gestational age 39 3/7 wks. Product of full-term pregnancy, NSVD, SROM epidural anesthesia, sl nuchal cord. Initial Apgar score 8/9.

Mother is 32-year-old G2 P1. Pregnancy was significant for maternal hypothyroidism and vanishing twin syndrome. See delivery note for labor course. EDC 24 Nov, initial prenatal care at 10 3/7 wks. Maternal labs: Blood type O positive, ABS neg, Rub immune, VDRL nonreactive, HIV neg, GBS neg, 1hr GTT 82, HBsAg neg, GC/Chlm neg.

Objective: Birth wt 7 lb 6 oz, head circ 14″, length 19 3/4″, head: normocephalic, fontanelles soft nonbulging. Mild caput, moderate molding. Skin: Pink and warm. Eyes: + red reflux × 2, PERRL. ENT: Nares patent, palate intact. TMs clear bilaterally. Lungs: Bilateral breath sounds equal, no accessory muscle use noted. Cardiovascular: Regular rate and rhythm, no murmur appreciated. Well-perfused, normal pulses. Capillary refill less than 2 seconds. Abdomen: Normal active bowel sounds, soft, no masses, three-vessel cord. No erythema or discharge at umbilical stump. Genitalia: Normal female, minimal engorgement, anus patent. Neuro: Lusty cry, good suck, reflexes: + rooting, + morrow, + grip, + Babinski reflex present bilaterally. Skeletal: Clavicle is intact. Spine: No dimples or defects noted. Hips: Normal range of motion, no click noted.

Assessment: Healthy, full-term infant. No defects noted.

Plan: Continue routine newborn care and monitoring. Hearing screen ordered. Check bili, ABO, CBC, and Coombs given Rh+ mother. Continue breast feeding, no supplemental feeding at this time.

Discharge Exam: 11/22/XX, 1000

Subjective: 2 d/o female infant. Breast feeding q. 2 h.r., 10 min ea breast; mother denies diff with latching on (+ breast fed previous infant), + lusty cry when hungry, easily consoled. + Wet diapers q. 2–3 hours, + meconium diapers × 3 since birth.

Objective: Wt 7 lbs 1.5 oz, afebrile throughout admission

See Newborn D/C Pe Form

Laboratory: Coombs neg, blood type B neg, bili 12, HTC 37, hearing screen pass, initial PKU pending

Assessment: Normal, healthy term infant, s/p SVD

Plan: D/C to home. Continue breast feeding. Follow up in clinic for wt check and repeat bili in 3 days. Hep B and 2nd PKU in 2 weeks. RT ER for temp >100.5°F, no wet diapers > 12 hours, lethargy, or resp distress. Education given to parents regarding use of car seat, + verbalized understanding.

Which of the following CPT code sets accurately represents the physician's services for this newborn hospital stay?

	11/20	11/21	11/22
a.	99460	99462	99238
b.	99460, 99464	99462	99238
c.	99460, 99360	99233	99238
d.	99464	99232	99238

9.69.   The following documentation is from the health record of a two-year-old boy.

Patient Name: Johnny Jones

CC: Routine checkup

HPI: Johnny is 2 1/2 years old and has Down syndrome and a ventricular septal defect, surgically corrected. Mother reports he is pulling at his ears and has been running a temp of 99 to 100°F in the past two evenings. Tylenol liquid has been effective in fever resolution according to mother. Development is coming along as expected. Walks with an ataxic gait but does not run. One-word speech pattern. No two-word sentences yet. Appetite is good. Child appears happy, well groomed, and well nourished. Mother reports no specific behavior or social-adjustment concerns.

Past History: Normal SVB, 8 lb 5 oz, 240 long. Heart surgery at 7 months. No known allergies. No medication at this time. Takes daily multivitamins.

Social: Lives at home with mother, father, and older brother. Receives physical, speech, and occupational therapy services from area education services in the home on a periodic basis.

Review of Systems: See patient data sheet and pediatric growth profile chart, not remarkable other than notation concerning recurrent ear infections. No cyanotic episodes, difficulty breathing, or other cardiac symptoms reported. Johnny had a follow-up visit to the cardiologist last month and his findings were reviewed; no significant problems. No voiding or digestive complaints by mother. Child still in diapers. All other systems negative (see detailed history).

Physical Exam: Weight 27 lb, Height 360. HEENT: Both ears positive for redness and otitis media with effusion evident on the left, eyes PERRLA, nose slightly congested clear discharge, neck supple without adenopathy. Throat slightly red. Temperature 99.6°F, blood pressure 108/82, R 15, P 72. Heart regular rate and rhythm; lungs clear to auscultation and percussion, no rales or wheezing. Abdomen soft without tenderness.

Extremities negative. (Detailed)

Assessment: Acute serous otitis media and slight throat infection, likely viral. Inject Bicillin L-A, 600,000 units and follow-up appointment in 3 days. No immunizations needed at this time. Fifteen additional minutes spent in counseling the mother concerning developmental expectations, reviewing cardiologist findings, and answering questions about future cardiac risks.

Which of the following code sets is assigned for reporting the pediatrician's services?

ICD-9-CM and CPT Code(s):

a. 381.01, 462, 758.0, V45.89, 99214, 96372, J0561
b. V20.2, 381.01, 462, 758.0, V45.89, 99392, 99214-25
c. 381.01, 462, 99214, 96372
d. 758.0, V45.89, 99213, J0561

ICD-10-CM Code(s): _____

9.70.   The following documentation is from the health record of a 10-year-old boy.

Preoperative Diagnosis: Status post palatoplasty, history of bilateral incomplete cleft palate with recurrent tonsillitis

Postoperative Diagnosis: Same

Operation: Second-stage palatoplasty with attachment of pharyngeal flap and incidental tonsillectomy

Indications: A 10-year-old patient scheduled for revision of palatoplasty with incidental tonsillectomy requested by pediatrician due to repeated infections

Description of Procedure: The patient was prepped and draped in normal sterile fashion. A midline incision was made through the soft palate, exposing the posterior pharyngeal wall. A flap was then taken by incising the mucosa, submucosa, and underlying muscle, and securely sutured to the soft palate.

Bilateral tonsillectomy was then performed by grasping with a tonsil clamp and capsule dissection. Bleeders were controlled with electrocautery and gauze packing. Sponge and instrument counts were taken and correct, and the patient was transferred to the recovery room in good condition. Follow-up in the office in 3 days.

Which of the following code sets will be reported?

ICD-9-CM and CPT Code(s):

a. 749.04, 42225, 42825
b. 749.04, 474.00, 42225
c. 749.04, 474.00, 42225, 42825-51
d. V50.8, 749.04, 474.00, 42200, 42826-51

ICD-10-CM Code(s): _____

9.71. The following documentation is from the health record of a 10-month-old baby.

Hospital Outpatient Services

A 10-month-old boy is seen in the Gastroenterology Lab to insert a gastrostomy tube. The child pulled out his previous G-tube during the night. He is being followed for congenital cytomegalovirus infection and GERD with erosion of the esophagus. Conscious sedation is provided by the anesthesiologist. The gastroenterologist positions the patient and probes the site with a catheter, injects contrast medium into the tract for assessment, and maneuvers a wire through the tract into the stomach under fluoroscopic guidance. The physician advances the gastrostomy tube over the wire and into position and then secures the device internally and externally. The system is put to gravity drainage and a sterile dressing is applied.

Which of the following code sets is reported by the pediatric gastroenterologist?

ICD-9-CM and CPT Code(s):

a. 536.49, 079.99, 530.81, 49440
b. 536.41, 771.1, 530.81, 530.89, 43760, 76000-26
c. V55.1, 530.81, 530.89, 771.1, 49450
d. V55.1, 530.81, 079.99, 49450, 76000-26

ICD-10-CM Code(s): _____

Pediatric Conditions

9.72. A three-year-old child was brought to the emergency department after inhaling a peanut. The child had a brassy cough that was not present prior to the incident. X-rays showed congestion in the lungs but no obvious foreign body in the larynx. The child was given Versed intravenously and placed on a papoose board. The ED physician could see the peanut on indirect laryngoscopy but could not grasp it with multiple attempts. An ENT specialist took the patient to surgery for removal under anesthesia. An expanded, problem-focused history, problem-focused physical exam, and medical decision making of low complexity were documented.

Give the correct CPT codes for reporting the independent ED physician's service.

a. 99281-25, 31505
b. 99281-25, 31511
c. 99282, 31505
d. 99281, 31511

9.73. The patient is a five-week-old male infant brought in by ambulance after the mother called 9-1-1. The baby was taking a bottle feeding normally and suddenly was blue in the face, appeared to stop breathing, and went limp. Breathing returned spontaneously as the mother moved the baby into various different positions but was still reportedly labored. A comprehensive history was obtained. A comprehensive physical exam in the emergency department revealed only mild tachycardia and increased work of breathing. The patient was transferred to the local pediatric hospital for continued evaluation, with a diagnosis of apparent life threatening event, cyanosis, apnea, rule out respiratory syncytial virus infection, rule out asphyxia by aspiration.

Which of the following diagnoses will be reported?

ICD-9-CM and CPT Code(s):

a. 770.83, 079.6, 933.1, E911, 99284
b. 782.5, 786.03, 799.82, 99285
c. 799.82, 99285
d. 782.5, 799.82, 99291

ICD-10-CM Code(s): _____

9.74. The following documentation is from the health record of a boy with a fracture.

Office Visits

3/31 Office Visit (Primary Care Physician)

S: Peter was playing basketball today, fell, and hurt his wrist.

O: Tenderness and swelling of the wrist, especially the volar aspect. There is a slight abrasion over the swelling. X-ray shows a fracture of the ulnar styloid and possibly the distal radius. There is some question of dorsal displacement of the epiphysis. Short arm cast is applied for comfort measures.

A: Fracture of the ulnar styloid

P: I am going to have the orthopedist look at the x-ray and obtain a consult to determine if reduction is necessary. Return to clinic in 2 days for ortho appt, sooner if problems.

4/1 Office Visit (Primary Care Physician)

S: Peter has pain inside his cast.

O: We thought this was pressure, so I split the cast and it really didn't relieve the pain much at all. I asked him what was hurting about it, and he said it was hurting further up his arm. Then he told me that at the time he had the injury he noticed a great big bulge there. He thought it was the bone poking through, pushed on it, and it sort of went down by itself. His x-ray clearly shows there is no bony injury at that area, but that he has the fracture down by the epiphyseal plate. This is probably a torn muscle.

A: Torn muscle left arm with fracture

P: Keep the appointment with ortho tomorrow. In the meantime, symptomatic care, and we left the cast split because it is probably going to have to be removed for adequate exam tomorrow anyway.

4/2 Office Visit (Primary Care Physician)

S: Peter injured the left wrist playing basketball. He is right-hand dominant. He is currently in a short arm cast, which had been split previously because it was a bit too snug. With the cast he has wrist in extension at least 15 degrees despite the fact that he has the epiphyseal plate fracture with slight posterior displacement of the distal fragment of about 4 mm. He has seen the orthopod in consultation, who felt that this did not require further reduction.

O: He has intact CMS today. Cast is removed, and he is placed in a short arm cast with anterior flexion of about 10 degrees with very slight ulnar deviation. The position of the distal epiphysis of the radius appears to be about the same as it was on the original x-rays taken 1 week ago. This position alignment should be quite satisfactory.

A: Distal radial fracture, Colles' type, with ulnar styloid fracture

P: We will continue with the short arm cast for a duration of 6 weeks. He is to return to see me in 2 weeks for repeat x-ray through the cast and follow up sooner if any problems.

Which of the following is the correct code set to report these visits with the primary care physician?

ICD-9-CM and CPT Code(s):

a. 3/31: 813.43, 25600, A4580
   4/1: 813.43, 840.9, 99024
   4/2: 813.44, 99024, A4580
b. 3/31: 813.43, 29075, A4580
   4/1: 840.9, 813.43, 99213
   4/2: 813.44, 25600, A4580
c. 3/31: 813.43, 25605, A4580
   4/1: 840.9, 813.43, 99213
   4/2: 813.44, 29075, A4580
d. 3/31: 813.43, 29075, A4580
   4/1: 840.9, 813.43, 99213
   4/2: 813.44, 25605, A4580

ICD-10-CM Code(s): _____

9.75.   The following documentation is from the health record of a 14-year-old male patient.

Admission Date:	2/2/XX
Discharge Date:	2/3/XX
Admission Diagnosis:	Peritonsillar abscess
Discharge Diagnoses:	1. Peritonsillar abscess
	2. Chronic tonsillitis
	3. Mononucleosis
	4. Type I diabetes

Reason for Hospitalization: This patient is a 14-year-old white male with a history of right peritonsillar abscess in December who presented with a 4- to 5-day history of progressively increasing sore throat. He had previously been started on amoxicillin as an outpatient, but the severity of his symptoms increased. He presented to the ER on 2/2 with findings consistent with a peritonsillar abscess.

Hospital Course: He was admitted and started on IV Unasyn. Blood glucose levels were drawn and showed only slight hypoglycemia, no doubt as a result of decreased intake due to throat pain. Insulin dosage was adjusted accordingly. An ENT consult was performed, and I&D was recommended. An endocrinology consult was obtained, and he was cleared for surgery. The patient was taken to the operating room that same day. An I&D of the right peritonsillar abscess was performed with a unilateral right tonsillectomy, given his history of recurrent peritonsillar abscesses. The patient was continued on IV antibiotics overnight. The following day, the patient reported significant improvement in his throat pain. He was noted to be afebrile. His Monospot was positive and consistent with acute infectious mononucleosis. Blood glucose levels were adequate. Later, on 2/3, he was seen by the surgeon, who thought he was doing well from a surgical standpoint. The patient was tolerating p.o. well, and the decision was made to discharge the patient home later that same day.

The patient is in satisfactory condition at the time of discharge. Discharge medications include Roxicet p.r.n. for throat pain, Augmentin, and insulin.

He was instructed to comply with a soft diet until further follow-up. Extra time was spent reviewing his insulin regimen and making adjustments (35 minutes with patient and family). Additionally, he was educated about activity restrictions, including no vigorous exercise or contact sports for the next 3 to 4 weeks because of his mononucleosis. The patient was instructed to follow up with the surgeon in 2 weeks.

Which of the following code sets is correct for reporting the attending physician's services on the day of discharge?

ICD-9-CM and CPT Code(s):

a. 475, 474.00, 075, 250.01, 99239
b. 475, 474.00, 075, 250.81, 99238
c. 475, 075, 250.01, 99238
d. 475, 474.0, 075, 250.81, 99239

ICD-10-CM Code(s): _____

Conditions of Pregnancy, Childbirth, and the Puerperium

9.76. The following documentation is from the health record of a female patient.

Discharge Summary

Admission Date: 03/12/XX

Discharge Date: 03/23/XX

Discharge Diagnoses:
1. Term intrauterine pregnancy, delivered, single liveborn
2. Maternal obesity
3. Iron deficiency anemia
4. Retained placenta
5. Endometritis

Procedures Performed: Right paramedian episiotomy, low outlet forceps vaginal delivery, repair of right paramedian episiotomy with repair of partial fourth-degree extension, manual removal of placenta 3/13/XX. Dilatation and suction curettage 3/22/XX.

Hospital Course: This patient presented at 39 weeks' gestation with rupture of membranes of clear fluid. She was not in active labor, her cervix was unfavorable for induction. She was initially managed expectantly, and oxytocin was used to facilitate labor. She progressed throughout the active phase of labor without complications. The fetal evaluations were reassuring throughout the labor process.

The fetal head presented on the perineum in the OA position; because of maternal exhaustion and inability to allow further descent because there was a single nuchal cord released, low outlet forceps were placed after right paramedian episiotomy was performed, and the fetal head was delivered without difficulty. Upon delivery, there was a partial fourth-degree extension just through the anal mucosa. There was retained placenta and manual extraction was required. The episiotomy was repaired by using 000 VICRYL suture, closing the rectal mucosa.

The postpartum course was complicated by the patient developing endometritis. The patient was placed on IV antibiotics and showed some sign of improvement with a dropping white blood cell count; however, her temperature continued to spike. An initial ultrasound revealed some intrauterine products that appeared to be retained placenta. The following day, however, she passed these retained products without difficulty, and her bleeding subsided. Her temperature, however, continued to develop intermittent fever, the antibiotics were switched to the IV, and she again showed a good clinical response with decreased uterine tenderness. Because of the fever continuing, however, a follow-up ultrasound was performed, and no placental products were appreciated. However, there were some clots and unidentifiable tissues still remaining in the intrauterine cavity. Thus, a dilatation and curettage was performed on 3/22/XX, and some amniotic membranes were removed, which appeared to be infected. There were no placental products noted in the curettage.

After removal of the amniotic membrane, her temperature defervesced, and she remained afebrile throughout the remainder of the hospitalization. On discharge, she was tolerating a regular diet, ambulatory without complaints, very scant vaginal spotting, and on oral antibiotics.

It should be noted that because of the excessive blood loss she was given two units of transfused blood to maintain hemoglobin levels from 8 to 9. She was asymptomatic with this hemoglobin, and thus was placed on iron and Colace therapy throughout the remainder of her hospitalization.

Discharge Medications: Include iron sulfate, Colace, and Augmentin

Which of the following is the correct code set, presuming this physician provided the antepartum and postpartum care?

ICD-9-CM and CPT Code(s):

a. 667.02, 670.02, 664.31, 663.31, V27.0; 648.22, 280.0, 59400, 59160-78
b. 667.04, 670.02, 664.31, 663.31, V27.0; 648.22, 280.0, 59400, 59300-51, 58120-78
c. 667.02, 664.31, 663.31, V27.0; 59400, 59300, 59160
d. 667.04, 670.02, 664.31, V27.0; 59400, 58120

ICD-10-CM Code(s): _____

9.77. The following documentation is from the health record of a female patient.

Anesthesia: IV sedation by CRNA, combined with paracervical block

Preop DX: Anembryonic gestation

Operation: Suction curettage

Postop DX: Anembryonic gestation

History: Problem list includes G4, P2, L2, and missed abortion. Patient has asthma with medications including albuterol p.r.n.

Findings: The laminaria that had been placed in the office yesterday had dilated the cervix, which easily fit a #20 Hanks dilator. The uterus sounded 12 cm. The uterus was 10-week size. There was a moderate amount of tissue obtained from the uterine cavity.

Procedure: Under satisfactory intravenous medication, the patient was prepped and draped in the dorsolithotomy position. A speculum was placed. Paracervical block was administered. The laminaria was removed. Using a #9 rigid curved Vacurette, curettage was performed. There was good clamping down effect of the uterus. The intrauterine contents were expelled. There were no complications of the procedure. There was a satisfactory amount of bleeding following the procedure. Estimated blood loss was negligible.

Path report demonstrates histological sections of the uterine contents, which show multiple chorionic villi. This is accompanied by fragments of decidualized tissue and gestational-type endometrium. These histological findings represent products of conception.

Which of the following code sets would be reported for this procedure?

ICD-9-CM and CPT Code(s):

a. 632, 493.90, 59820, 59200-51
b. 630, 493.90, 59870
c. 631, 59856, 59200
d. 631, 493.90, 59820

ICD-10-CM Code(s): _____

Disorders of the Respiratory System

9.78. A patient is seen in the office with increasing shortness of breath, weakness, and ineffective cough. This patient is seen frequently for this chronic condition. Orders were given for a chest x-ray and lab work. Antibiotics were also prescribed. This patient already is on oxygen at home. The physician will try to manage this patient at home, according to his wishes. A detailed history was done with an expanded problem-focused exam and medical decision making of moderate complexity. Diagnoses were listed as acute respiratory insufficiency and acute exacerbation of COPD. Which of the following is the correct code assignment?

ICD-9-CM and CPT Code(s):

a. 491.21, 518.82, 99214
b. 518.81, 491.21, 99213
c. 518.82, 491.21, 99203
d. 491.21, 99214

ICD-10-CM Code(s): _____

9.79. A patient has recurrent polyposis with right pansinusitis and left anterior polyposis with blocked maxillary ostiomeatal units on both sides. The surgeon performs a bilateral intranasal sphenoethmoidectomy and maxillary antrostomy with polypectomy.

The patient was placed under general anesthesia and appropriately prepped and draped. The nose was anesthetized with cocaine flakes, 200 to 300 mg, and topical adrenaline 1:1000. A large polyposis on the right side was removed to gain access for more vasoconstriction using a Robert's snare. Injections of Xylocaine and epinephrine were also used, and the procedure was essentially the same on both sides.

On the left side, there was extensive scarring of the middle turbinate, so through-cutting punches were used to open up the ethmoidectomy bilaterally. While manipulating the left middle turbinate, there was a small CSF leak noted at the junction of the turbinate with the equivaform area. No instrumentation had been done in this area, and it was only a slitlike small leak. This was packed with topical Gelfoam and topical thrombin with Gelfoam at the end of the case and held onto the pack. The nasal antral windows were opened bilaterally and were cannulated, using the right-angle ethmoid curet until palpation showed the natural ostium of the maxillary sinus. The uncinate process was still there from the previous surgery, and this was removed with back-biting forceps and opened into the maxillary sinus widely.

Both sphenoides were widely opened. There was an adhesion from the head of the middle turbinate to the nasal septum on the left side, and this was lysed. A Cottle speculum and the through-cutting forceps were used throughout the case as well as the 1.7-power-magnification operating microscope. The patient had a moderate bout of bleeding bilaterally that was controlled with towel clip pledgets of 1:10,000 of adrenaline. Silastic splints were placed on both sides of the nose to prevent adhesions and were sewn in with 4-0 Prolene sutures. Expandable foam packs were then placed and expanded with 1 g and 10 cc of Ancef. The procedure was then terminated with estimated blood loss at 300 cc for the entire case. The patient tolerated the procedure well and there were no CSF leaks found at the end of the procedure.

Which diagnosis and procedure codes are assigned for this procedure performed in the outpatient surgical department of the hospital?

ICD-9-CM and CPT Code(s):

a. 473.8, 471.8, 349.81, 31201-50, 31051-50, 31020-50
b. 473.8, 471.8, 998.2, E870.0, E849.7, 31201-50, 31051-50, 31020-50
c. 478.19, 473.8, 31267-50, 31288-50, 31254-50
d. 473.8, 471.8, 998.11, 998.2, E870.0, E849.7, 31090-50

ICD-10-CM Code(s): _____

9.80. A patient with bilateral partial vocal cord paralysis requires removal of the arytenoid cartilage to improve breathing. Following a temporary tracheostomy, a topical anesthetic is applied to the oral cavity, pharynx, and larynx, and the laryngoscope with operating microscope is inserted. After adequate visualization is established, the arytenoid cartilage is exposed by excision of the mucosa overlying it. The procedure is performed in the outpatient surgery center of the hospital. Which diagnosis and procedure codes are going to be reported for this procedure?

ICD-9-CM and CPT Code(s):

a. 478.33, 31561, 31600
b. 478.30, 31560
c. 478.33, 31561
d. 478.33, 31560, 69990

ICD-10-CM Code(s): _____

9.81. A 54-year-old male patient with bronchial carcinoma, right lower lobe, has an obstructed bronchus in the right lower lobe of the lung. The pulmonologist views the airway using a bronchoscope introduced through the oral airway following administration of conscious sedation. Thirty minutes of moderate sedation services were performed. The obstruction is identified with the assistance of fluoroscopic guidance. A laser probe is introduced through the bronchoscope to eradicate the obstruction and relieve the stenosis. The procedure was performed in the physician's clinic/surgery center. What codes are reported for physician services for the procedure performed at the outpatient ambulatory surgery center?

ICD-9-CM and CPT Code(s):

a. 162.5, 31641, 99144
b. 162.5, 31641, 76001
c. 239.1, 31640, 99144-51
d. 239.1, 31641, 99144, 76001

ICD-10-CM Code(s): _____

9.82.   A 78-year-old-patient is scheduled for a transbronchial needle aspiration biopsy with fluoroscopic guidance for a lung mass. Following the administration of conscious sedation by the anesthetist, the patient experiences a run of atrial fibrillation, and the physician elects to terminate the procedure before the biopsy is obtained. The procedure is done in the hospital's same-day surgery department.

Which of the following shows correct code assignment for physician services?

ICD-9-CM and CPT Code(s):

a. 239.1, V64.1, 31629, 76000
b. 786.6, 427.31, 31629-52
c. 786.6, 427.31, V64.1, 31628-53
d. 786.6, 427.31, V64.1, 31629-53

ICD-10-CM Code(s): _____

9.83.   A patient is admitted to have a thoracoscopic lobectomy performed. The patient has a malignant neoplasm of the left lower lobe. Because of extensive pleural effusion, the physician was unable to complete the endoscopic procedure. They converted to an open technique, and a successful lobectomy was performed. What are the correct procedure codes?

a. 32480, 32663-53
b. 32663, 32480
c. 32480
d. 32484, 32663-52

9.84.   The following documentation is from the health record of a two-year-old boy seen in the pediatric clinic.

Chief Complaint: Difficulty breathing.

History of Present Illness: Patient is a two-year-old black male with a one-day history of difficulty breathing and a cough. No fever or chills. He otherwise has been acting normally.

Past Medical History: Unremarkable. No history of asthma.

Medications: Over-the-counter cough medicine.

Allergies: None.

Physical Examination

General:	Alert, playful black male in no apparent distress.
Vitals:	Temperature 98.5°F; pulse 125; respiration 28; blood pressure 95/64.
Head, Ears, Eyes, Nose, and Throat:	Conjunctivae clear. Pupils are equal and reactive to light. Tympanic membranes normal. Oropharynx negative.
Neck:	Supple without adenopathy.
Heart:	Regular. No murmurs or gallops noted.

| Lungs: | Breath sounds equal bilaterally with mild wheezing. Minimal retractions. |
| Abdomen: | Benign. |

Diagnosis: Acute bronchitis with bronchospasm.

Disposition and Plan: The patient was given two breathing treatments and his wheezing cleared. He was no longer retracting. He was discharged home on albuterol syrup 3/4 teaspoon q 8 hours; Amoxil 250 mg per 5 mL one teaspoon three times a day. Follow-up in two to three days with primary care physician. Return if worse.

Which of the following is the correct code set for this physician?

ICD-9-CM Code(s):

a. 466.0
b. 466.0, 519.11
c. 519.11
d. 466.19

ICD-10-CM Code(s): _____

Trauma and Poisoning

9.85.   An adult patient is seen in the emergency department after sustaining second- and third-degree burns of the chest and both upper and lower arm after pulling a pan of boiling soup out of the microwave onto his right side while cooking dinner at home. The burn size was documented as 18 cm × 24 cm on the chest, and 26 cm × 8 cm on the right arm. The chest burn was full thickness and the arm burn was partial thickness. The total size was estimated to be about 11% third degree of the total body surface area. Due to the associated pain, local anesthesia, including IM Demerol, was administered. The wound was debrided, and a sterile dressing was applied. The patient was transferred to a local burn unit for further treatment.

What are the correct code assignments for this procedure as reported and billed by the ED physician, who performed a detailed medical history, performed an expanded problem-focused physical examination to rule out other injuries, and rendered moderately complex medical decision making before undertaking the burn care?

ICD-9-CM and CPT Code(s):

a. 942.32, 943.29, 948.10, E924.0, E849.0, E015.2, E000.8, 99283-25, 16030
b. 942.32, 948.00, E924.0, E000.8, 16025
c. 942.23, 942.33, E924.0, E015.2, 99284, 16025
d. 942.22, 943.20, 948.10, E924.0, 11000, 11001

ICD-10-CM Code(s): _____

9.86.   A motorcyclist is brought into the emergency department after a motorcycle accident. The ED physician confirms an open tibia (proximal) fracture and performs extensive debridement of gravel, glass, and other matter, down to and including part of the muscle, at the site of the fracture in preparation for surgery. The orthopedic surgeon then takes the patient to surgery to perform the reduction of the fracture, and the patient is subsequently admitted to the hospital.

In addition to the evaluation and management service, what is the correct code assignment for the ED physician's services?

ICD-9-CM and CPT Code(s):

a. 823.10, E819.2, 27535, 11011-51
b. 823.12, E819.2, 11043
c. 823.10, E819.2, 11011
d. 823.90, E819.2, 27535, 11043-51

ICD-10-CM Code(s): _____

9.87.   A 35-year-old patient was a passenger on a motorcycle involved in an accident and sustained three severely broken ribs and a fractured femur. Chest x-ray showed a 45 percent collapse of the left lung and air in the pleural space. The patient complained of increasing shortness of breath and was cyanotic. A chest tube was inserted into the third intercostal space by the emergency department physician. A subsequent chest x-ray showed marked improvement to only 5 percent collapse. The patient was thoroughly evaluated by the ED physician for possible internal injuries. The ED physician documented a comprehensive history, comprehensive physical examination, and complex medical decision making. The final diagnosis was tension pneumothorax; fractured femur, midshaft; and multiple rib fractures. The patient was taken to surgery by the on-call orthopedic surgeon to care for the fractured femur sustained in the accident.

Which of the following is the correct code set for reporting the ED physician's services?

ICD-9-CM and CPT Code(s):

a. 512.0, 821.01, 807.03, E819.3; 99284-25, 32551
b. 860.0, 821.01, 807.03, E819.3; 99285-25, 32551
c. 860.0, 821.00, 807.09, E819.3; 99285, 32405
d. 512.0, 821.00, 807.09, E819.3; 99284, 32405

ICD-10-CM Code(s): _____

9.88. A patient was seen in the emergency department for an intentional overdose of barbiturates and acetaminophen. The patient was stabilized medically and transferred to the psychiatric unit for further treatment.

Excluding External Cause Status, Activity, and Place of Occurrence codes, what diagnosis codes would be reported by the ED physician?

ICD-9-CM Code(s):

a. 965.4, E950.0
b. 968.3, E950.4
c. 969.3, E938.3, 965.4, E950.0
d. 967.0, E950.1, 965.4, E950.0

ICD-10-CM Code(s): _____

9.89. A patient arrived in the emergency department in full cardiopulmonary arrest following a gunshot wound to the chest. He was intubated, and large-bore IVs of lactated Ringer's solution were started in each arm. A STAT type and cross-match was ordered, along with six units of PRBCs. Dr. Jones, a private trauma surgeon, was on call and was present in the ED when the patient arrived. The patient's chest was opened, and cardiac massage was begun. Despite all efforts at resuscitation, the patient expired of massive blood loss after approximately 85 minutes in the ED.

What CPT codes will be reported by Dr. Jones?

a. 99291, 99292, 32160, 31500
b. 99291, 99292, 32160
c. 99291, 99292, 31500-51
d. 99291, 32160, 31500

9.90. A surgeon performs an evacuation of an epidural hematoma. The physician incises the scalp and peels it away from the area to be drilled. After drilling a burr hole in the cranium and identifying the hematoma via CT scan, the hematoma is decompressed and bleeding is controlled. The hematoma is located outside the dura just under the periosteum. The scalp is repositioned and sutured into place. The patient tolerates the procedure well and is sent to recovery.

What is the correct code set for physician reporting of this procedure?

ICD-9-CM and CPT Code(s):

a. 852.40, 61154
b. 853.00, 61108
c. 852.40, 61156
d. 853.00, 61156

ICD-10-CM Code(s): _____

9.91. The following documentation is from the health record of a 19-month-old with a burn.

Preoperative Diagnosis: Full-thickness burn with deep necrosis and limb loss involving bilateral lower extremities and posterior buttocks area

Postoperative Diagnosis: Full-thickness burn with deep necrosis and limb loss involving bilateral lower extremities and posterior buttocks area and a small portion of the left flank

Procedure Performed: Cultured skin placement to bilateral lower extremities and right buttock with autografting to bilateral buttocks and left flank and a small portion of the left stump. Total area covered was 1,030 cm², of which 720 cm² was cultured skin.

Anesthesia: General

Estimated Blood Loss: 100 mL

IV Fluids: 250 mL of Normosol
140 mL of blood
350 mL of Pitkin

Urine Output: 42 mL

Indications for Procedure: The patient is a 19-month-old male who has undergone multiple excision and grafting procedures in the past for a 72 percent total body surface area (TBSA) burn (50% third degree). He most recently underwent removal of allograft on his bilateral extremities and buttocks area in preparation for skin grafting today. He also has a small area on his left flank where he has not received grafting in the past for which he will also receive skin if sufficient skin is available. His grandmother is present and knows the initial attempt will be to see if the cultured skin is sufficient to cover everything without donor site. However, given the recent fact that 900 cm² was reduced to 700 cm² and 20 cm², this may not be sufficient and the donor site will then be taken from the scalp and lower abdomen. The grandmother is aware of risks and we are proceeding today.

Description of Procedure: After successful induction of general anesthesia, time out for patient identification and surgery planned, the patient was placed in the supine position. His dressings were removed to level of the red rubber catheter.

A 0 Prolene was placed into the bilateral stumps in order to allow for easy access to the lower extremities with elevation. The dressings were removed down and revealed a nice healthy base. Hemostasis was obtained using Epinephrine-soaked laparotomy pads as well as electrocautery. Cultures were taken from the left lower extremity for the cultured skin study as well as biopsies from the past autograft of the lower abdomen and cultured skin. The cultured skin was placed in serial fashion along each of the lower extremities with coverage attained with all but a small portion of the left lower extremity stump. Three pieces remained which will be placed on the abdomen, but since donor site will be necessary, the skin was then harvested from the upper scalp and lower abdomen after Pitkin infiltration using the Padgett dermatome at a thickness of 0.015 inches. Once complete, this was meshed

2:1 and the donor sites were covered with Kaltostat and dry gauze. The patient was then flipped into the prone position. Dressings were removed and patient was re-prepped and draped and then the final dressing lying over the base was removed revealing a nice healthy base. Hemostasis was obtained again with electrocautery and Epinephrine-soaked laparotomy pads. When complete, the meshed skin was placed over the defect and the remaining three pieces of cultured skin on the right upper buttock area. These were all secured with surgical staples and covered with a layer of fine mesh gauze, burn gauze, red rubber catheters, burn gauze and a spandex stent. A small piece of skin was placed onto the left flank where Bacitracin and sterile nonadherent dressing was used as coverage due to the small size. The patient was then returned to the supine position with no shearing of the cultured skin. The distal area on the left stump was covered with meshed graft with a final dressing being attained using a layer of fine mesh gauze, burn gauze, red rubber catheter, burn gauze, and Ace wrap for the right lower extremity, then a Spandex stent for the left lower extremity in order to keep the upper thigh protected and avoid maceration.

Which codes does this surgeon assign?

ICD-9-CM and CPT Code(s):

a. 945.50, 942.44, 942.43, 11100-59, 15150, 15151, 15152 × 7, 15100, 15101 × 3
b. 945.50, 942.49, 11100-59, 15150, 15151, 15152 × 7, 15100, 15101 × 3
c. 945.50, 942.44, 942.43, 11100, 15150, 15151, 15152 × 7, 15100, 15101 × 3
d. 945.50, 942.44, 942.43, 11100-59, 15150, 15151, 15152, 15100, 15101 × 3

ICD-10-CM Code(s): _____

Part IV
Coding Challenge

Chapter 10

Coding Challenge: Nonacute Settings; ICD-10-CM and ICD-10-PCS Code Sets; CPT Modifiers, HCPCS Level II Modifiers

Note: Even though the specific cases are divided by setting, most of the information pertaining to the diagnosis is applicable to most settings. If you practice or apply codes in a particular type of setting, you may find additional information in other sections of this publication that may be pertinent to you.

Every effort has been made to follow current recognized coding guidelines and principles, as well as nationally recognized reporting guidelines. The material presented may differ from some health plan requirements for reporting. The ICD-9-CM code sets utilized are the 2013 codes that are in effect October 1, 2012, through September 30, 2013. The ICD-10-CM/PCS code sets utilized are the 2013 draft codes published in 2012, and the HCPCS (CPT and HCPCS II) codes are in effect January 1, 2013, through December 31, 2013. The current standard transactions and code sets named in HIPAA have been utilized, which require ICD-9-CM Volume III procedure codes for inpatients.

Instructions: Assign all applicable codes appropriate for the setting for the case studies presented. Some of the cases provide multiple-choice answers, and the reader must select the appropriate code set. In other instances, the reader is expected to assign codes without any prompts.

The scenarios are based on selected excerpts from health records without reproducing the entire health record. However, in practice, the coding professional should have access to the entire health record. Health records are analyzed and codes are selected only with the physician's complete and appropriate documentation available. According to coding guidelines, codes are not assigned without physician documentation.

The objective of the cases and scenarios reproduced in this publication is to provide practice in assigning correct codes, not necessarily to emulate actual health record analysis. For example, the reader may be asked to assign codes based only on an operative report or discharge summary. Labeled excerpts are used as source documentation for coding skill practice.

Home Health

10.1. A patient is being followed for postoperative care after surgery for a bleeding gastric ulcer. What code would be assigned in M0230?

a. V code for aftercare of surgery
b. Bleeding gastric ulcer
c. Traumatic wound of abdomen
d. None of the above

10.2. This 85-year-old female lives alone. She recently was in the hospital with aspiration pneumonia. There are infiltrates still present on the chest x-ray, and home healthcare is focused on the treatment of the pneumonia. She also has type II diabetes mellitus. She had partial colectomy last year for acute diverticulitis. What diagnosis would be reported in M0240?

a. Aspiration pneumonia
b. Diverticulitis
c. Diabetes mellitus
d. Acute diverticulitis and diabetes mellitus

10.3. This patient had colon resection because of carcinoma of the transverse colon. He has skilled nursing services for management of the surgical wound, which has a surgical drain not scheduled to be removed for several days. He lives alone and has right hemiplegia after a stroke. What code is reported in M0230?

a. 438.20
b. 153.1
c. V58.42
d. V58.31

10.4. A 72-year-old female patient recently had rectal resection for rectal cancer. She is scheduled for radiation and chemotherapy treatments. Home health services will provide visits four times per week to teach colostomy care and assess compliance with medication. What coding is the best?

a. M0230: V58.42; M0240: 154.1, V55.3
b. M0230: V55.3; M0240: 154.1, V58.42
c. M0230: 154.1; M0240: V55.3, V58.42
d. M0230: V55.3; M0240: V10.06, V58.42

10.5. What code is assigned for a patient who had thyroid cancer two years ago? She underwent a thyroidectomy and received chemotherapy. She has had no treatment in the past year. How is the cancer reported in M0240?

a. 193
b. V10.87
c. V16.8
d. The status of the cancer would not be reported.

10.6. This 80-year-old female patient recently had cholecystectomy for chronic cholecystitis and cholelithiasis. She developed postoperative infection and is being seen for monitoring of antibiotics, vital signs, and observation of the wound, with frequent surgical wound dressing changes. What code is assigned in M0230?

    a. 998.59
    b. V58.31
    c. 879.2
    d. 574.10

10.7. Patient is status post left total hip replacement secondary to localized osteoarthritis and was experiencing problems with ambulation and gait following hip surgery. The patient was discharged with home health services twice weekly. Home care was ordered for wound care. The patient also received physical therapy for gait training and strengthening to increase the patient's ability to ambulate. How should this encounter be coded? Note: Include codes for M0230, M0240, and M0246 (if applicable).

ICD-9-CM Diagnosis code(s): _____
ICD-10-CM Diagnosis code(s): _____

10.8. The patient is a 75-year-old man with varicose veins and ulcer of the right calf (with the fat layer exposed), but he also has two diabetic toe ulcers of the left foot (limited to breakdown of skin) at this time. Patient has chronic lower extremity edema, CHF, HTN. He has daily caregivers through the Medicaid program. The nurse is seeing him four times per week to change leg dressings (using Polymem and covering with stretch bandage), monitor/adjust medications, teach medication management, teach caregivers to provide a low-sodium diet, and keep leg elevated. The nurse hopes to teach a neighbor to change the dressing at least once per week. Physical therapy is ordered every other week for exercise, transfer training, and gait training. Patient ambulates minimally, only with close assistance and a walker. He needs assistance with all ADLs. What codes are assigned? Note: Include codes for M0230, M0240, and M0246 (if applicable).

ICD-9-CM Diagnosis code(s): _____
ICD-10-CM Diagnosis code(s): _____

10.9. A 69-year-old right-handed woman is discharged from the hospital four days after a left modified radical mastectomy for breast cancer of the lower-outer quadrant. Her only medications are oral tamoxifen and pain medications. She is scheduled to begin chemotherapy in the next two weeks. Skilled nursing is prescribed for management of the surgical wound, including dressing changes. The surgical drain is not scheduled to be removed for several days. The patient lives alone and has residual dysfunction of her right arm due to monoplegia after a stroke. The nurse will also supervise the patient's performance of the exercises ordered to improve her shoulder range of motion on the affected side and to monitor for the development of lymphedema in her arm. What codes are assigned? Note: Include codes for M0230, M0240, and M0246 (if applicable).

ICD-9-CM Diagnosis code(s): _____

ICD-10-CM Diagnosis code(s): _____

10.10. Section I of the *Official Guidelines for Coding and Reporting* must be followed for:

    a. Hospital inpatients
    b. Physician services
    c. Home health agencies
    d. All of the above

10.11. A 74-year-old patient was discharged from the hospital after surgical amputation of the right foot due to diabetic osteomyelitis. The patient has type II diabetes. She was admitted to home healthcare for wound care consisting of assessment for signs and symptoms of a wound infection, instructing the patient and her husband on wound care, and surgical wound dressing changes. She will also receive physical therapy to improve her gait. What codes are assigned? Note: Include codes for M0230, M0240, and M0246 (if applicable).

ICD-9-CM Diagnosis code(s): _____

ICD-10-CM Diagnosis code(s): _____

10.12. An 89-year-old man fell in his home, sustaining a right hip fracture. An open reduction with internal fixation was performed six days ago. The patient was discharged home, where his daughter now cares for him. The patient does not bear weight on the right lower extremity but can perform supervised pivot transfers with contact guard assistance in and out of bed. The physician orders the agency to provide physical therapy for gait training and exercise three times per week for five weeks. What codes are assigned? Note: Include codes for M0230, M0240, and M0246 (if applicable).

ICD-9-CM Diagnosis code(s): _____

ICD-10-CM Diagnosis code(s): _____

10.13. What code(s) is/are assigned for a patient receiving home care after a kidney transplant?

    a. V58.44
    b. V58.44, V42.0
    c. 585.6
    d. V42.0

10.14. How many categories are there for skin disorders in the HH-PPS?

    a. One
    b. Two
    c. Three
    d. Four

ICD-10-CM and ICD-10-PCS

Introduction

HIM professionals across the country will lead the transition from ICD-9-CM to ICD-10-CM and ICD-10-PCS. In preparation they need to take steps to become experts on how ICD-10-CM and ICD-10-PCS differ from ICD-9-CM. Coding professionals will need to become proficient in coding with the ICD-10 systems. The following exercises are designed to increase your familiarity with ICD-10-CM and ICD-10-PCS.

Selected sections of the code sets are included with the exercises where possible. Current drafts of the ICD-10-CM index and tabular volumes are available on the website for the National Center for Health Statistics (NCHS). You may download the volumes at http://www.cdc.gov/nchs/icd/icd10cm.htm.

The current draft of both the ICD-10-CM and ICD-10-PCS coding system and Official Coding Guidelines are available on the website for the Centers for Medicare and Medicaid Services (CMS). You may access this information at http://www.cms.gov/ICD10/.

ICD-10-CM

10.15. A myocardial infarction is considered acute for _____ weeks according to the ICD-10-CM *Official Guidelines for Coding and Reporting*.

    a. 2
    b. 4
    c. 6
    d. 8

10.16. Which of the following conventions means that a condition is "not included here"?

    a. Excludes1
    b. Excludes2
    c. Includes
    d. NEC

10.17. ICD-10-CM codes will be utilized by all healthcare settings to assign diagnosis codes.

    a. True
    b. False

10.18. What would be the appropriate ICD-10-CM code for lumbar stenosis?

    a. M48.00
    b. M48.06
    c. M48.07
    d. M48.26

10.19. Assign the appropriate ICD-10-CM diagnosis code(s) for cataract due to hypoparathyroidism.

    a. E88.9, H28
    b. H28
    c. E20.9, H28
    d. H28, E20.9

10.20. Assign the appropriate ICD-10-CM diagnosis code for aspiration pneumonia due to inhalation of food.

    a. J15.9
    b. J69.0
    c. J18.9
    d. J69.1

ICD-10-PCS

10.21. ICD-10-PCS is based on a seven-character alphanumeric code. The meaning of each individual character changes according to the needs of the clinical section.

    a. True
    b. False

10.22. Recall that the first character of an ICD-10-PCS code specifies the section within ICD-10-PCS. Using the list of ICD-10-PCS sections provided below, identify the first character that would be assigned to the following procedures.

Sections of ICD-10-PCS

0	Medical and surgical	B	Imaging
1	Obstetrics	C	Nuclear medicine
2	Placement	D	Radiation oncology
3	Administration	F	Physical rehabilitation and diagnostic audiology
4	Measurement and monitoring	G	Mental health
5	Extracorporeal assistance and performance	H	Substance abuse treatment
6	Extracorporeal therapies		
7	Osteopathic		
8	Other procedures		
9	Chiropractic		

    a. ____ Cranioplasty
    b. ____ Cholecystectomy
    c. ____ Gait training
    d. ____ Computerized tomography, spine
    e. ____ Application of lower extremity pressure dressing
    f. ____ Acupuncture

10.23. Using the list of ICD-10-PCS root operations provided below, identify the root operation used to describe each of the procedures in items a through k.

ICD-10-PCS Medical and Surgical Root Operations

0	Alteration	H	Insertion
1	Bypass	J	Inspection
2	Change	K	Map
3	Control	L	Occlusion
4	Creation	M	Reattachment
5	Destruction	N	Release
6	Detachment	P	Removal
7	Dilation	Q	Repair
8	Division	R	Replacement
9	Drainage	S	Reposition
A	Alteration	T	Resection
B	Excision	U	Supplement
C	Extirpation	V	Restriction
D	Extraction	W	Revision
F	Fragmentation	X	Transfer
G	Fusion	Y	Transplantation

a. _____ Kidney transplant

b. _____ Total nephrectomy

c. _____ Diagnostic bronchoscopy

d. _____ Lithotripsy, bladder stone

e. _____ Varicose vein stripping

f. _____ Fallopian tube ligation

g. _____ Cosmetic face lift

h. _____ Pyloromyotomy

i. _____ Adhesiolysis

j. _____ Adjustment of hip prosthesis

k. _____ Removal of coin from trachea

10.24. Match the approach term with the correct definition.

ICD-10-PCS Character-Approach

0   Open

3   Percutaneous

4   Percutaneous endoscopic

7   Via natural or artificial opening

8   Via natural or artificial opening endoscopic

F   Via natural or artificial opening with percutaneous endoscopic assistance

X   External

Definitions

a. _____ Entry, by puncture or minor incision, of instrumentation through the skin or mucous membrane and any other body layers necessary to reach the site of the procedure.

b. _____ Entry of instrumentation through a natural or artificial external opening to reach the site of the procedure.

c. _____ Cutting through the skin or mucous membrane and any other body layers necessary to expose the body site of the procedure.

d. _____ Entry of instrumentation through a natural or artificial external opening to reach and visualize the site of the procedure, and entry, by puncture or minor incision, of instrumentation through the skin or mucous membrane and any other body layers necessary to aid in the performance of the procedure.

e. _____ Entry, by puncture or minor incision, of instrumentation through the skin or mucous membrane and any other body layers necessary to reach and visualize the site of the procedure.

f. _____ Entry of instrumentation through a natural or artificial external opening to reach and visualize the site of the procedure.

g. _____ Procedures performed directly on the skin or mucous membrane and procedures performed indirectly by the application of external force through the skin or mucous membrane.

10.25. Using the definitions listed in item 10.24 above, match the following:

Procedure	Approach
a. ____ Total abdominal hysterectomy	1. Via natural or artificial opening
b. ____ Needle biopsy of the liver	2. Open
c. ____ Endotracheal intubation	3. Percutaneous endoscopic
d. ____ Laparoscopy	4. Percutaneous

10.26. What is the correct ICD-10-PCS code for a total right knee arthroplasty with insertion of total knee prosthesis? _____

ICD-10-CM/PCS Application Exercise

10.27. You are a coding professional at General Medical Center. One of your responsibilities includes responding to requests for coded data. Facility data in the registry has been coded in ICD-10-CM and ICD-10-PCS for two years. Prior to that, data was coded in ICD-9-CM. You receive requests for data that spans the most recent five years for the following cases. How will you find all applicable cases in the registry for these two requests?

a. Request for cases with an initial acute myocardial infarction of the anterior wall: _____

_____

b. Request for cases with exploration of the common bile duct during an open cholecystectomy: _____

_____

10.28. Code the following operative report using ICD-10-CM and ICD-10-PCS.

Preoperative Diagnosis: Left breast mammographic abnormality

Postoperative Diagnosis: Fibrocystic disease of the left breast

Operation: Left breast biopsy with needle localization

Estimated Blood Loss: Minimal

Complications: None

Procedure: The patient was taken to the Operating Room and placed in the supine position and after induction of endotracheal anesthesia, the left breast was prepped using Betadine solution and draped in a sterile fashion.

A transverse incision was made in the left breast medial to the insertion point of the needle. Incision was taken to the subcutaneous layers and the tissue surrounding the guidewire was excised using electrocautery. The amount of tissue excised measured approximately 3 × 2 cm and was submitted for specimen radiography. This was performed and demonstrated a portion of the nodule in question to be in specimen and this was further submitted for a frozen section diagnosis.

With this in mind, the deeper layers of the incision were closed with interrupted 000 Vicryl. The skin was closed with subcuticular 0000 Vicryl and a sterile dressing was applied.

The patient was taken to PACU in good condition after having tolerated this procedure well.

Code(s): _____

10.29. Code the following using ICD-10-CM and ICD-10-PCS.

Preoperative Diagnosis: Carcinoma of prostate

Postoperative Diagnosis: Carcinoma of prostate

Operation: Transurethral resection of the prostate

Anesthesia: Spinal

Procedure: After operative consent, the patient was brought to the operating room and placed on the table in the supine position. With spinal anesthesia induced, the patient was converted to the dorsolithotomy position. The genital area was prepped and draped in the usual and sterile fashion. A 26 French continuous flow resectoscope sheath was inserted per urethra into the bladder with the obturator in place. The obturator was removed and the resectoscope was seated within its sheath. The bladder was visualized. The ureteral orifices were identified. The resectoscope was pulled to the distal portion of the verumontanum and turned to the 12 o'clock position and resection was begun. Resection was carried circumferentially around the glans channeling a large channel. Hemostasis was obtained by means of electrocoagulation. There were no major venous sinuses or capsular perforations encountered. The verumontanum was left intact. After completion of resection, the bladder was evacuated of residual prostatic chips using the Ellik evacuator. The bladder was then visualized. There were no residual chips identified. Ureteral orifices were intact and uninjured. The bladder neck and prostatic fossa were widely patent. Final hemostasis was obtained by means of electrocoagulation and the resectoscope was removed. A 22 French, 3 way, 30 cc Foley catheter was inserted per urethra into the bladder with ease. It was irrigated until clear. It was placed on light traction with continuous bladder irrigation with sterile water and the patient was transported to the recovery room in stable condition.

Code(s): _____

10.30. Code the following operative report using ICD-10-CM and ICD-10-PCS.

Preoperative Diagnosis: Immediately postpartal; desiring sterility

Postoperative Diagnosis: Same

Operation: Tubal ligation

Blood Loss: Negligible

Blood Replaced: None

Drains: None

Procedure: With the patient under an adequate epidural anesthetic, the periumbilical area was prepped with Betadine and sterile drapes were applied.

The abdomen was entered through a small umbilical incision. The fallopian tubes were identified bilaterally and traced to their fimbriated ends. A knuckle of tube was ligated bilaterally with 0 chromic. The tubes were also ligated proximally and distally with 00 Ethibond. A small portion of tube was resected bilaterally. Hemostasis was adequate.

The peritoneum and fascia were closed together with 00 Vicryl. The skin was closed with 000 Vicryl. A sterile dressing was applied.

The patient tolerated the procedure well and was sent to the PACU in good condition.

Code(s): _____

10.31. Code the following using ICD-10-CM and ICD-10-PCS.

Preoperative Diagnosis: Bronchial alveolar cell carcinoma of the left upper lobe of the lung

Postoperative Diagnosis: Same

Operation: Exploratory left thoracotomy. Left pneumonectomy.

Procedures: This patient was operated on under general endotracheal anesthesia. We had a double lumen tube in where we could selectively ventilate both lungs. He was in the lateral decubitus position. We used a standard posterior lateral left thoracotomy incision and the chest was opened. There was one adhesion to the apical area which was not neoplastic in any manner. I took this down and we were able to easily mobilize the lung. There was a large diffuse lesion in the left upper lobe periphery. I really did not know what to do with this. The lesion had previously been biopsied, and we thought we were dealing with a bronchial alveolar cell.

The man did have a past history of non-Hodgkin's lymphoma years ago which was presumably cured. I began dissecting on the pulmonary artery to look at things to see what kind of fissure I had developed, but the inner lobar branches were just too dense, that is, there was no fissure basically and I knew if I did a lobectomy it was really entering the tumor area peripherally. I therefore went ahead and elected to do a left pneumonectomy since his pulmonary function studies were satisfactory pre-op, and this was the best thing I thought. The main pulmonary artery was divided between a vascular staple gun. Dissection was a little tenuous. The artery seemed quite friable but it held nicely. I then reinforced this with a large Chromic tie. We divided the superior and inferior pulmonary vein and prepared for clamping of the bronchus. This completed the pneumonectomy. He lost some blood due to a bleeding adhesion up above which was not recognized until he had about a half a unit of blood in the left upper chest. This was suctioned clean and we transfused him with 2 units of packed cells. He tolerated the procedure well. He had some hypotension but he was hypotensive on induction throughout the entire procedure. Blood gases were satisfactory during clamping of the mainstem bronchus, and he seemed to be reacting well. We closed the chest in layers with Dexon pericostal sutures, approximated clips on the skin.

Code(s): _____

CPT Modifiers

10.32. Dr. Raddy, staff radiologist, interprets a chest x-ray that was obtained in the hospital radiology department. Dr. Raddy is contracted with the hospital to read radiographs. The equipment and staff are owned and/or employed by the hospital. What modifier, if any, should Dr. Raddy report with the chest x-ray code?

    a. No modifier is necessary because Dr. Raddy interpreted the x-ray under contract with the hospital. The hospital will bill the global and pay Dr. Raddy from the reimbursement.

    b. Modifier -26, Professional component

    c. Modifier -TC, Technical component

    d. Modifier -59

10.33. Tiny Patti Sue Smith, 15 days old, currently weighs 1,652 g. She is taken to the operating room for small bowel resection for necrotizing enterocolitis, a frequent complication of prematurity. The remaining portions of the small bowel were anastomosed end-to-end. CPT code 44120 reports a small bowel resection with anastomosis. Is a modifier necessary, and if so, which modifier?

    a. No modifier is needed for the surgery, although the anesthesiologist might need a modifier.

    b. Modifier -63 is reported because the baby weighs less than 4 kg and thus is a higher surgical risk than a larger neonate.

    c. No modifier is needed because code 44120 already applies to neonates who are very low weight.

    d. A modifier is optional and may or may not be assigned depending on the departmental coding guidelines.

10.34. A patient is seen in the emergency department because of hyperkalemia due to an inadvertent overdose of his potassium medication. Over the course of the next six hours he receives infusions and his potassium is measured three times. What is/are the appropriate modifier(s) to report with the second and third potassium determinations?

    a. Modifier -59, to show that these were not duplicate charges but indeed separate incidents.

    b. No modifier is necessary for repeat laboratory tests, only for repeat surgical procedures.

    c. Modifier -91

    d. Modifiers -91 and -59 should be reported for the second and third determinations.

10.35. A patient who was high on PCP stabbed himself in the chest, causing a pneumothorax. He was seen in the emergency department, and Dr. Jones inserted a chest tube. Approximately one hour later, despite soft restraints, the patient managed to free himself and pull out his chest tube. Dr. Jones reinserted the chest tube via a fresh incision. What modifier should be reported on each procedure?

    a. Modifier -76, Repeat procedure by the same physician, should be reported for each chest tube insertion.

    b. Modifier -76 should be reported with the second procedure; no modifier is needed on the first procedure.

    c. Modifier -59 should be reported with the second procedure; no modifier is needed with the first procedure.

    d. Either modifier -59 or -76 may be reported on the first and second procedures.

10.36. A patient underwent gallbladder removal by Dr. Pitts on 4/1 and was discharged home on 4/2. On 4/16, he developed right lower quadrant abdominal pain and evaluation was strongly suggestive of acute appendicitis. Dr. Pitts performed an exploratory laparotomy and appendectomy for an acutely inflamed appendix. What modifier, if any, should be reported with the appendectomy code?

    a. No modifier is needed because the ICD-9-CM diagnosis code and the CPT procedure code clearly identify that this was a procedure not related to the cholecystectomy.

    b. Modifier -79, Unrelated procedure or service by the same physician during the postoperative period, should be reported with the appendectomy code.

    c. Modifier -78, Return to the operating room for a related procedure during the postoperative period, should be reported with the appendectomy code.

    d. Modifier -58, Staged or related procedure or service by the same physician during the postoperative period, should be reported with the appendectomy code.

HCPCS Level II Modifiers

10.37. A patient is brought to the emergency department of Community Hospital following a motor vehicle accident. He appears to have an avulsion of the aortic root and is rushed to the operating room where repair is attempted. The patient expires on the operating room table just as the surgery is being completed and before he can be admitted to the hospital. The CPT code for repair of avulsion of the aortic root is designated as an "inpatient only" code under the outpatient prospective patient system (OPPS). Is there a modifier that the hospital can report to obtain reimbursement for this procedure when performed as an outpatient?

   a. No. If an "inpatient only" procedure is performed on an outpatient basis, the hospital cannot obtain reimbursement under any circumstances.
   b. Modifier -CA, Procedure payable only in the inpatient setting when performed emergently on an outpatient who expires prior to admission, may be appended to the CPT procedure code.
   c. Modifier -ST, Related to trauma or injury, may be appended and a 50 percent reimbursement will be available to the hospital.
   d. Modifier -SC, Medically necessary service or supply, may be appended and a 25 percent reimbursement will be available to the hospital.

10.38. A patient undergoes a bunionectomy on the big toe of the right foot. What modifier is appended to report the location of this procedure?

   a. No modifier. By definition, bunionectomy is performed on the big toe.
   b. Modifier -T5
   c. Modifier -RT
   d. Modifier -TA

10.39. A hospice patient, under hospice care for terminal COPD, falls out of bed and fractures his wrist. He is taken to the emergency department at the local hospital and has a cast applied to the nondisplaced fracture. What modifier is reported to show that these services are not related to the patient's hospice-qualifying condition?

   a. Modifier -GW
   b. Modifier -AT
   c. Modifier -GZ
   d. Modifier -SC

10.40. HCPCS Level II modifiers can be used with which of the following code sets?

   a. CPT codes
   b. HCPCS Level II codes
   c. ICD-9-CM Volume III codes
   d. Both a and b

10.41. Modifiers -G1 through -G5, which report the levels of Urea Reduction Ratio (URR) in the blood, are reported with codes for _____ and measure the efficacy of this modality.

    a. Laboratory tests
    b. Dialysis codes
    c. Coronary artery interventional procedures
    d. Oxygen therapy

10.42. Match the HCPCS Level II modifier in column 2 with its application in column 1.

1. The patient was pronounced dead after the ambulance was called. Ambulance company is entitled to reimbursement.	a. -KA
2. Left hand, fourth digit	b. -SG
3. The beneficiary has been informed of rent/purchase option and has decided to rent the item.	c. -GH
4. Service furnished in an ambulatory surgery center	d. -QY
5. Left circumflex coronary artery	e. -E4
6. Monitored anesthesia care	f. -QL
7. Diagnostic mammogram converted from screening mammogram same day	g. -F3
8. Add-on option or accessory for wheelchair	h. -QS
9. Lower right eyelid	i. -BR
10. Medical supervision of one CRNA by an anesthesiologist	j. -LC

10.43. After a tragic accident where a 75-year-old patient's eye was injured, the patient received a court order for provision of an extended-wear, hydrophilic contact lens. What HCPCS Level II modifier(s) should be appended to code V2523?

_____

Long-term Acute Care (LTAC) Coding

10.44. Patient Julie Jones suffers a massive intracerebral hemorrhage due to right basilar artery bleed. She is admitted to City Acute Hospital where she remains for eight days undergoing acute care and regulation of anticoagulation.

Following her acute hospital stay, she is transferred to City LTAC for continued management. Treatment at City LTAC will focus on continued management and intensive physical, occupational, and speech-language therapy for rehabilitation from the following sequelae of her intracranial bleed:

Left (dominant-sided) hemiplegia involving her upper and lower extremities

Expressive aphasia

Severe dysphagia with impaired swallowing and risk for aspiration

Assign the admission diagnoses that City LTAC will report.

a. 433.00, 438.21, 438.11, 438.82
b. V57.89, 438.21, 438.11, 438.82
c. V58.9, 438.21, 438.11, 438.82
d. V57.2, V57.3, V57.89

10.45. The patient developed buttock and heel decubiti, both stage II, following an extended stay in the acute hospital. He has had resolution of the underlying acute condition that occasioned his admission there and is transferred to the LTAC for treatment of the decubitus ulcers. While in LTAC, he undergoes nonexcisional debridement of the decubiti. He also has underlying diabetes without documented complications and COPD. Assign the appropriate ICD-9-CM diagnoses and procedural codes for this admission.

a. 707.05, 707.07, 707.22, 250.00, 496, 86.28
b. V57.89, 707.05, 707.07, 707.22, 250.00, 496, 86.28
c. 707.05, 707.07, 707.22, 86.28
d. 707.05, 707.07, 707.22, 86.22

10.46. This patient is admitted for pulmonary rehabilitation in a setting of advanced COPD. She also has ASHD and type II diabetes mellitus with peripheral neuropathy. She has been ventilator-dependent at the local acute hospital but was weaned from the ventilator prior to transfer to LTAC. What are the principal diagnosis and secondary diagnoses that the LTAC personnel will report for her stay?

a. 496, 414.00, 250.60, 337.1
b. V57.0, 496
c. V57.89, 496, 414.00, 250.60, 337.1
d. V57.89

10.47. This patient underwent an above-knee amputation of her left leg for severe vascular trauma with transaction of the posterior tibial artery just below the level of the knee and loss of viability of the distal leg, after a motor vehicle accident. She has had continued stump infections and healing has not occurred, now four weeks after amputation. She is transferred to the long-term acute care hospital for management of the stump infection, eventual rehabilitation, and possible prosthetic fitting. What is the principal diagnosis that the LTAC personnel should report for this admission?

a. V57.89
b. V52.1
c. 904.53
d. 997.62

Outpatient Rehabilitation Cases

10.48. Physician Order

Diagnosis: Congenital CP, scoliosis, bilateral congenital dislocated hips

Treatment Goals: Increase in ADLs, strengthening

Therapy Provided

PT: ROM exercises, strengthening, stretching

OT: ADLs, upper extremity strengthening/ROM

What are the correct diagnosis codes for this outpatient therapy visit? (Procedure codes are captured via the chargemaster.)

ICD-9-CM: _____
ICD-10-CM: _____

10.49. Physician Order

PT to evaluate and treat IT band syndrome of left leg

Therapy Provided

PT: Evaluation and treatment in the weight room

What are the correct diagnosis codes for this outpatient therapy visit? (Procedure codes are captured via the chargemaster.)

ICD-9-CM: _____
ICD-10-CM: _____

Inpatient Rehabilitation Cases

10.50. History and Physical for Inpatient Case

Purpose of Consultation: Physical medicine and rehabilitation evaluation at the request of Dr. Brown, status post trochanteric femoral nailing of left IT fracture on 5/19 with touch weight-bearing restrictions.

History of Present Illness: Joe is a 52-year-old male with a history of mental retardation. He resides at home with parents whom I believe are near their 70s. Joe apparently fell in the home setting and sustained a left intertrochanteric femur fracture and was admitted to Regional Hospital on 5/16. He was evaluated by Dr. Smith and then operated on 5/19 with trochanteric femoral nailing, Synthes type, placed by Dr. Brown.

The patient has been followed by Dr. Smith secondary to difficulties with prior arrhythmia and A Fib flutter with him having been on Coumadin chronically until this admission. His INR today is 2.7, his platelets are 283,000, and his hemoglobin preoperative on 5/16 was 15.6 g/dL. His hemoglobin on 5/22 was 13.2 g/dL.

Chemistries of today, 5/25, are sodium 138, potassium 4.3, chloride 99, CO_2 31, BUN 20, creatinine 0.8, glucose 105, magnesium low at 1.4.

He has been working with a physical therapist and has been very slow to progress until significantly improving and tolerating activities and instructions yesterday on 5/24. At that time, he was able with touch to non-weight bearing on the left lower limb with walker ambulate 15 to 20 feet to the doorway and back with contact-guard assistance. He is tall in stature at 6'2". His admission weight was recorded at 119.3 kg; weight today is 138.5 kg, with a discrepancy likely in his admission weight recording. Pain scores have ranged from a 1 to 2 of 10 today. He has noted some cramping and tightness in his calf, although nontender. He has been working on stretching this out. His medications are as per MAR. He currently remains on telemetry.

Past Medical History:
1. As above, notable for mental retardation and living with parents. He lives in a trilevel home, which he describes as having no stairs to enter the main floor or second level. He lives in the lower level with stair access and frequently is at the upper or higher level. Please refer to the occupational therapy evaluation of tub and difficulties with transfers therein.
2. History of A Fib flutter as above
3. History of gastroesophageal reflux
4. History of chronic Coumadin

Allergies: No known drug allergies

Current Medications: Per MAR, as above

Family History: Noncontributory

Social History: As per above. His care is monitored by his parents. His father has stated that he needs to be more mobile and able to care for himself before returning home. He has been very concerned about his disposition at this time. There is a history of tobacco use approximately 10 years ago. He has a dental bridge prosthesis. He wears glasses for vision and has had a history of night terrors. He is disabled. He is single. His primary care physician is Dr. Allen Smith.

Review of Systems: As per admission H&P of Dr. Brown, as well as ER evaluation of Dr. Canter. See also Dr. Smith evaluation and ongoing care. He has recommended telemetry until discharged from Regional Hospital.

Physical Examination: Admission height: 6'2"

Admission Weight: As above I believe is in error at 119.3 kg

Most Recent Weights: These have been in the 130 to 140 kg range. Today is 138.5.

Vital Signs: BP 133/73, afebrile at 97.6, heart rate in the mid-70s

General: He is alert and conversant. He is sitting up in a chair. He is reading a magazine. He has his lenses in place. He is able to demonstrate functional range of the shoulders and upper extremities and denies any aggravation or irritation with use of the walker for the touch or no weight-bearing on the left. He does have a saline lock.

He has significant ecchymotic change about the left posterior elbow and forearm; this is nontender. He is able to demonstrate good strength, and this limits symmetric reflexes.

Lungs: Clear to auscultation

Cardiovascular: Regular rate and rhythm without A Fib at this time

Abdomen: Soft, normoactive bowel sounds

GU: He is voiding spontaneously.

Extremities: Lower limbs demonstrate +1 reflexes, left knee jerk does evoke some left hip discomfort. He is able to ankle plantar flex, somewhat pain-inhibited on the left. There is no distal swelling. He has TED hose in place, knee high. He is able to follow instructions.

Assessment:
1. Status post fall with left intertrochanteric femur fracture on 5/16 in the home setting
2. Status post 5/19 ORIF with trochanteric femoral nailing
3. Touch weight-bearing limitations, left lower extremity
4. History of arrhythmia and A Fib flutter; on chronic Coumadin
5. Gastroesophageal reflux disorder
6. Mild mental retardation; living with parents
7. Pain issues
8. Slow progress but now improving and tolerating therapies per my discussion with his physical therapist

Plan/Comment: I had the pleasure of evaluating Joe today. He appears to be a good candidate for rehab intervention to maximize his functional status so that he can return home with his parents. We will anticipate his admission therein on 5/27 if he continues to progress as well.

Discharge Summary

Date of Discharge: 6/21/20XX

Date of Admission: 5/28/20XX

Discharging Diagnoses:
1. Status post fall with left intertrochanteric femur fracture 5/16/XX, in home setting
2. Status post open reduction and internal fixation with intertrochanteric femoral nailing 5/19/XX, by Dr. Brown, with touch weight-bearing restrictions left lower limb
3. History of arrhythmia and atrial fibrillation flutter, on Coumadin chronically
4. Gastroesophageal reflux disorder
5. Postoperative pain issues
6. Mild cognitive issues, chronic
7. Mobility and self-care deficits

History of Present Illness: The patient is a 52-year-old Caucasian male. He has a history of some mild mental retardation and resides with his parents who are in their 70s.

His primary physician is Dr. Smith, and he is being followed by Dr. Brown in current hospitalization since being admitted on 5/16/XX, at Regional Hospital.

The patient was evaluated by myself in consultation on 5/25/XX, for rehabilitation needs with him coming to the Rehabilitation Hospital on 5/28/XX. Please refer to my consultation of 5/25/XX for specifics.

Hospital Course: The patient was brought to Rehabilitation Hospital for comprehensive therapy programming. He and his parents were in agreement with this.

He is a large Caucasian male who is pleasant and cooperative. He has had problems with pain limitations and some swelling in the left leg. He has remained on Coumadin and was on this chronically before. He has been followed by cardiology and is scheduled to see Dr. Smith in follow-up on 6/22/XX, at 11:15 a.m. He remains on Coumadin, which is followed by his primary physician with him to have further pro time/INR on 6/23/XX, Thursday.

His physical mobility has continued to progress. He has been maintaining touch weight bearing much better with contact guard assistance for gait using front-wheeled walker for 50-feet distances × 2. He has been able to perform total hip arthroplasty exercise program and is independent in 10 repetitions of each.

He has been followed for lymphedema of the left lower limb and has been issued Juzo garments, and his parents were instructed by the physical therapist on his day of discharge on how to don and doff these garments.

With self-care skills, his upper extremities remained with 4/5 strength and active range of motion. Sensation was intact. Somewhat slower on the right side than the left side for 9-hole peg coordination: 38 seconds right, 24 seconds left. Sitting balance was good. Endurance was within functional limits. He has some mild problems with cognition in terms of problem solving and judgment. Visual perceptive skills were thought to be good using his lenses. FIM-level scores were improved by 2 levels for all tasks except for toileting, which improved from a 3 to a 4. He is independent in feeding and dressing. Dressing lower extremities FIM level 5, grooming 6, toileting 4, showering 5. Discharge equipment includes commode.

Medications at Discharge:

1. Fentanyl patch 25 mcg per hour with this having been decreased the day prior to discharge from 50 mcg to 25 mcg with him noting no substantial change in pain levels. He is provided with refill for 5 patches or 15 days with these to be changed every 72 hours with it to then be discontinued.
2. He has also been using oral medications for pain relief, using Percocet (oxycodone/acetaminophen) 5/325 with 10.100 provided for 1 to 2 p.o. every 4 to 6 hours p.r.n. No refills.
3. Coumadin 3 mg daily currently with 2-week supply issued on 6/21/XX.
4. Durable medical equipment includes:

    Front-wheeled walker with large fixed wheels

    Bedside commode

Rental wheelchair, 20 inches wide. This gentleman is 6′2″ or 6′3″ in height and weighs 116 kg secondary to left hip fracture and mobility defects with limited weight bearing.

5. Ferrous sulfate 650 mg p.o. b.i.d. with meals
6. He has been on Prevacid, but will resume his previous proton pump inhibitor at home for which he has a prescription. His home PPI is Aciphex.
7. He is on Betapace 160 mg p.o. b.i.d.
8. Lanoxin 0.25 mg p.o. every evening
9. Cardizem CD 120 mg p.o. daily
10. He may use over-the-counter stool softeners as needed.

Discharge Instructions:

1. He is to wear his Juzo stockings on the left leg, being placed initially in the morning, removed at bedtime.
2. Fall precautions should be in place.
3. Patient and family chose Regional Hospital Home Health Care for ongoing home health PT, OT, visiting nurse, and aid, with his parents involved in all care decisions.

His prognosis is fair for continued compliance and ongoing follow-up care.

a. What are the correct diagnosis codes (admit, principal, and secondary) for reporting on the UB-04? _____
b. What are the correct diagnosis (etiology and comorbidities) codes for the Patient Assessment Instrument (IRF-PAI)? _____

10.51. Neurology Rehabilitation H&P for Inpatient Case

Date of Consultation: 4/10/XX

Introduction: Rehabilitation consultation is requested to evaluate this 30-year-old man who was injured in a motorcycle accident on 4/3. At that time, he was thrown from his bike and apparently sustained a transient loss of consciousness consistent with concussion. He also apparently had quadriparesis at the scene. He was transported to Regional Hospital where he was ultimately found to have, I believe, a significant hyperflexion injury without major fracture dislocation. He did not require emergency stabilization surgery.

He was clinically and radiographically diagnosed with a cervical spinal cord contusion. This was most prominent at the C3–4 level. There was some initial respiratory impairment, and he was transiently placed on a ventilator. He has since been extubated.

The patient's clinical course has been consistent with a central type of spinal cord contusion such that he has had paralysis of his arms and paresis of the legs. The sensory deficits follow similarly. Patient is now being considered for eventual transfer to the Rehab Hospital.

Current Medications

1. Insulin by sliding scale
2. Bacitracin
3. Dulcolax, p.r.n.

4. Decadron, 4 mg q.6 h. and eventually will be tapered according to protocol
5. Lovenox, 90 mg subcutaneously q.12 h.
6. Prevacid, 30 mg p.o. b.i.d.
7. Claritin, 10 mg p.o. daily
8. Senokot, 8.6 mg p.o. b.i.d.
9. Tylenol, p.r.n.
10. Benadryl, 25 mg p.o. q. 6 h. p.r.n.
11. Ativan, 0.5 mg was used 1 time only
12. Percocet, 5/325, 1 to 2 hours p.o. q. 4 to 6 h. p.r.n.
13. Ambien, p.r.n.
14. Zofran, p.r.n.

Allergies: He has no known medication allergies but has a history of intolerance to morphine and to Motrin. These tend to cause significant itching. He is having some mild itching with his Percocet, but this is relieved with Benadryl.

Past Medical History: He has a torn anterior cruciate ligament.

Review of Systems: Prior to admission, the patient has had no fever, chills, sweats, or weight loss. No change in his vision. No ear, nose, or throat complaints. No chest pains or palpitations. No shortness of breath, coughing, or wheezing. No nausea, vomiting, diarrhea, or constipation. No bladder or kidney dysfunction. No bone or joint problems outside of the anterior cruciate tear. No skin lesions such as rash. No mental illness. No other neurologic problems. No diabetes, thyroid disease, blood or bleeding problems, swollen lymph nodes, or allergic or asthmatic problems.

Family History: Parents are in good health. No neurologic problems.

Social History: He is divorced. Lives in Watson. He is a corrections officer for County Jail. Parents live in Plainsville. He has two children; however, they do not reside with him.

General Exam: Appearance: The appearance is that of a well-developed, athletic-appearing young man who is lying on his back. He has a rigid cervical collar in place. The rigid collar is not to be removed.

Vital Signs: His temperature reached a maximum of 100.3°F but is now down to 99°F. Blood pressure 121/68, pulse is at 72. Respirations 18.

General: He appears normocephalic. The left arm is swollen and wrapped with an ACE-type wrap. No obvious head trauma.

Heart: Is beating at a regular rate and rhythm without murmur. Carotid pulsations cannot be examined at this time. Peripheral pulses cannot easily be examined at this time.

Neurological Exam: He is a bit sleepy. He has received some narcotics and Benadryl. He arouses easily to voice. He is oriented to place and person and thought the date was 4/17. His recent and remote memory is grossly intact, although he has some amnesia for the accident when he was rendered unconscious. His attention span and concentration is grossly normal. Receptive expressive language normal. Fund of knowledge appropriate. His pupils are equal, round, and reactive to light.

Funduscopic exam is benign. Visual fields are intact. Visual acuity is grossly normal. Eye movements are intact. Facial sensation, corneal responses, muscles of mastication are normal. Facial movement symmetrical and normal. Hearing intact. Tongue and palate move normally. The sternocleidomastoid is not examined at this time due to the rigid collar. Trapezius testing was not attempted because of his immobilized neck.

He has complete plegia of the upper extremities bilaterally. In the legs, he does have some leg extension, hip extension, and thigh adduction with abduction. He has some ability to extend the legs bilaterally. There is a limited ability to lift the heels off the bed. There is virtual absence of foot dorsiflexion bilaterally; however, there is a weak plantar flexion response bilaterally. Muscle tone slightly increased in the legs. Babinski responses were not attempted. The muscle stretch reflexes are absent in the upper extremities and hyperactive at the knees and ankles. Sensation grossly intact to light touch and temperature in the legs bilaterally. There is anesthesia of the arms bilaterally and reduced sensation of the lower abdomen. The chest sensation and upper shoulders have essentially normal light touch sensation.

Coordination cannot be attempted. Patient obviously not ambulatory at this time.

Lab Studies: Most recent lab studies of note: Glucose is 137, BUN is at 23, creatinine 1.1. Sodium is at 136. The other chemistry parameters are normal. White count is elevated at 12,100, hemoglobin normal at 15.

Imaging Studies: Are most pertinent for the MRI scans. The MRI is most noteworthy for the abnormal signal within the spinal cord, primarily at the C3–C4 disk space level. An additional small area of signal abnormality noted at the C5–C6 disk level. The abnormality within the spinal cord is consistent with spinal cord edema and contusion. There is an additional abnormality in the soft tissues with interspinous ligamentous edema at C3–C4 and C5–C6. Patient coincidentally also has a relatively small spinal canal that appears congenital.

Assessment: Thirty-year-old man with spinal cord injury without significant fracture but is associated with severe cervical spinal cord contusion, primarily at the C3–C4 disk level. Clinically patient has a "central cord" syndrome with paralysis of his arms and paresis of the legs.

Plan: 1. Patient should be an excellent candidate for comprehensive rehabilitation.
2. We will follow along and facilitate transfer when needed.

Interim Discharge Summary for Inpatient Rehab Case

Discharge Diagnosis

1. Cervical instability with plans for cervical fusion and stabilization procedure by Dr. Johnson, neurosurgery
2. Status post motor vehicle accident with cervical trauma and cord myelopathy
3. Quadriparesis and central cord syndrome
4. Neurogenic bowel and neurogenic bladder
5. Dysesthetic pain and numbness
6. Mobility and self-care deficits

John is a 30-year-old Caucasian male who was involved in motor vehicle trauma with subsequent spinal injury and quadriparesis. Please refer to admission H&P for details. He was admitted in transfer from Regional Hospital for comprehensive rehabilitation programming given his quadriparesis. He has been undergoing spinal recovery program with comprehensive therapies and intervention to include neuropsychology.

He has remained somewhat unrealistic and has deferred many of the spinal education efforts that have been offered to him. He is returning on 5/13/XX to Regional Hospital for cervical stabilization procedure, with Dr. Johnson planning a C3 through C6 anterior cervical diskectomy and fusion.

He has had significant motor recovery from his initial presentation, with his lower extremity strength now +3/5 at the hip extensors and knee extensors. Quadriceps +3/5 bilaterally. Knee flexors, hamstrings were 2/5. Ankle dorsiflexion +1/5. Plantar flexion 3/5. Spasticity and tone does interfere with gait patterning and does limit his ability to progress, with him needing assistance. Bed mobility is rolling with minimal assistance to his stronger right side. Sliding board transfers to bed and chair were with moderate assistance of 1. Supine to sit was with moderate to maximum assist of 1. Gait with ARJO Walker with heavy truncal support is 75 feet with moderate assistance of 1, knee brace on the right, and AFO on the right. Steps and stairs have not yet been attempted.

In terms of self-care skills, the patient remains essentially dependent although he is beginning to show almost antigravity strength being −2 to +2 in the upper limbs with some flicker of hand movement. Palmer grasp on the right 3 lb and left 1 lb. He continues to have a greater degree of sensation proximally than distally, although deep pressure is intact. Light touch is impaired. He is unable to complete a 9-Hole Peg Test and is unable to functionally use the hands bilaterally. Visual perceptive skills are intact.

Medications as per MARS

Plans are for return within 72 hours to the Rehabilitation Hospital if medically stable to resume acute rehabilitation program.

Plan: Disposition is home with support of family and possible spinal cord attendant program via state services. Equipment needs are still to be determined. The patient remains optimistic.

a. What are the correct diagnosis codes (admit, principal, and secondary) for reporting on the UB-04? _____
b. What are the correct diagnosis (etiology and comorbidities) codes for the Patient Assessment Instrument (IRF-PAI)? _____

10.52 Interim History and Physical for Inpatient Case

Subjective: This is an interim history and physical for a 73-year-old woman who sustained an acute right hemisphere ischemic stroke on 03/30/XX. The patient was actually in preadmission at Regional Hospital where she was planning to undergo an orthopedic procedure when she developed acute left hemiparesis. She was transported immediately to the emergency department. It was determined that she had an acute ischemic stroke and received TPA. Despite the TPA, however, the patient was left with severe residual deficits in the form of left hemineglect, left facial weakness, left arm plegia, left leg paresis, and inability to walk. In the course of her workup, she was found to have atrial fibrillation but no significant stenosis of the internal carotid arteries. She was determined to be a suitable candidate for chronic Coumadin therapy.

The patient was fairly stable neurologically, although she had chronic debilitation prior to her admission. This debilitation was related to multiple medical problems, but she was ambulatory, I believe, with a walker. Because of her severe deficits, the patient is now being transferred to the Rehabilitation Hospital for a complete rehabilitation program.

The patient has several comorbid medical problems, including atrial fibrillation, diabetes mellitus, morbid obesity, hyperlipidemia, and degenerative arthritis to include a particular problem with her hip, which was being considered for replacement.

At the time of transfer, she has a temperature of 97.8°F, pulse 108, respirations 20, and blood pressure 134/93. She is awake, alert, and oriented. Her speech is fluent. Her eyes tend to gaze to the right. There is left facial droop consistent with central-type facial weakness. There is left upper extremity plegia, left neglect, and left lower extremity paresis. She is unable to walk.

Assessment:	1. Right hemisphere ischemic infarction with severe residual deficits
	2. There are several complicating comorbid problems, which are likely to aggravate her stroke deficit. In particular, these include degenerative arthritis, diabetes, heart disease, and chronic mobility problems.
Plan:	1. Transfer to Rehabilitation Hospital
	2. Physical therapy, occupational therapy, speech therapy, and therapeutic recreation
	3. Primary goals of therapy will be to improve her ability to ambulate and take care of herself with regard to independence of ADLs.
	4. It is anticipated the patient will require 3 to 4 weeks of inpatient rehabilitation.
	5. It is anticipated disposition would be to home with the care of family, if possible.

Rehab Hospital Discharge Summary for Inpatient Rehab

Date of Admission:	4/7/XX
Date of Discharge:	5/10/XX
Admission Diagnosis:	Right hemisphere infarction with severe residual deficits
Secondary or Comorbid Conditions:	1. Degenerative arthritis
	2. Diabetes
	3. Coronary artery disease
	4. Chronic mobility problems
Discharge Diagnoses:	1. Right hemisphere infarction with severe residual deficits
	2. Degenerative arthritis

3. Diabetes
4. Coronary artery disease
5. Chronic mobility problems

History of Present Illness: Patient is a 73-year-old female who sustained a right hemisphere infarction on 3/30/XX. Patient apparently was in the process of undergoing preadmittance for orthopedic procedure when she developed acute left hemiparesis. She was transferred to the emergency room. She received TPA. However, she was left with severe left deficits in the form of left hemineglect, left facial weakness, left arm plegia, and left leg paresis, and an inability to walk.

In the course of her workup, she was found to have atrial fibrillation. It was thought that she was a suitable candidate for chronic Coumadin. Patient was stabilized in the Regional Hospital setting, and it was thought that she would be an appropriate rehabilitation candidate. Her examination at the transfer to the Rehabilitation Hospital showed her general medical exam to be stable. Neurologically, she was awake, alert, and oriented on mental status, and her speech was fluent. The cranial nerves showed a right gaze preference with a left facial droop that was central in nature. There was left upper extremity plegia and left neglect and left lower extremity paresis, and the patient was unable to walk.

During the course of her rehab stay, the patient did undergo some laboratory workup. This consisted of a series of PT and INR values. Initial PT/INR from 4/8/XX showed PT of 24.0 with an INR of 2.2. Prior to discharge on 5/01/XX, the PT was 26.7 with an INR of 2.5. The patient did undergo some limited metabolic profiles including one from 4/22/XX, showing elevated glucose of 143 with a sodium low at 123, chloride low at 88. Uric acid was 6.2. The osmolality was 0.273. On repeat metabolic profile from 4/23/XX showed an elevated glucose of 126 with a sodium low at 123, and a low chloride at 88. On 4/26/XX, glucose was 131. Sodium was 127, chloride 92. On 5/5/XX, patient had sodium level checked and it was at 130. It had improved to 134. Patient had a series of Glucometer checks done throughout the course of her rehabilitation stay. These levels appeared to have remained fairly consistently elevated with values at times near 190, but no values were noted below grossly 120.

During the course of her rehabilitation stay, she underwent some radiographic imaging including a swallowing study from 4/8/XX, which showed some delay in oral phase of swallowing, likely the result of sensory issues. She had a right hip x-ray from 4/10/XX, showing relatively severe arthritic involvement of the right hip. Right shoulder x-ray from 4/10/XX showed a degenerative change with history of previous surgery. A CT of the right shoulder from 4/19/XX showed previous surgery with screws in the proximal right humerus. There were arthritic changes with subluxation of the humeral head superiorly, suggesting a chronic degenerative rotator cuff tear.

During the course of her rehabilitation stay, the patient was seen by the various therapy services. This included speech therapy, who felt that she had trouble swallowing; the patient was to undergo dysphagia management techniques and diet texture modification and full supervision with p.o. She had speech trouble and was to undergo oromotor exercises. She had communication and language deficits and was to undergo standard speech therapy protocol assessment. She had memory trouble and was to undergo assessment, and she was to be 79 percent accurate with auditory and visual memory exercises. The occupational therapy team thought she had decreased independence with ADLs, and she was to be seen three to five times per week to be educated in ADL techniques and in AE. She had decreased use of the left lower extremity and was to be seen for education and weight-bearing techniques and self-range of motion. She had decreased independence with functional transfers and was to be educated in safety with functional transfers. She had decreased independence with leisure participation and was to be seen for education in leisure exploration. The therapeutic recreation team thought she had decreased leisure participation due to hospitalization and was to be provided an opportunity for successful leisure involvement in an activity of choice. The physical therapy team thought that the patient was dependent on transfers and was to undergo transfer training. She had decreased lower extremity strength and was to undergo strengthening exercise. She had dependence with standing and gait and was to undergo standing and gait training.

Rehab Hospital Course: Patient was admitted for an aggressive inpatient rehabilitation stay. The patient was able to participate with rehabilitation efforts and did make slow but steady progress throughout the course of her rehabilitation stay. She was followed by internal medicine during her stay, and various medical issues were addressed in that regard. Patient had no major setbacks during the course of her stay. She was seen by Dr. Benson for a chronic rotator cuff tear and physical therapy was recommended. The patient's hyponatremia gradually improved throughout the course of her rehabilitation stay.

By 5/10/XX, it was thought that the patient had optimized her rehabilitation hospital benefits. As of that date, the various therapy services noted as follows. Occupational therapy thought that the patient had met some but not all of her goals due to inconsistency and poor attention to task. Physical therapy felt that the patient had met almost all of her goals except the first goal of bed mobility and also her standing goal because she still needed moderate assistance. Therapeutic recreation felt that she had met her established goals with recommendations to continue with social and leisure interest and community involvement. Speech therapy staff thought her condition had improved.

On 5/10/XX, the patient was discharged home with outpatient physical therapy, occupational therapy, speech therapy, and nursing. She was on a diabetic, pureed food, full-supervision diet and was to be encouraged to eat a consistent diet. Her activity was as tolerated, and she was not allowed to drive. She was to transfer with 2 on a sliding board, and she was to continue with her knee-high T.E.D. hose. She was to get a PT/INR on 5/11/XX. She was to check her blood sugar before breakfast and evening meals. She was to have a drop-arm shower and transport in a commode. She was to get a hospital bed with rails and a slide board.

Discharge Medications
1. Baby aspirin daily
2. Lemon juice b.i.d. to t.i.d.
3. Over-the-counter stool softeners
4. Novolin insulin subcu b.i.d. on a sliding-scale basis
5. Sinemet 25/100 at bedtime for restless legs
6. Coreg 6.25 mg b.i.d.
7. Klonopin 0.5 mg at bedtime
8. Lanoxin 0.125 mg daily

9. Surfak 240 mg b.i.d.

10. Zetia 5 mg b.i.d.

11. Neurontin 600 mg b.i.d. and then 900 mg at 10 p.m.

12. Prevacid 30 mg b.i.d.

13. Levothyroxine 100 mcg at bedtime

14. Cozaar 100 mg at 8 a.m.

15. Magnesium oxide 400 mg at 8 a.m.

16. Glucophage 1000 mg b.i.d., 500 mg at noon

17. Singulair 10 mg at 10 p.m.

18. Actos 45 mg at 8 a.m.

19. Zoloft 50 mg b.i.d.

20. Zocor 80 mg at 6 p.m.

21. Coumadin 1 mg at 4 p.m.

a. What are the correct diagnosis codes (admit, principal, and secondary) for reporting on the UB-04? _____

b. What are the correct diagnosis (etiology and comorbidities) codes for the Patient Assessment Instrument (IRF-PAI)? _____

Skilled Nursing Facility (SNF) Cases

10.53. The patient was admitted to the acute hospital with a pathological fracture of the left femur due to underlying metastatic cancer from the breast (resected years ago). She underwent percutaneous fixation in the hospital. She had been largely nonambulatory prior to the injury, and remains so. She is admitted to the skilled nursing facility for continued healing of the fracture and for general conditioning. Assign the appropriate diagnosis codes for the skilled facility to report.

ICD-9-CM: _____
ICD-10-CM: _____

10.54. This patient had been residing at home until an episode of pneumonia resulted in his hospitalization. While there, it was determined that he really was not able to remain in his home on his own due to rapidly advancing Alzheimer's dementia and episodes where he tried to wander away from the hospital. He was transferred to the skilled nursing facility because of this condition, although no specific therapy was ordered. The pneumonia had completely resolved in the acute hospital, and no further treatment was needed in the skilled nursing facility. The patient does have underlying chronic obstructive pulmonary disease, hypertension, and ASHD that require daily medication. Assign the appropriate diagnosis for this long-term admission.

a. 486, 496, 401.9, 414.00
b. 331.0, 294.11
c. 331.0, 294.11, 496, 401.9, 414.00
d. V57.89, 331.0, 294.11, 496, 401.9, 414.00

10.55. This patient underwent a subtotal colectomy in the acute hospital for resection of a carcinoma of the transverse colon. She was left significantly weak and debilitated following her surgery and was admitted to the skilled nursing facility for conditioning. The surgery appears to have been successful in eradicating the malignancy, and she was receiving no chemotherapy or radiation therapy at the time of her transfer. Assign the appropriate codes for the skilled nursing facility to report for this admission.

a. V58.75, 780.79, V10.05
b. V58.75, 997.99, 780.79, V10.05
c. V10.05, 780.79
d. V58.75, 780.79, 153.1